Free Will and the Brain

Neuroscientific evidence has educated us in the ways in which the brain mediates our thought and behavior and, therefore, forced us to critically examine how we conceive of free will. This volume, featuring contributions from an international and interdisciplinary group of distinguished researchers and scholars, explores how our increasing knowledge of the brain can elucidate the concept of the will and whether or to what extent it is free. It also examines how brain science can inform our normative judgments of moral and criminal responsibility for our actions. Some chapters point out the different respects in which mental disorders can compromise the will and others show how different forms of neuromodulation can reveal the neural underpinning of the mental capacities associated with the will and can restore or enhance them when they are impaired.

Walter Glannon is Professor of Philosophy at the University of Calgary. His research interests are primarily in the areas of bioethics and neuroethics and he has published on free will and moral and criminal responsibility, with a focus on how cognitive and clinical neuroscience has influenced how we conceive of and assess these concepts and associated practices. His publications include *Brain, Body and Mind: Neuroethics with a Human Face* (2011), *Bioethics and the Brain* (2007) and *Biomedical Ethics* (2005). In 2010 he was the recipient of a grant from the John Templeton Foundation for the project 'Diminishing and Enhancing Free Will'. *Free Will and the Brain* is the product of this project.

Free Will and the Brain

Neuroscientific, Philosophical, and Legal Perspectives

Edited by
Walter Glannon

CAMBRIDGE
UNIVERSITY PRESS

CAMBRIDGE
UNIVERSITY PRESS

University Printing House, Cambridge CB2 8BS, United Kingdom

Cambridge University Press is part of the University of Cambridge.

It furthers the University's mission by disseminating knowledge in the pursuit of education, learning and research at the highest international levels of excellence.

www.cambridge.org
Information on this title: www.cambridge.org/9781107036031

First published 2015

A catalogue record for this publication is available from the British Library

Library of Congress Cataloguing in Publication data
Free will and the brain : neuroscientific, philosophical, and legal perspectives / edited by Walter Glannon
pages cm
Includes index.
ISBN 978-1-107-03603-1 (Hardback)
1. Free will and determinism. 2. Brain–Research. I. Glannon, Walter, editor.
BF621.F74 2015
123′.5–dc23 2014038618

ISBN 978-1-107-03603-1 Hardback

Contents

Preface

The chapters from an international group of researchers and scholars in this book explore how our increasing knowledge of the brain can elucidate the concept of the will and whether or to what extent it is free. They also examine how brain science can clarify our normative judgments of moral and criminal responsibility without explaining them away. The book is distinctive in its interdisciplinary approach to free will, showing that we can gain a better understanding of it when philosophy, clinical neuroscience, cognitive psychology, and criminal law inform and are informed by each other in the study of human thought and behavior. The volume is also distinctive in that a number of the authors are both neuroscientists and philosophers, which gives them expertise in and a unique perspective from which to examine the normative aspects of free will and responsibility as well as the neurobiological underpinning of the mental capacities associated with them. Some of their insights into free will come from treating actual patients with mental disorders that impair the will. Many of the chapters are written by authors from overlapping or complementary disciplines, resulting in a book that is more richly textured than other works addressing these questions solely from the view of philosophy. Another prominent feature of the book is that many of the authors are at the forefront of research in psychology, clinical and forensic psychiatry, functional neurosurgery, and legal theory. All of this makes the volume a valuable source of information, analysis, and discussion of how brain function enables and how brain dysfunction disables the capacity for reasoning, decision-making, and action.

I thank my editors at Cambridge University Press, Hetty Marx and Rebecca Taylor, for supporting this project as well as for their guidance and excellent advice. I am also grateful to the three reviewers commissioned by Cambridge University Press for their constructive comments on the book proposal – Jonathan Lowe, Peter Clarke, and Steven Quartz. I regret that Professor Lowe, who died in January 2014, did not live to see this book. The following comments he made on the book concisely capture its aim: "Recent developments in neuroscience, drawing on findings from brain-imaging experiments and the like, have prompted exaggerated and philosophically naïve claims about the 'illusory' character of free will, and have been met with equally ill-conceived criticisms from some scientifically uninformed philosophers. The present volume promises to be a valuable corrective to such fruitless debates and a genuine meeting of minds." Most of all, I am grateful to the authors for their contributions to the book. This project was made possible in part through the support of a grant from the John Templeton Foundation. The opinions expressed in this publication are those of the editor and authors and do not necessarily reflect those of the John Templeton Foundation.

Contributors

ADRIAN CARTER, PhD, NHMRC Postdoctoral Fellow, University of Queensland Centre for Clinical Research, Australia

SANNEKE DE HAAN, PhD, Department of Psychiatry, Academic Medical Center, University of Amsterdam, The Netherlands

DAMIAAN DENYS, MD, PhD, Department of Psychiatry, Academic Medical Center, University of Amesterdam, and The Netherlands Institute for Neuroscience, The Royal Netherlands Academy of Arts and Sciences, Amsterdam, The Netherlands

FARAH FOCQUAERT, PhD, Bioethics Institute Ghent, Department of Philosophy and Moral Sciences, Ghent University, Belgium, Research Foundation Flanders, Belgium Visiting Professor of Public Health Ethics, HoWest, Belgium

GRANT GILLETT, MBChB, DPhil, Professor of Medical Ethics, Bioethics Centre, University of Otago Medical School, former Neurosurgeon, Dunedin, New Zealand

WALTER GLANNON, PhD, Professor of Philosophy, University of Calgary, Canada

ANDREA L. GLENN, PhD, Assistant Professor of Psychology, Center for the Prevention of Youth Behavior Problems, University of Alabama, Tuscaloosa, USA

WAYNE HALL, PhD, NHMRC Australia Fellow in Addiction Neuroethics, University of Queensland Centre for Clinical Research, Queensland Brain Institute, National Drug and Alcohol Research Centre, University of New South Wales, Australia, National Addiction Centre, Kings College London

STEVEN E. HYMAN, MD, Director of the Stanley Center for Psychiatric Research, Broad Institute of MIT and Harvard University,

Department of Stem Cell and Regenerative Biology, Harvard University, USA

AXEL LINDNER, PhD, Department of Cognitive Neurology, Hertie Institute for Clinical Brain Research, University of Tubingen, Germany

NIR LIPSMAN, MD, Neurosurgery Resident, Division of Neurosurgery, Toronto Western Hospital, University of Toronto, Canada

ANDRES M. LOZANO, MD, PhD, Dan Family Chair in Neurosurgery, Tasker Chair in Stereotactic and Functional Neurosurgery, Canada Research Chair in Neuroscience, Division of Neurosurgery, Toronto Western Hospital, University of Toronto, Canada

GERBEN MEYNEN, MD, PhD, Assistant Professor, Faculty of Philosophy, VU University Amsterdam, Endowed Professor of Forensic Psychiatry, Tilburg Law School, The Netherlands

STEPHEN J. MORSE, JD. PhD, Ferdinand Wakeman Hubbell Professor of Law, Professor of Psychology and Law in Psychiatry, Associate Director of the Center for Neuroscience & Society, University of Pennsylvania, USA

GEORG NORTHOFF, MD, PhD, EJLB-CIHR Michael Smith Chair in Neurosciences and Mental Health, Canada Research Chair for Mind, Brain Imaging and Neuroethics, University of Ottawa Institute of Mental Health Research

ADRIAN RAINE, PhD, Professor, Departments of Criminology, Psychology and Psychiatry, University of Pennsylvania, USA

ERIK RIETVELD, PhD, Professor of Philosophy, University of Amsterdam, the Netherlands

MAARTJE SCHERMER, MD, PhD, Endowed Chair in Philosophy of Medicine, ErasmusMC University Medical Center, Rotterdam, the Netherlands

MATTHIS SYNOFZIK, MD, Center for Neurology and Hertie Institute for Clinical Brain Research, University of Tübingen, Germany

NICOLE A VINCENT, PhD, Associate Professor of Philosophy, Law, and Neuroscience, Georgia State University, USA; Chief Investigator of the Enhancing Responsibility Project, Technische Universiteit Delft, the Netherlands

GOTTFRIED VOSGERAU, PhD, Professor of Philosophy, Heinrich-Heine-University, Düsseldorf, Germany

Part I

Introduction

1 Free will in light of neuroscience

Walter Glannon

ABSTRACT

In this chapter, I provide a historical overview of the main philosophical positions on free will. Neuroscience has motivated a shift in the debate on free will from an external to an internal focus, from features of the external world to features of the brain and how it enables the mental capacities necessary for free and responsible agency. Neither neuroscientific determinism nor mechanism poses a real threat to these capacities and whether or how they are exercised. Neurological and psychiatric disorders may impair the will by disabling the neurobiological structures and processes that mediate the ability to reason and make decisions. But nothing about a normally functioning brain challenges the conviction that we have this ability and can act freely and responsibly. I provide summaries of the other chapters in this volume and the authors' perspectives on how our knowledge of the brain influences how they analyze theoretical and practical aspects of free will and moral and criminal responsibility.

Introduction

For centuries, philosophers have attempted to explain how human agents can choose and act freely and have an impact on events in the physical universe. The most serious challenge to the conviction that we have free will has come from causal determinism. This is the thesis that a complete description of the state of the world at some time T, in conjunction with a complete formulation of the natural laws, entails every truth about the physical state of the world at later times. Causal determinism implies that any action one performs at a given time is the only action one could have performed at that time. Insofar as free will requires the ability to do otherwise and causal determinism rules out this ability, it seems to follow that we lack free will. And insofar as moral responsibility presupposes free will, it also seems to follow that we cannot be morally responsible for any of our actions if causal determinism is true.

There have been different philosophical responses to causal determinism. While some of the authors in this volume describe and discuss some of these responses, it will be helpful to summarize them here. Philosophers who believe that free will is incompatible with causal determinism can be divided into two groups. Hard incompatibilists, or as William James described them, "hard determinists" (1956, pp. 145ff.) argue that causal determinism is true and therefore we have no free will. Libertarian incompatibilists argue that we do have free will and that causal determinism is false. They can be divided further into event-causal libertarians and agent-causal libertarians. The first group maintains that the decisions and actions of human agents are physically caused, but in an undetermined way. The second group maintains that human agents can perform some actions that are not caused by any physical events. The agent is the sole cause or originator of the action. All incompatibilists claim that the control of actions identified with free will requires that we be their source and that alternative possibilities be open to us when we act (van Inwagen 1983; Kane 1996; Strawson 2010). This depends on whether certain features of the universe obtain or fail to obtain. To use a metaphor from Jorge Luis Borges' 1941 short story, "The Garden of Forking Paths," alternative possibilities are the forking paths extending from the present to the future and among which we choose when we act (Fischer 1994, p. 3). If causal determinism is true, however, then there are no forking paths but only one path to the future, a path we cannot create or choose. This is what the hard incompatibilist believes. Compatibilists argue that free will and responsibility are compatible with causal determinism because the relevant sort of control does not require these types of alternative possibilities (Dennett 1984, 2003; Frankfurt 1988; Fischer 1994; cf. Berofsky 2012) Instead, we can control our thought and behavior when we have the capacity to respond to reasons for acting or refraining from acting (Fischer and Ravizza 1998). It is not natural laws and events in the past that impair or undermine this capacity but instead different forms of coercion, compulsion, or constraint. The control associated with free will does not depend on metaphysical features of the universe but on mental capacities of agents. The alternative possibilities necessary for one to act or refrain from acting are not possible states of affairs waiting to be actualized by us. Instead, they are functions of different sets of desires, beliefs, reasons, and intentions leading to actions. Like the actual sequence of mental and physical events that results in action, any alternative sequence that might have resulted in a different action is not external but internal to the agent and a function of his or her own mental simulation of future possibilities in adapting to the environment.

The will is not a single faculty associated only with volition but a deliberative and executive process extending from beliefs and motivational states to actions. The will is free when one has the capacity to recognize and react appropriately to reasons in forming and executing intentions in actions that accord with one's considered desires and values. We have free will when we can control the sorts of mental states we have and whether and how they issue in our actions. A psychological conception of the will based on mental capacities rather than a metaphysical conception based on features of the universe is more in line with our normative practices and institutions, especially the criminal law's view of persons as agents with the capacity for rationality. Legal theorist Stephen Morse notes that "libertarian free will is not an element of any crime or of any affirmative defense. To establish prima facie guilt, the prosecution *never* needs to prove that the defendant had [libertarian] free will" (2013, p. 38). What is needed to establish guilt or excuse is whether the defendant was capable of responding to reasons. This may be described as a broadly compatibilist sense of free will. That is, even if causal determinism were true, persons would still have free will if they had the capacity for deliberation and rational reflection, to respond to reasons and translate them into appropriate actions. Morse further says that "compatibilism is the only metaphysical position that is consistent with both the criminal law's robust conception of responsibility and the contemporary scientific worldview" (2013, p. 41. See also Chapter 13 in this volume).

Neuroscientific determinism

Neuroscience has a critical role in the psychological conception of free will because of the brain's capacity to represent different courses and outcomes of action and to generate and sustain the mental capacities that enable decisions and actions. Neuroscientific findings in the last thirty years have motivated a gradual shift in the focus of free will from external factors associated with natural laws and events in the past to internal factors associated with the relation between our brains and minds (Mele 2014b). This shift has not defused all possible threats to free will. Neuroscience may show that the mental processes on the basis of which we explain our actions may be determined by or reducible to neurobiological processes. This could undermine conscious control of our thought and behavior. As neuroscientist and philosopher Adina Roskies puts it: "The underlying worry is that those things that once seemed to be forever beyond the reach of science might soon succumb to it: neuroscience will lead us to see the 'universe within' as just part and parcel of the law-bound machine that is the universe without" (2006, p.420). So, moving the locus of agency inside the agent may just introduce another medium for determinism. There are differences between deterministic and mechanistic processes in the brain regarding their implications for agency, and I will discuss the implications of each for free will in turn. The main point here is that neuroscientific determinism challenges the psychological conception of free will because it implies that neural processes alone ensure that we perform particular actions at particular times.

There is insufficient evidence from neuroscience to prove a deterministic relation between neural processes and mental processes associated with behavior. Because of limitations in functional neuroimaging and other neurophysiological measures of brain activity, neuroscience at best can show correlations between brain activity and the mental activity involved in decision-making and action. Correlation is not causation, and accordingly there is no warrant for claiming that neural processes cause us to have particular mental states and to choose and act in particular ways. The blood-oxygenation-level-dependent (BOLD) signal in fMRI is an indication of blood flow and increased metabolic demand in the brain. A more active BOLD signal in certain regions of the brain indicates more activity in those regions. If a subject in an experiment using fMRI is asked to perform a cognitive task such as choosing between two options, then presumably there will be increased activity in the prefrontal cortex and anterior cingulate cortex, two structures associated with executive functions such as planning and conflict resolution. But there is no way of telling whether the activity is due to excitatory or inhibitory effects in these brain regions and whether these effects determine that the subject chooses one of these options over the other. Moreover, it cannot be known whether or to what extent the changes in blood flow and increased metabolic demand were caused by the subject's consciously forming and executing an intention to choose, or whether these mental acts were caused by the neural activity. We cannot conclude from the activity displayed on fMRI that it caused the subject to choose as he did. Choice cannot be reduced to activation in a particular area of the brain. The BOLD signal and images displayed on fMRI or other forms of functional imaging are at best approximations of brain activity. They are visualizations of statistical analyses based on a large number of images and are more accurately described as scientific constructs than "pictures" or "snapshots" of what is actually occurring in the brain. The signal-to-noise ratio in fMRI requires that images be averaged over many trials to yield statistically significant results. Functional imaging generates group data, and one cannot draw a direct inference from information about the brains of groups to information about the brains of individuals and how they affect their mental states (Poldrack

2011). Roskies points out that this "raises a major concern ... about the degree to which functional data about individuals can be interpreted, and whether and how scientific generalizations about brain function can be rendered applicable to individual cases" (2013, p. 45). The epistemic gap between what we know about neuroimaging and what we know about individual brain function warrants caution in drawing inferences from our limited knowledge of the brain to ontological claims about events and processes occurring within it. This pertains especially to the relation between brain activity and human thought and behavior.

There is also insufficient evidence to prove that brain functions can be explained in terms of indeterministic or stochastic processes. Some event-causal libertarians (Kane 1996, pp. 129ff.) appeal to this idea to motivate their arguments for free will. Moreover, some neuroscientists have explained free will in terms of fluctuating background noise in the brain that generates an element of randomness in our decisions to act (Bengson et al. 2014). Conceptually, it is unclear whether quantum stochasticity or any sort of randomness could provide us with the control of our behavior required for free will, since randomness is at odds with the idea of control. Empirically, it is plausible to assume that quantum stochasticity operates at the micro-level of subcellular information transfer in neurons. It is also plausible to assume that determinism operates at the meso-level of neural ensembles and at the macro-level of neural networks. But it is not known whether presumed indeterminate micro-level processes influence or cancel out and become irrelevant at meso- and macro-levels of brain activity. There is no convincing empirical evidence for the claim that brain activity is either completely deterministic or completely indeterministic. This casts doubt on claims that deterministic neural processes rule out or that random neural processes support the idea of free will. It is an oversimplification to assume that external deterministic or indeterministic processes go straight through the brain to action in a direct input-output relation, as though the behavioral outputs were nothing more than a function of the inputs. Neuroscientists Harald Atmanspacher and Stefan Rotter assert: "The intricate relations between determinacy and stochasticity raise strong doubts concerning inferences from neurobiological descriptions to ontological statements about the extent of determinism in the brain" (2011, p. 98). They further state: "Our bottom line is that pretentious claims as to deterministic or indeterministic brain activity are unfounded, and so are the consequences drawn from them" (2011, p. 99. See also Roskies 2006, 2010; and Balaguer 2010).

There are conceptual and practical difficulties with neuroscientific determinism apart from the empirical difficulties just considered. If brain events determined mental events in a way that ruled out free will and responsibility for all human agents, then there would be no normative difference between a person who commits premeditated murder and one who kills another because of an uncontrollable violent impulse. Nor would there be any difference between a drunk driver who kills a pedestrian and a driver who has an unforeseeable seizure resulting in the same outcome. Those who assassinate others in the name of religion could not be responsible for their actions because they "could not have done otherwise." Neuroscientific determinism is also at odds with the fact that some therapies can cause changes in the minds and brains of some criminal offenders and rehabilitate them. The different normative judgments we make of these individuals reflect the understanding that the control of thought and behavior associated with free will is not an all-or-nothing capacity but one that comes in degrees. There is a continuum of control corresponding to the extent to which one has the mental capacity to respond to reasons for or against actions. As some of the authors in this volume point out, if neuroscientific determinism were true, then these differences would be irrelevant to questions about control and responsibility. No one could control their behavior and be responsible for it. There would be no basis for distinguishing between and among full responsibility, mitigation, or excuse in the criminal law, differences based on the understanding that individuals possess and exercise cognitive, affective, and volitional control of their actions to varying degrees. But there is no need to revise our moral and legal concepts and practices in light of neuroscientific determinism because this thesis has yet to be – and may never be – proven.

Neuroscientific mechanism

Mechanism may pose a more serious threat to free will. This thesis says that mental phenomena can be explained entirely in terms of their component neurobiological parts and the organization of and interactions between these parts (Craver 2007). If reductive mechanism is true, then neural processes obviate the need for psychological explanations of our behavior (Nahmias 2006, 2010). This can be described as the "causal exclusion problem" (Bayne 2011, p. 39). Mental properties are excluded from having a causal role in agency because the causal efficacy of neural properties underlying them provides a complete explanation of agency. If free will requires that our mental states play a causal role in our decisions and actions, and if mechanism shows that these states, *qua* mental, play no such role, then it seems that we lack free will.

In the early 1980s, neuroscientist Benjamin Libet conducted a series of experiments in which he used electroencephalography (EEG) to detect and measure activity in motor, premotor, and prefrontal cortices and supplementary motor areas of the brain when subjects were asked to flex their fingers or wrists (1985). These were a further development of similar experiments conducted in the 1960s (Kornhuber and Deecke 1965). Libet's experiments demonstrated that neural activity in the form of readiness potentials in these motor regions preceded the subjects' conscious awareness of their intention to act by several hundred milliseconds. The results of Libet's experiments suggested the epiphenomenal view that conscious mental states are the effects of neural mechanisms but have no causal influence on these mechanisms, which provide a complete account of our actions (Gallagher 2006, p. 110). Libet did not explicitly say that his experiments demonstrated that free will is an illusion, but he did say that they would have "a profound impact on how we view the nature of free will" (2004, p. 201) The challenge posed by the results of these experiments is how we could have free will if unconscious events in the brain rather than conscious mental states initiate actions. Psychiatrist Sean Spence spells out the apparent upshot: "If this is the case, then what space is left for freedom?" (2009, p. 6) It is difficult to sustain the view that we can be free and responsible agents if we are "merely victims of neuronal circumstances" (Greene and Cohen 2004, p. 1785).

But the idea that our conscious mental states or events do not initiate our actions does not mean that they have no causal role in our performing them. The fact that an unconscious neural event initiates an action does not imply that it can account for all the events in the process that extends from the formation of an intention to act to its execution in action. Philosopher Alfred Mele distinguishes proximal intentions from distal intentions. While the first type refers to intentions occurring just before action, the second refers to intentions to act at later times. These intentions may be either conscious or unconscious. Regarding bodily movements, Mele explains that from the datum that some neural events "begin before a conscious proximal intention emerges, one cannot legitimately infer that any of the following play no role in producing the movement: the acquisition of the proximal intention, the agent's consciousness of the intention, or the physical correlates of either of these items" (2009, p. 71). Events occurring unconsciously in motor or other areas of the brain may be the basis of an urge or inclination to act; but these might not lead to a decision to act (Mele 2009; Bayne 2011). The formation and execution of a conscious intention may be necessary to complete this process. Many of our actions result not only from proximal intentions to perform them but also from distal intentions involving long-range planning. Even if neural events initiate particular actions, conscious distal intentions may influence neural events and their causal role in these actions. Libet's experiments at most show that certain neural events are necessary, not sufficient, for the occurrence of decisions to act (Mele 2014b). This is one example of the limitations of Libet's experiments. The actions the subjects performed involved a very narrow time frame and did not reflect the fact that many of our actions are the result of a broader temporal process of planning and decision-making. This process may involve many hours, days, weeks, or even years. Moreover, finger- and wrist-flexing are relatively trivial motor tasks that have little bearing on the types of actions for which free will is worth wanting. They are not the types of actions that make us candidates for praise, blame, responsibility, or punishment (Roskies 2006, 2010; Bayne 2011). These actions and the deliberation that precedes them do not occur as isolated neurological or mental events but are "embedded in a pragmatically or socially contextualized situation" (Gallagher 2006, p. 120. See Gillett's discussion of Chapter 3 in this volume).

The conclusions drawn from Libet-type studies cannot be generalized to the broader class of actions that figure in our normative judgments. This is at least partly because these studies involved only basic cognitive and motor tasks and focused mainly on prefrontal, premotor, and motor cortices and the supplementary motor area mediating these tasks. While the basal ganglia are also mentioned by some of the neuroscientists conducting these studies, there is little discussion of the role of these nuclei in planning and motor tasks (Haggard 2008, 2011, p. 11). The capacity for reasoning and decision-making is mediated by a broader network of interacting neural circuits in cortical, limbic, and subcortical regions of the brain (See Lipsman and Lozano's discussion in Chapter 10 of this volume). This network consists of re-entrant loops projecting from the prefrontal and parietal cortices to the thalamus, basal ganglia, and cerebellum, which then project back to the cortex (Spence 2009, p. 154). The basal ganglia and cerebellum are not only critical for motor control but also for the cognitive and affective processes necessary to coordinate action plans. While the prefrontal cortex plays a critical role in the formation and execution of intentions, higher- and lower-level neural circuits projecting to and from each other are all engaged in a normal healthy brain when a person makes a decision. Still, it seems plausible to say that neural events alone underdetermine our decisions and actions, and that both neural and mental events and states are necessary to explain thought and behavior and assess whether or to what extent a person has free will and can be responsible for what he or she does or fails to do.

Many neuroscientists who have expressed skepticism about free will base their claims on dualism about neural and mental properties. Some assume that free will presupposes substance dualism, the thesis that the brain and mind are distinct material and immaterial substances. These neuroscientists question the causal efficacy of the mental because an immaterial mind or soul cannot have any causal power of its own. But the assumption that the mind is independent of the brain may beg the question in favor of the causal irrelevance of the mind and the idea that free will is an illusion. Seizing upon this idea, biologist Anthony Cashmore says that "if we no longer entertain the luxury of a belief in the 'magic of the soul,' then there is little else to offer in support of the concept of free will" (2010, p. 4499). One philosophical response to this challenge relies on a very different interpretation of substance dualism. For example, philosopher Richard Swinburne claims that it is metaphysically possible that we could exist without a brain, which presumably supports the idea that we are essentially souls or minds. He adopts an agent-causal view of free will purportedly immune to the constraints imposed on agency by any form of materialism (Swinburne, 2013). Given current knowledge about the brain–mind relation, these claims against all forms of materialism and for free will are questionable because substance dualism is not a tenable thesis. It may be metaphysically possible for the mind to exist independently of the brain, but not empirically possible.

A number of philosophers of mind accept some form of property dualism. This says that there is only one kind of substance, the physical kind, but two distinct kinds of properties, physical and mental (Chalmers 1996, 2010). Mental properties depend on physical properties of the body or brain. Some of these philosophers argue that property dualism implies epiphenomenalism. They concede the existence of conscious mental properties but claim that they have no causal effects in the brain (Jackson 1982). Consistent with this interpretation of property dualism, some neuroscientists seem to hold that a mechanistic explanation of behavior in terms of neural processes implies epiphenomenalism. Neuroscientist Patrick Haggard suggests this idea in his comment that "Although consciousness may be part of brain activity, consciousness cannot cause brain activity, nor can it cause actions" (2011, p. 18).

Yet studies in psychiatry and neurology show that conscious mental states can cause brain activity and can at least partly explain behavior. Cognitive behavioral therapy (CBT) can rewire circuits in cortical-limbic pathways of the brains of patients with major depressive disorder (Goldapple et al. 2004). Reframing one's conscious and unconscious beliefs about external stimuli can cause changes in brain regions mediating thought and mood. Neurofeedback may also enable subjects to modulate brain activity and symptoms in a range of disorders through their visualization of and response to this activity as displayed on EEG or fMRI. Patients with intractable pain can attenuate their perception of pain by modulating perceived activity in brain regions mediating pain, such as the rostral anterior cingulate cortex (de Charms et al. 2005). Producing effects similar to those in CBT, patients with major depression can alter brain activity regulating mood through neurofeedback as well (Linden et al. 2012). In addition, at least one study has shown that patients with Parkinson's disease who expected to receive a dopamine agonist but instead received a placebo produced endogenous dopamine in the basal ganglia (de la Fuente-Fernandez et al. 2001). In a similar study, Parkinson's patients receiving a placebo modulated neural activity in the subthalamic nucleus, a component of the basal ganglia, which in turn relieved some of their motor symptoms (Benedetti et al. 2004; Benedetti et al. 2011). While unconscious conditioning mechanisms based on neural processing partly explain these phenomena, they do not provide a complete explanation of them. Conscious expectation in the type of top-down processing involved in placebo responses also plays a causal explanatory role in the effects in the brain. These examples illustrate that psychological properties can have physical effects in the brain and that these properties have an important role in behavior control. Insofar as the content of the relevant mental states is shaped by interaction between the patient and physician, or the research subject and investigator, the examples also show that a biopsychosocial model including factors internal and external to the brain may provide the most satisfactory explanation of behavior.

If neuroscientific skepticism about free will is driven by a mechanistic model of human agency, and if this model cannot provide a satisfactory explanation of agency, then such skepticism is not on solid ground. Like neuroscientific determinism, the failure of neuroscientific mechanism to rule out free will and responsibility leaves our normative practices and institutions such as the criminal law unscathed. This lends support to the psychological account of free will. Morse implicitly appeals to this account and its application to the law when he states: "The law's view of the person is a creature capable of practical reason, an agent who forms and acts on intentions that are the product of the person's desires and beliefs. The law does not treat persons generally as non-intentional creatures or mechanical forces of nature" (2007, p. 205). Our increasing knowledge of the neurobiological underpinning of mental disorders may lead to a more humane criminal justice system in which deterrence and rehabilitation are given more weight than retribution in the treatment of criminal offenders (Burns and Bechara 2007). However, it does not warrant replacing a psychological model with a mechanistic model as the basis of this system. There would be no point to rehabilitation, for example, if it did not enable a person to become more responsive to moral reasons for certain actions. Neuroscience can inform our practices of holding people morally and criminally responsible without explaining away these practices and the idea of rationality on which they are based.

The brain–mind relation and the will

The mind emerges from the brain when it reaches a certain degree of complexity to promote the adaptability of the organism to the environment. Explanatory emergence says that although conscious mental states are not themselves distinct from physical states in the brain, appeal to physical models or theories alone cannot explain them. Neurons alone cannot fully represent the environment to the organism because they lack the property of intentionality, or directedness to stimuli or states of affairs in the external world. Together with the neural networks that generate and sustain them, the content of conscious mental states includes information about the world that enables the subject to interpret and respond to it appropriately. The concept of emergence does not imply property dualism or epiphenomenalism. Rather than becoming independent of neural processes, emergent mental states are constrained by these processes and in turn constrain them in what neuropsychiatrist Todd Feinberg calls a "nested hierarchy" (Feinberg 2001, pp. 127–129; 2011). Higher-level processes associated with the conscious mind are not identical to but are compositionally dependent on, or nested within, lower-level processes associated with cortical, limbic, and subcortical circuits in the brain. Brain and mind are interacting, interdependent components of one system. Feinberg uses the idea of constraint to describe how the brain–mind relation promotes homeostasis of systems within the organism. Constraint refers to the control that one level of a system exerts over a different level. It operates not just in a top-down way but in a bottom-up way as well, with normal functioning neural circuits ensuring that the content of mental states accurately reflects the external world. By accurately representing the world to the organism, beliefs and other mental states promote homeostasis by ensuring that the neural circuits underlying these mental states are neither underactive nor overactive. Chronic psychological stress can negatively influence one's beliefs about stimuli and over-activate the amygdala in the fear system. This can disable cortical constraint on this system and result in the pathological behavior in generalized anxiety, panic, and major depressive disorders, all of which can impair or undermine free will. The hallucinations and delusions of a person with schizophrenia result from dysregulation of information processing due to disabled constraints on the mind by dysfunctional auditory and prefrontal cortices. Failure of the critical brain regions to constrain the mind results in this disorder of the will.

Any form of constraint on the conscious formation and execution of intentions in action presumably would impair rather than promote free will. Indeed, earlier I noted that, together with compulsion and coercion, constraint is one of the conditions that can impair or undermine control of choice and action on a traditional compatibilist account of free will. Also, Spence suggests that we have free will to only a limited degree when he asserts: "The human capacity for volition, for voluntary control, or the apparent expression of 'willed' actions, is subject to multiple constraints" (2009, p. 363). He adds: "If the human agent possesses any 'freedom' at all, then it is a freedom that is expressed under certain 'optimal' conditions, be they structural, neurochemical, interpersonal, or situational" (2009, p. 378). Spence's use of "constraints" and "optimal" in these passages is significant. Together they suggest that some degree of neural constraint on conscious mental states is not only compatible with but also necessary for free will. The control that gives us this freedom requires a balance between interacting conscious and unconscious mental processes and the brain circuits that mediate them. As paradoxical as it may sound, free will requires limits on the conscious deliberation that leads to action.

Control of thought and behavior presupposes a balance between deliberative and automatic behavior. If most of our actions were automatic, then that would threaten our intuitive sense of agency. By the same token, too much conscious thought can impair control by interfering with many basic actions that we ordinarily perform as a matter of course without having to give much thought to them. This is one hypothesis for the pathology in obsessive-compulsive disorder. (See the discussion by de Haan, Rietveld, and Denys in Chapter 5 of this volume). Unconscious proceduralized actions regulated by subcortical regions of the brain release prefrontal areas from attending to them and allow these areas and the cognitive functions they mediate to attend to more demanding executive tasks. Balanced conscious and unconscious processing at the mental level is grounded in balanced activity between cortical and subcortical circuits regulating motor and executive functions. This balance contributes to what Spence calls the "optimal" conditions in the brain enabling behavior control. Hyperactivity or hypoactivity in a critical neural circuit or its connections with other circuits can disrupt this balance and result in pathologies causing mental paralysis that disables the will.

Antonio Damasio is another neuroscientist who criticizes the dualistic separation of conscious and unconscious processes promoted by Libet, Haggard, and psychologist Daniel Wegner (2002) in their skeptical claims about free will. Damasio asserts that "the reality of nonconscious processing and the fact that it can exert control over one's behavior are not in question . . . nonconscious processes are, in substantial part and in varied ways, under *conscious* guidance" (2010, p. 285). He comments further: "Consciousness came of age by first restraining part of the nonconscious executives and then exploring them mercilessly to carry out preplanned, predecided actions. Nonconscious processes became a suitable and convenient means to execute behavior and give consciousness more time for further analysis and planning" (2010, p. 286). Damasio goes on to say that "the conscious-unconscious cooperative interplay also applies in full to moral behaviors. Moral behaviors are a skill set, acquired over repeated practice sessions and over a long time, informed by consciously articulated principles and reasons but otherwise 'second-natured' into the cognitive unconscious" (2010, p. 287). These comments support the view that nondeliberative, unconscious behavior frees the conscious mind from motor tasks so that it can attend to more demanding cognitive tasks. This division of labor in agency between conscious and unconscious processes promotes flexible behavior and adaptability. Damasio's use of "restraining" is the concept of constraint used by Feinberg and Spence to describe the checks and balances between different circuits and functions in the brain and mind that enable us to choose and act freely.

Nothing about normal brain function supports skepticism about free will or the claim that it is an illusion. Different types of brain dysfunction can undermine or impair free will to varying degrees. This occurs in mental disorders such as addiction, schizophrenia, OCD, and psychopathy, which are discussed by some of the authors in this volume. These can be described as disorders of the will. Still, what matters is not brain dysfunction as such, but how it affects the mental capacities necessary for reasoning and decision-making. One of the distinctive features of this book is that many of its chapters demonstrate how studying neuropsychiatric disorders and their neural underpinning can elucidate whether or to what extent the will is or is not free. They analyze and discuss how brain function enables control of thought and behavior, as well as how brain dysfunction can disable this control. Many of the authors show how psychiatry, cognitive psychology, neurology, and neurosurgery can inform our understanding of how the brain–mind relation regulates agency in actual people. Some of the authors discuss the idea of a disordered will within a framework of forensic psychiatry and consider the degree to which it can impair the capacity to be criminally responsible and liable to punishment. There is also discussion of how what Spence calls "interpersonal" and "situational" factors in the external world influence brain function and the mental processes associated with deliberating and acting. A satisfactory explanation of the brain's role in our thought and behavior requires recognition of the fact that human agents act and interact with other agents in the natural and social environment.

Neuroscience, philosophy, and criminal law

The authors in Part II analyze the conceptual foundations of free will in the context of neuroscience. In the first chapter of this section, Georg Northoff discusses the theoretical question of whether a neurophilosophical conception of free will is more observer-based than brain-based. Claims about the causal role of neural mechanisms on our behavior may reflect extrinsic properties associated with our observation of the brain more so than intrinsic properties of the brain itself. Northoff distinguishes between the brain's resting state and stimulus-induced activity in the brain to illustrate the epistemic gap between what we observe and what actually occurs in the brain. This has important implications for claims by some neuroscientists that neural mechanisms rule out free will. If we can only approximate knowledge of what occurs at the neural level, then we cannot definitively state that neural mechanisms completely explain our behavior. Northoff maintains that brain processes fall along a continuum and may be neither completely deterministic nor indeterministic. Nevertheless, neuro-experimental and neuroepistemological constraints on our knowledge of the brain may make free will more of an observer-based than a brain-based concept.

Grant Gillett follows by combining Aristotle's account of the will as the ability to translate reasons into actions with John Hughlings Jackson's account of the will as one component of consciousness in the neural evolution of sensorimotor functions. Gillett describes OCD and psychopathy as disorders of the will resulting from failure to translate reasons into actions. Consistent with the views of Aristotle and Nietzsche as well as those of Hughlings Jackson and neuropsychologist Alexander Luria, Gillett points out that the meaning of freedom and responsibility depends on a marriage of neuroscience and philosophy based on a conception of human agents as beings-in-the-world-with-others.

In the last chapter of this section, Matthis Synofzik, Gottfried Vosgerau, and Axel Lindner focus on free will as an experience grounded in self-attributions of agency. Free will is tightly connected with responsibility in terms of the feeling and judgment of agency. They analyze how the "positive" symptoms of delusions and hallucinations in schizophrenia undermine free will by disturbing the neurocognitive underpinnings of self-attribution of actions, where one feels that one is no longer in control of them. The authors argue that free will and responsibility depend on but are not reducible to these underpinnings. They are primarily social phenomena resulting from an internalization of social norms and expectations. Like Gillett, Synofzik, Vosgerau, and Lindner maintain that free will and responsibility depend on factors both inside and outside the brain. These three chapters move the debate on free will beyond the dialectical stalemates about the implications of causal determinism and mechanism for our decisions and actions.

Part III focuses more closely on psychiatric disorders and how they can compromise the will and responsibility for one's behavior. Challenging the traditional assumption that one is freer the more conscious control one has over one's actions, Sanneke de Haan, Erik Rietveld, and Damiaan Denys examine the phenomenology of OCD and argue that increased conscious control of actions can diminish agency and free will. They maintain that too much deliberation can disturb the flow of unreflective agency and impede actions that ordinarily are performed in an unreflective "second-nature" way. Hyper-reflectivity and excessive cognitive monitoring can at least partly explain the psychopathology of OCD. One hypothesis these authors consider for the pathophysiology of this disorder is that excessive frontal-striatal connectivity disturbs the balance between conscious and unconscious processes regulating thought and behavior. Their description of the experiences of patients with OCD highlights the shortcomings of the conception of free will as requiring complete conscious control.

Farah Focquaert, Andrea Glenn, and Adrian Raine discuss the implications of psychopathy for free will and moral and criminal responsibility. They argue for the "pragmatic value" of a compatibilist account of reasons-responsiveness in conceptualizing free will and responsibility. Their integration of this account with empirical literature from neuroscientific studies provides a helpful framework for analyzing how the cognitive and affective deficits of the psychopath impair his or her capacity to act freely and be responsible for his or her actions. These authors maintain that offenders with severe psychopathy should not be held criminally responsible, and that mild psychopathy should be a mitigating factor making the agent at most partly responsible. They also explore experimental interventions that might modulate abnormal brain function in cortical-limbic pathways as potentially effective treatments for psychopathy in the future.

Gerben Meynen considers a range of psychiatric disorders and explains how they can impair different mental capacities that constitute free will. One especially significant feature of his chapter is Meynen's discussion of how a mental disorder can weaken a person's insight into his or her condition and his or her volition to seek and follow up on treatment for it. He emphasizes the critical role of the psychiatrist in motivating the patient to begin or continue treatment. This shows how an understanding that one's will is disordered can lead to therapeutic interventions. Meynen concludes by commenting on future directions for research in areas such as neuroimaging that can clarify the dysfunctional neurobiological correlates of disorders of the will. His chapter demonstrates how forensic psychiatry can contribute to a deeper understanding of the role of mental capacities in behavior control.

Wayne Hall and Adrian Carter describe two competing models of addiction. According to the brain disease model, chronic drug use produces changes in brain function that reduce addicted persons' capacity to control and be responsible for their behavior (Koob and Volkow 2010). According to the moral model, drug use is always a free choice for which persons are and should be held fully morally and legally responsible. Addiction is not a disease but a disorder of voluntary choice. Addicts stop taking drugs when the costs of continued use become too great. There is nothing compulsive or out of control in seeking and taking addictive substances (Heyman 2009). The fact that many addicts stop using substances without treatment casts suspicion on the disease model. Still, the question of behavior control in addiction is one area in which there is considerable disagreement between neuroscientists and philosophers. After analyzing the neuroscientific and epidemiological research on addiction, Hall and Carter point out that the justice system in many countries operates on a compromise between the brain-disease and moral models. The accepted view is that addicted persons are not fully responsible for their criminal acts because their decision-making is impaired, but not to a degree sufficient to exculpate them (Hyman 2007). Addicted persons are treated as responsible; but their condition can be a mitigating factor in setting penalties. Hall and Carter also consider the argument for compulsory treatment of severely addicted persons for paternalistic reasons and argue that it requires a stronger justification than it has received in the literature.

In the last chapter of this part, Nicole Vincent uses a broadly compatibilist theory that focuses on mental capacities in analyzing the influence of cognitive neuroscience and behavioral genetics in the debate on free will and moral and criminal responsibility. Vincent points out that it is unclear how we should understand the normative notion of "capacity" and that some mental incapacities could be interpreted as character flaws. This makes it ambiguous whether the neurological or genetic features associated with mental incapacities should diminish or mitigate guilt or excuse one from it. Such ambiguity needs to be addressed before we consider intervening in the brain to modify the relevant capacities. Vincent proposes ways of clarifying how empirical data about the brain can inform our normative assessments of people's behavior.

The two chapters in Part IV discuss how some interventions in the brain can inform our understanding of the neural basis of decision-making, as well as how other interventions can restore, enhance, or impede it. Lipsman and Lozano describe how functional neurosurgery can elucidate how a heterogeneous set of cortical and subcortical structures in the brain regulate the capacity for decision-making. This intervention can also show how dysfunction in these structures causes neuropsychiatric disorders that impair this capacity. They distinguish primary from secondary disorders of will (Lozano and Lipsman 2013). In the first type of disorder, patients have impaired or distorted perception of reality and often attribute their decisions and actions to external sources or influences. In the second type of disorder, there is incongruity between the way patients actually think and behave and the way they want to think and behave. They do not doubt that they are the source of their actions but report a loss of control over them. The thought and behavior described by Synofzik, Vosgerau, and Lindner in their discussion of schizophrenia in Chapter 4 are symptomatic of a primary disorder of the will. Lipsman and Lozano demonstrate that by allowing privileged access to the brain, functional neurosurgery can provide insight into how neurological and psychiatric disorders can disable the will. They also show how modulating techniques such as deep-brain stimulation (DBS) can restore the will by restoring function of its underlying neural circuits.

Maartje Schermer then discusses how existing and emerging neuromodulation techniques affect individual autonomy, defined as the capacity to govern oneself. "Autonomy" can be used interchangeably with "free will" insofar as both concepts pertain to the control that persons have of their actions and the mental states from which they issue. Schermer explains how these techniques can restore or even enhance autonomy by restoring or improving normal brain function. However, they can also reduce autonomy by causing adverse side effects such as mania or compulsive behavior, as has occurred in some cases of DBS. She argues that non-invasive techniques such as neurofeedback do more to promote autonomy than invasive techniques such as DBS. In neurofeedback, the subject has a more active role in modulating brain activity and controlling thought and behavior through a mental response to images of his or her brain without having to rely on a device implanted in the brain.

In Part V, Steven Hyman and Stephen Morse examine the legal implications of neuroscience. Hyman points out how contemporary neuroscience is yielding increasingly detailed knowledge of the involuntary causal mechanisms underlying cognitive, emotional, motivational, and executive functions. This mechanistic view of human behavior conflicts with moral intuitions about free will that form the basis of responsibility and retributive punishment in the criminal justice system. While a causal mechanistic view supports a shift from a retributive to a consequentialist model of punishment, it runs the risk of explaining away the moral intuitions and emotions that form the basis of our sense of justice, which includes both models of punishment. Even if neuroscience alters our understanding of criminal responsibility, assessment of the scientific evidence will be influenced by public opinion, politics, and social conditions. Hyman concludes by claiming that there is no one correct theory to guide our conception of criminal justice and that we are left with a healthy tension between moral intuition and causal mechanism, where each informs and is informed by the other in shaping legal practices.

In the last chapter of the book, Morse argues that the new cognitive, affective, and social neuroscience does not pose a serious challenge to theoretical and practical aspects of criminal responsibility. These are based on the folk-psychological conception of the person as a partial but fundamental explanation of human behavior, which is not threatened by but is consistent with the truth of determinism. Legal rules are action-guiding within this conception. Morse acknowledges that there is a metaphysical problem of free will. But he argues that the libertarian conception of free will defended by some philosophers and questioned by many neuroscientists is not foundational for the legal conception of responsibility. While he notes that there have been major advances in neuroscience and is open to the possibility that it could have an impact on legal policy and practice, in the near to intermediate term neuroscience will likely make modest contributions to them. Morse offers an incisive critique of the view that neuroscience will cause us to radically change our conception of ourselves as rational agents and our legal doctrines and practices. Neuroscience findings do not replace but need to be translated into the law's folk-psychological framework. There are limits to what neurolaw can tell us about how we should regulate our lives in a complex society.

REFERENCES

Atmanspacher, H. and Rotter, S. 2011. On determinacy or its absence in the brain. In Swinburne (ed.), pp. 84–101.

Balaguer, M. 2010. *Free Will as an Open Scientific Problem*. Cambridge, MA: MIT Press.

Bayne, T. 2011. Libet and the case for free will scepticism. In *Swinburne* (ed.), pp. 25–46.

Benedetti, F., Colloca, L., Tome, E., Lanotte, M., Melcarne, A., et al. 2004. Placebo-responsive Parkinson's patients show decreased activity in single neurons of subthalamic nucleus. *Nature Neuroscience* 7: 587–588.

Benedetti, F., Carlino, E., and Pollo, A. 2011. How placebos change the patient's brain. *Neuropsychopharmacology* 36: 339–354.

Bengson, J., Kelly, T., Zhand, X., Wang, J.-L., Mangun, G. 2014. Spontaneous neural fluctuations predict decisions to attend. *Journal of Cognitive Neuroscience* 26: 2578–2584.

Berofsky, B. 2012. *Nature's Challenge to Free Will*. New York: Oxford University Press.

Burns, K. and Bechara, A. 2007. Decision making and free will: a neuroscience perspective. *Behavioral Sciences and the Law* 25: 263–280.

Cashmore, A. 2010. The Lucretian swerve: the biological basis of human behavior and the criminal justice system. *Proceedings of the National Academy of Sciences* 107: 4499–4504.

Chalmers, D. 1996. *The Conscious Mind*. New York: Oxford University Press.

2010. *The Character of Consciousness*. New York: Oxford University Press.

Craver, C. 2007. *Explaining the Brain: Mechanisms and the Mosaic Unity of Neuroscience*. New York: Oxford University Press.

Damasio, A. 2010. *Self Comes to Mind: Constructing the Conscious Brain*. New York: Vintage Books.

de Charms R., Maeda, F., Glover, G., Ludlow, D., Pauley, J., et al. 2005. Control over brain activation and pain learned by using real-time functional MRI. *Proceedings of the National Academy of Sciences* 102: 18626–18631.

De la Fuente-Fernandez, R., Ruth, T., Sossi, V., Schulzer, M., Calne, D., and Stoessl, A. J. 2001. Expectation and dopamine release: mechanisms of the placebo effect in Parkinson's disease. *Science* 293: 1164–1166.

Dennett, D. 1984. *Elbow Room: The Varieties of Free Will Worth Wanting*. Cambridge, MA: MIT Press.

2003. *Freedom Evolves*. New York: Penguin Books.

Feinberg, T. 2001. *Altered Egos: How the Brain Creates the Self*. New York: Oxford University Press.

2011. The nested neural hierarchy and the self. *Consciousness and Cognition* 20: 4–15.

Fischer, J. M. 1994. *The Metaphysics of Free Will: An Essay on Control*. Cambridge, MA: Blackwell.

Fischer, J. M. and Ravizza, M. 1998. *Responsibility and Control: A Theory of Moral Responsibility*. New York: Cambridge University Press.

Frankfurt, H. 1988. *The Importance of What We Care About*. New York: Cambridge University Press.

Gallagher, S. 2006. Where's the action? Epiphenomenalism and the problem of free will. In W. Banks, S. Pockett, and S. Gallagher (eds.), *Does Consciousness*

Cause Behavior? An Investigation of the Nature of Volition. Cambridge, MA: MIT Press, pp. 109–124.

Goldapple, K., Segal, Z., Garson, C., Lau, M., Bieling, P., et al. 2004. Modulation of cortical-limbic pathways in major depression: treatment-specific effects of cognitive behavior therapy. *Archives of General Psychiatry* 61: 34–41.

Greene, J. and Cohen, J. 2004. For the law, neuroscience changes nothing and everything. *Philosophical Transactions of the Royal Society of London* 359: 1775–1785.

Haggard, P. 2005. Conscious intention and motor cognition. *Trends in Cognitive Sciences* 9: 290–295.

2008. Human volition: towards a neuroscience of will. *Nature Reviews Neuroscience* 9: 934–946.

2011. Does brain science change our view of free will? In Swinburne (ed.), pp. 7–24.

Heyman, G. 2009. *Addiction: A Disorder of Choice*. Cambridge, MA: Harvard University Press.

Hyman, S. 2007. The neurobiology of addiction: implications for voluntary control of behavior. *AJOB Neuroscience* 7 (1): 8–11.

Jackson, F. 1982. Epiphenomenal qualia. *Philosophical Quarterly* 32: 127–136.

James, W. 1956. *The Will to Believe*. New York: Dover.

Kane, R. 1996. *The Significance of Free Will*. New York: Oxford University Press.

Koob G. and Volkow, N. 2010. Neurocircuitry of addiction. *Neuropsychopharmacology* 35: 217–238.

Kornhuber H. and Deecke, L. 1965. Hirnpotentialanderungen bei Willkurbewegungen undpassiven Bewegungen des Menschen: Bereitschaftspotential und reafferente Potentiale. *Pflugers Archiv fur die gesamte Physiologie des Menschen und der Tiere* 284: 1–17.

Libet, B. 1985. Unconscious cerebral initiative and the role of conscious will in voluntary action. *Behavioral and Brain Sciences* 8: 529–566.

2004. *Mind Time: The Temporal Factor in Consciousness*. Cambridge, MA: Harvard University Press.

Linden D., Habes, I., Johnston, S., Lindon, S., Tatineni, R., et al. 2012. Real-time self-regulation of emotion networks in patients with depression. *PLoS ONE*, June 4. Doi: 10.1371/journal.pone.0038115.

Lozano A. and Lipsman, N. 2013. Probing and regulating dysfunctional circuits using deep brain stimulation. *Neuron* 77: 406–424.

Mele, A. 2009. *Effective Intentions: The Power of Conscious Will*. New York: Oxford University Press.

2014a. *Free: Why Science Hasn't Disproved Free Will*. New York: Oxford University Press.

2014b (ed.). *Surrounding Free Will: Philosophy, Psychology, Neuroscience*. New York: Oxford University Press.

Morse, S. 2007. The non-problem of free will in forensic psychiatry and psychology. *Behavioral Sciences & the Law* 25: 203–220.

2013. Common criminal law compatibilism. In N. Vincent (ed.), *Neuroscience and Legal Responsibility*. New York: Oxford University Press, pp. 27–52.

Nahmias, E. 2006. Folk fears about freedom and responsibility: determinism versus reductionism. *Journal of Cognition and Culture* 6: 215–237.
2010. Scientific challenges to free will. In T. O'Connor and C. Sandis (eds.), *A Companion to the Philosophy of Action.* Cambridge, MA: Wiley-Blackwell, pp. 345–356.
Poldrack, R. 2011. Inferring mental states from neuroimaging data from reverse inference to large-scale decoding. *Neuron* 72: 692–697.
Roskies, A. 2006. Neuroscientific challenges to free will and responsibility. *Trends in Cognitive Sciences* 10: 419–423
2010. How does neuroscience affect our conception of volition? *Annual Review of Neuroscience* 33: 109–130.
2013. Brain imaging techniques. In S. Morse and A. Roskies (eds.), *A Primer on Criminal Law and Neuroscience.* New York: Oxford University Press, pp. 37–74.
Spence, S. 2009. *The Actor's Brain: Exploring the Cognitive Neuroscience of Free Will.* Oxford University Press.
Strawson, G. 2010. *Freedom and Belief*, revised edn. Oxford: Clarendon Press.
Swinburne, R. (ed.). 2011. *Free Will and Modern Science.* Oxford University Press.
2013. *Mind, Brain, and Free Will.* Oxford University Press.
Van Inwagen, P. 1983. *An Essay on Free Will.* Oxford: Clarendon Press.
Wegner, D. 2002. *The Illusion of Conscious Will.* Cambridge, MA: MIT Press.

Part II

Conceptual issues

2 Is free will an observer-based concept rather than a brain-based one? A critical neuroepistemological account

Georg Northoff

ABSTRACT

How are the brain and our observation of it in neuroscientific investigation related to each other? I here distinguish between brain-based and observer-based concepts. Brain-based concepts mean that they are very much in accordance with the way the brain functions and processes neural activity independent of our observation of it. In contrast, observer-based concepts refer to the dependence of our observations on the observer and his or her particular experimental (and technological and other) requirements. Since in observer-based concepts the observer intrudes into the observations and ultimately into the brain itself, I also speak of 'observer-related intrusions'. I distinguish between extrinsic and intrinsic observer-related intrusions: extrinsic observer-related intrusions can in principle be avoided and minimized while intrinsic ones cannot in principle be overcome. This is so because they concern, as I assume, intrinsic design features of the brain, and do therefore define the brain as brain. I conclude that the intrinsic observer-related intrusions pose 'neuro-experimental and neuroepistemological constraints' on our possible knowledge of the brain. Extrinsic observer-related intrusions pose methodological fallacies that are to be avoided, as, for instance, the projection of the concept of free will onto the brain.

Introduction

There is an intense debate about free will in current philosophy and neuroscience. Philosophical discussion often focuses on the metaphysical question of whether human agents can choose and act freely in light of causal determinism. Neuroscientific discussion focuses on the neural mechanisms underlying the will and what they imply about whether or to what extent it is free. If these mechanisms are part of a process in which they do all or most of the causal work in producing actions, then this seems to rule out free will. On this view, our behavior is controlled not by what occurs at the mental level of beliefs, desires and intentions but instead by what occurs at the neural level (Farah 2005; cf. Walter 2001). The main question is whether the demonstration of neural activity is a sufficient condition to opt for neural determinism and the implication that we lack free will.

My approach in this chapter will be different. Rather than taking the concept of free will for granted and then projecting a definition of it onto the brain, I opt against such a 'mapping strategy'. Instead, I focus on the epistemological presuppositions on which the application of the concept of free will to the brain is based. For that I will discuss at length epistemological considerations like the distinction between observer- and brain-based concepts as well as intrinsic vs. extrinsic observer-related intrusions. These imply that the current philosophical models and concepts of free will, including their mapping onto the brain, may be conceptual artifacts produced by the observer that as such are projected upon the brain. Hence, I designate free will as primarily an observer-based concept, as distinguished from empirically plausible concepts that then would need to be described as brain-based concepts.

This opens new lines of inference. Traditionally, it is assumed that neuroscientific results have direct implications for the question of determinism or indeterminism and hence whether there is free will or not. Independently of whether one opts for determinism or indeterminism, one draws a direct inference from the neuroscientific data to the conceptual question of determinism versus indeterminism. One thus implicitly presupposes the concepts of determinism or indeterminism to be brain-based, since otherwise one could not draw direct inferences from brain to concept. This changes once one associates the concepts of indeterminism and determinism and especially the apparently mutually exclusive character of these concepts being observer-rather than brain-based. Then a direct inference from brain to concept seems no longer plausible. Instead, in the first instance, one would then investigate the relationship between observer and brain rather than the one between brain and concept. If it turns out that the concepts of indeterminism and determinism can be located towards the observer end of the continuum between brain- and observer-based concepts, then any inference from brain to concept may be even more distant and problematic. If, in contrast, the concepts of indeterminism and determinism can be located towards the brain end (being brain-based to a higher degree) of the continuum, an inference from and direct relationship between brain and concepts seems to be more plausible. In other words, I claim that the possibility of drawing inferences from our current neuroscientific data to either determinism or indeterminism very much depends on the characterization of these concepts as either observer- or brain based. The empirical plausibility of our neurophilosophical assumptions about free will may thus need to take into account the epistemological characterization of the concept itself as either brain- or observer-based.

Neuroepistemological remark: distinction between brain- and observer-based concepts

Neuroscience acquires data and ultimately facts to describe the brain (the distinction between data and facts may by itself be worth discussing from a philosophical point of view, though it is not pursued here; see Northoff 2012). Thereby it uses concepts to describe those data and facts. Usually, one would expect the concepts to correspond to and thus match the data and facts. In this case, there is a one-to-one relation with one particular datum being the only and exclusive content the concepts describe.

Life is not that easy, though, especially the life of a neuroscientist. Concepts are usually more general and vague than particular data and facts. This means that concepts usually include more than one particular content and thus by definition are general. That in turn makes them less specific when compared to data and facts. The concepts the neuroscientist (and any scientist) uses (or must use) remain consecutively unable to completely match and correspond to the data and facts in a one-to-one way. Instead, the concepts may also refer to contents other than the ones from particular data and facts in question. This implies a one-to-many relationship where one concepts stands for (or codes) many data/facts. Hence, rather than coding data and facts in either a local (even sparse) way, concepts seem to encode data and facts in a rather dense way. This means that there is almost certainly a certain degree of mismatch between concepts and data/facts.

This all sounds very philosophical, the neuroscientist may want to say. Let the philosophers discuss this, but leave me alone in generating data and facts. As noted, life is not that easy. Because of the almost certain mismatch between concepts and data/facts with the former encoding the latter in a dense way, we are prone to confusion. More specifically, we can never be completely sure (or know as the epistemologist may want to say) whether the concept we use to describe our data and facts really matches and corresponds to the latter. And where there is uncertainty, there is the possibility of mismatch and confusion. This applies to both the neurophilosopher and the neuroscientist. Given the need to start our experimental investigation with concepts and terminate it with the interpretation of the data via concepts, there is no way of avoiding concepts even in neuroscientific investigation. However, the seemingly unavoidable (or necessary) presence of concepts in the interpretation that are often not distinguished from the one used to describe the data themselves suggests intrusion of the observer into the neuroscientific investigation. There seems to be almost no way of avoiding the observer's intrusion even in the seemingly most objective investigation. There is thus a neuroepistemological constraint, the intrusion of the observer via the use and definition of concepts, inherent in our neuroscientific and neurophilosophical methodology. The only way to minimize that intrusion may be to introduce methodological and epistemological distinctions like the one introduced here: brain-versus observer-based concepts and intrinsic versus extrinsic observer-related intrusions (see below).

How can we now describe such possible confusion between concepts and data/facts in further detail? Concepts are generated by the observer. The very same observer who conducts the experiments also needs to generate concepts to describe his or her data/facts and to formulate his or her hypotheses. Yielding hypotheses and data/facts is possible only when considering certain requirements that need to be fulfilled within the experimental context. One such experimental requirement is the careful distinction between different experimental variables that need to be treated in a segregated and independent way. This makes necessary the introduction of concepts describing these segregated and independent variables.

So far, so good. The problem starts once the very same concepts that describe these segregated and independent experimental variables are also assumed to describe the brain itself. More specifically, based on the experimental data/facts, the concepts describing the respective experimental variables are assumed to describe one-to-one the processes and mechanisms in the brain itself. Thereby the concept is supposed to match and correspond to the brain's neuronal processes as they are independent of the observer's observation. The concept is thus supposed to refer to the brain as it is by itself. However, one could also imagine instances where the concept does not match or correspond to the brain's neuronal processes and mechanisms as they are by themselves. In that case, the concept is more related to the observer and his or her experimental requirements than to the brain itself and its neuronal processes and mechanisms considered independently of the observer. This means the concept is more observer-based than brain-based. I hence distinguish between what I describe as observer- and brain-based concepts.

The distinction between observer- and brain-based concepts is not an All-or-Nothing distinction but rather a More-or-Less distinction. This means that a particular concept may be based on both the observer's experimental requirements and the brain's neuronal processes thus reflecting a continuum between brain- and observed-based concepts (see Figure 2.1a). It may thus be just a matter of degree and balance between the two ingredients, observer and brain, that determine the concept in question. A concept is thus either more or less strongly based on either the observer and his or her experimental requirement or the brain's neuronal processes. There is thus a continuum with its two extreme poles describing purely observer- and brain-based concepts. The neuroscientist seeks of course concepts where the balance is tilted strongly towards the brain-based pole of the continuum and away from the observer-based pole.

Neuroepistemological remark: examples of observer-versus brain-based concepts

In neuroscience, we encounter several examples of suspicious concepts where the balance seemed to be more strongly tilted towards the observer than the brain itself. In the following I want to briefly mention some of them.

Central neurotransmitters in the brain are glutamate and GABA (gamma-aminobutyric acid). Experimentally, we need to segregate glutamate and GABA and correspondingly neural excitation and inhibition from each other. In order to measure, for instance, glutamate and neural excitation, we need to experimentally parse both variables from any traces of GABA and neural inhibition. Otherwise we cannot be sure whether our data really tell us about glutamate and neural excitation themselves. This means ultimately that GABA and glutamate and hence neural inhibition and excitation are treated as segregated and independent experimental variables. The designation of GABA and glutamate as segregated and independent variables occurs on purely experimental grounds and is therefore strongly observer-based. Based on the data whose acquisition presupposes such experimental segregation and independence, one would assume GABA and glutamate to also act segregated and independently in the brain itself. One consecutively assumes that certain levels of GABA and neural inhibition are necessary for a specific neuronal process. While these levels may be open to (secondary) modulation by glutamate and neural excitation, they are considered (primarily) as independent and segregated (in a constitutive rather than merely modulatory sense.

What does this imply for our distinction between brain- and observer-based concepts? This means that now the observer's concepts are transferred to the brain itself. The initially observer-based characterization of GABA and glutamate as independent and segregated experimental variables is now projected onto the brain itself and assumed to accurately

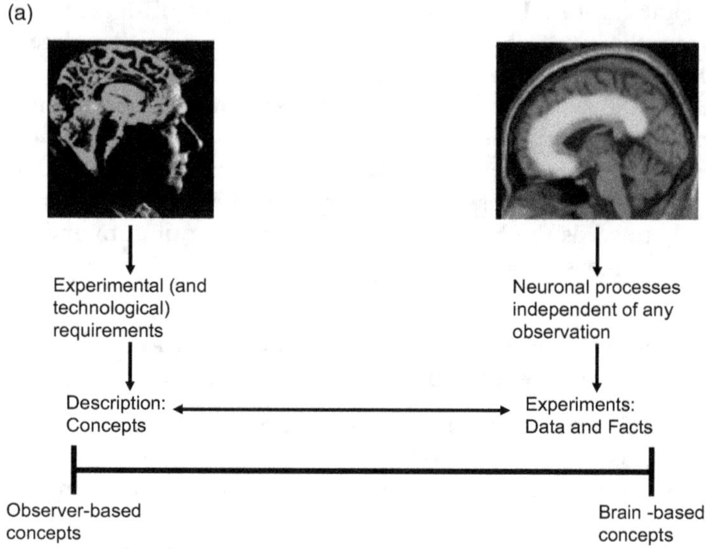

Figure 2.1a The figure describes two key features in the relation between brain and observer, the continuum between brain- and observer-based Caption for Figure 2.1 (*cont.*) concepts (a) and the distinction between intrinsic and extrinsic observer-related intrusions (b). (a) Observer-based concepts are those concepts that describe the brain but rely on us as observers and or abilities to observe the brain. Hence, we cannot be fully sure whether these concepts are related more to us as observers or the brain itself. In contrast, brain-based concepts describe the brain as it is by itself independent of our observation of it. The data reflect the brain itself rather than us as observers. I assume a continuum between brain- and observer-based concepts (lower part) with both being extreme cases in their pure forms on a continuum.

describe its neuronal processes. In short, it is no longer regarded as observer-based but rather as brain-based.

Does such experimentally based segregation and independence between GABA/neural inhibition and glutamate/neural excitation really correspond to the empirical data? I deny that. Instead, I assume that both GABA and glutamate can be characterized by difference-based coding with each coding the relative relation between the two rather than their absolute value independent of this relation (see Northoff 2014a). This is empirically manifest in the excitation–inhibition balance (EIB) that is

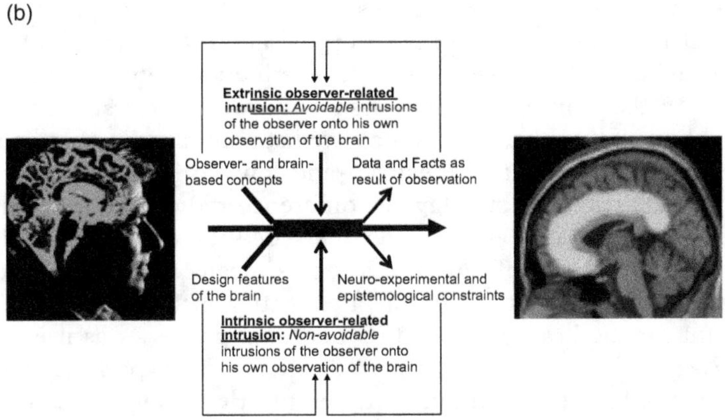

Figure 2.1b Extrinsic observer-related intrusions (upper part) are those intrusions of the observer into the brain's neural activity that can in principle be avoided by better experiments, etc. In contrast, intrinsic observer-related intrusions (lower part) are those that can in principle not be avoided because observation is supposed to be possible only on the basis of the brain's intrinsic features without which observation would remain impossible. Hence, observation cannot but intrude into the brain and its intrinsic design features because otherwise it would remain impossible in principle.

supposed to provide the measure for the subsequent generation of neural activity. Yet such coding of the difference to the respective other puts the assumption of (primary and constitutive) segregation and independence between glutamate and GABA into doubt. The characterization of GABA and glutamate by (primary and constitutive) segregation and independence may be relevant (and even required) for the observer (and his experimental approach). It may not apply to the brain as such independently of the observer. This means that such characterization is more strongly related to the observer and his or her experimental requirements than to the brain's neuronal processes as they are by themselves independent of the observer's observation. In other words, assuming segregation and independence between GABA and glutamate may turn out to be more observer-based than brain-based.

Another example is the distinction between different types of stimuli according to their origin in either the brain, i.e. neuronal stimuli, the body, i.e. interoceptive stimuli or the world, i.e. exteroceptive stimuli. Based on these distinct origins, different anatomical structures and pathways have been assumed as it is well reflected in the radial-concentric threefold anatomical organisation (see Northoff 2014a). However, on a functional level, the distinction between the different origins of the stimuli and their respective anatomical structures seems to be blurred: this was, for instance, well apparent in the observed neural activity, i.e. functional connectivity and low- to high-frequency fluctuations, and the coding strategy, i.e. difference-rather than stimulus-based coding, that operated across and superseded the underlying anatomical structure (See Northoff 2014a). Yet this means that the distinction of stimuli according to their origin, i.e. matter of origin, may be not as relevant for the brain itself and its neuronal processes as it is for us as observers and our experimental requirements: the experimental requirement is not to confuse stimuli of different origins. Otherwise we cannot say anything about, for instance, exteroceptive stimuli and their underlying neuronal processes.

However, as important as the question of the origin of stimuli is for us as observers, it does not seem important for the brain itself. The brain seems to be more 'interested' in varying degrees of statistically based differences between different stimuli (and itself) than the stimuli themselves and their respective origins. Hence my characterization of the brain's neural operation as a 'matter of degrees and differences' rather than a 'matter of origins and stimuli'. This means, though, that the characterization of the brain's neural processing by 'matter of origin and stimuli' may be more strongly related to the observer him- or herself than the brain itself. I assume that the 'matter of degrees and differences' is tilted more towards the brain-based pole in the continuum between the extremes of purely observer- and brain-based concepts.

Let us provide a final example where brain- and observer-based concepts may be confused: the distinction between resting-state and stimulus-induced activity. Experimentally, we clearly need to segregate and delineate both since otherwise we will never be able to know the contributions of the stimulus and that of the brain itself in stimulus-induced activity. One may consecutively assume segregation between resting-state and stimulus-induced activity. Yet as the empirical data suggest, both cannot principally be distinguished from each other, let alone segregated.

Resting-state activity and stimulus-induced activity are not categorically distinct but can be distinguished from each other only on the basis of degrees. This means that the principal distinction between resting-state and stimulus-induced activity is more strongly based on the observer than the brain itself. One may thus formulate what can be described as a 'continuity hypothesis' that assumes neuronal continuum and discontinuum between resting-state and stimulus-induced activity. If the stimulus-induced activity does not alter much the pre-existing resting-state activity, the latter may shift towards the brain end of the continuum between brain- and observer-based concepts. If, in contrast, the extrinsic stimulus and its stimulus-induced activity exert major changes to the brain's intrinsic activity, e.g. its resting-state activity, the increasing discontinuum between the two may go along with a shift towards the observer end on the continuum. Why? Because the observer is always already involved in the extrinsic stimuli he or she applies, be it directly as part of that stimulus itself, or indirectly as the applicant or cause of that stimulus. In other words, the investigation of extrinsic stimulus-induced activity may be more prone to intrusions by the observer and thus to the consecutive development of observer-rather than brain-based concepts (Northoff 2014a and 2012).

How can we escape the possible confusion between brain- and observer-based concepts? In order to shift concepts away from the observer-based pole towards the brain-based pole, we thus need to also shift our perspective. More specifically, we need to abandon our observer-based perspective and imagine how it is for the brain itself independent of our observation to generate the kind of neuronal processes we observe. We should aim to move from the observer's perspective to the brain's perspective, taken in a figurative sense because the brain itself has no perspective. Metaphorically one may consequently say that we need to replace the 'What it is like for the observer' by the 'What it is like for the brain'

Taken together, I here demonstrated various examples of concepts that seem to be more strongly based on the observer himself and his experimental requirements than on the brain's neuronal processes independent of any observation. We may want to sharpen the point even further: is an observer-free and thus truly objective (in an absolute rather than relative sense) investigation of the brain possible at all for us? Or are there always already some intrusions which we cannot avoid by all means, e.g. intrinsic observer-related intrusions? And one may argue that already raising this question is possible only on the basis of an observer. Hence no data about the brain can be interpreted without an observer and the possibility of intrusion. Diagnosis of the more strongly observer-based component in these concepts led me to search for other concepts that are presumably more brain-based. This in turn was accompanied by a shift in experimental variables and hypotheses in order to test these more brain-based concepts experimentally and lend empirical support to them. That also makes it clear that the distinction between observer- and brain-based concepts is not a mere philosophical-conceptual exercise but highly relevant both experimentally and empirically.

Neuroepistemological remark: extrinsic observer-related intrusions

How can we be sure that the concepts we apply are more brain-than observer-based? The only way for us to know is to develop corresponding hypotheses and conduct the appropriate experiments. If the data are in accordance with the characterization implied by these concepts, the assumption of them being more brain-based may be justified. If, in contrast, the data do not support them, my concepts may turn out to be as observer-based as the ones I replaced.

If the data are in accordance with the concepts, then the latter are empirically plausible. They are thus to a higher degree based on the brain than the observer. The opposite case of no empirical support suggests that they are based more on the observer than the brain. Hence, the degree of empirical plausibility, the accordance of the concept with the empirical data, may be regarded as a measure of the degree to which the concept is more strongly brain- or observer-based. This also implies that purely brain-based concepts seem more of an ideal than reality. What further supports this view is the problem of drawing valid inferences from brain images to the data, given that there is no direct correspondence between them (Roskies 2008). To formulate it in even stronger terms, purely brain-based concepts may in principle be impossible. However, alternative experimental designs should also be applied using different experimental variables. If they yield the same or analogous results, the likelihood of both data sets being confounded by the experimental requirements of segregation and independence of experimental variables is rather low. The data may then provide an excellent basis for being associated with a concept that shows a high probability of being brain-based rather than observer-based.

How is such low empirical plausibility with a more strongly observer-based concept possible? In that case the observer and his or her experimental (and technological and other) requirements seem to intrude too much into the concept and the subsequent experimental design to yield more brain-based concepts. The observer thus intrudes into the brain and imposes him- or herself, thereby manipulating what he or she can observe from the brain's neuronal processes according to his or her own stance and needs. I call such intrusion 'observer-related intrusion'.

The concept of the 'observer-related intrusion' refers to the intrusion or imposition of the observer him- or herself into/onto his or her own observation of the brain's neuronal processes (see Figure 2.1b). In short, observer-related intrusions describe that the observer him- or herself confounds his or her own observations. Observer-related intrusions do consecutively lead to low degrees of empirical plausibility and more observer-than brain-based concepts.

How can we deal with observer-related intrusions? We can try out alternative concepts and conduct the respective experimental designs. Then we can compare the results from both experimental lines and see how much they accord with the respectively presupposed concept. The experimental line with the higher degree of accordance, i.e. empirical plausibility, may then be the one where the concept is less observer-based when compared to the respective other one. We have to try out different alternative concepts and put them to rigorous experimental testing (see chapter 3 in Northoff 2011 for such methodology, which I describe as 'concept-fact iterativity'). This means that we are not at the mercy of observer-related intrusion and that we do have methodological tools to minimize and ultimately avoid it. We can minimize the degree to which an observer intrudes and imposes himself onto our concepts. In the best case, we can avoid observer-related intrusions altogether; respective concepts are strongly brain-based approaching the one extreme end of the continuum between brain- and observer-based concepts. Since we are in principle able to minimize the degree of observer-related intrusion, I characterize them as extrinsic. The concept of 'extrinsic observer-related intrusion' suggests that the observer's intrusion and imposition can in principle be minimized and at best be avoided thus remaining extrinsic to both observation and concept.

Neuroepistemological remark: intrinsic observer-related intrusions

I assume that extrinsic observer-related intrusions can in principle be minimized and at best avoided altogether. This is possible by refining our concepts, as described, and developing better and more precise technological tools for measuring and acquiring data (as, for instance, higher resolution brain scanning). There may be instances where we remain unable to minimize observer-related intrusion. This, to be clear, does not concern the individual observer as distinct from other individual observers; rather, it pertains to all possible observers.

Let me start with Buszaki and his emphasis on rhythms and oscillations. He argues in his excellent book *Rhythms of the Brain* (2006) that rhythms and oscillations are a hallmark feature of the brain. To prove his point, though, he would need to experimentally investigate a brain without oscillations and see whether it does not show the kinds of effects for which he assumes oscillations to be necessary. Yet that remains impossible since we cannot even imagine a brain without oscillations, let alone test it experimentally, as Buszaki himself remarks (see Buszaki 2006, 360).

Even pathological cases like schizophrenia, depression or vegetative states that may help in overcoming extrinsic observer-related intrusions do not provide an option here. Why? Because they still show rhythms and oscillations which, despite being distorted, are nonetheless present and thus not completely absent as experimentally required. There is thus a limit to the possible experimental testing that in principle cannot be overcome or avoided. More specifically, to gain experimental proof of the causal role of oscillations in specific psychological processes and even consciousness, we would need to eliminate them completely. This is not the case even in neuropsychiatric disorders. There oscillations are still present, though in a distorted way. From those abnormalities we may gain some clues about the possible role of oscillations for particular psychological processes, especially if the latter are also altered in the psychiatric patients. However, this is not sufficient to demonstrate a causal role of oscillations for the respective psychological processes but only a modulatory or correlational role. Mere modulation or correlation is not to be equated with causality since the alterations in the patients' psychological processes may be modulated by the oscillations yet caused by other neuronal processes completely different from the oscillations. Hence, neuropsychiatric disorders can help in our understanding of the brain as distinct from the observer but not overcome our epistemological limits, e.g. intrinsic observer-related intrusions, as I will call them below.

We can describe such limits in further detail. The limits consist in the fact that we remain in principle unable to prove whether our concepts of rhythms and oscillations are ultimately based on the brain itself independent of us as observers or whether they reflect how we can (and cannot) observe the brain. We are thus stuck in our own intrusion, i.e. the concept of rhythms and oscillations, without being able to ever free ourselves from them. I therefore speak of an 'intrinsic observer-related intrusion' as distinguished from an 'extrinsic observer-related intrusion'.

How is it possible that 'observer-related intrusions' are intrinsic rather than extrinsic? This amounts to the question for the different concepts associated with intrinsic and extrinsic observer-related intrusions. The concepts of rhythms and oscillations refer to a feature that characterizes the brain's designs and, even stronger, defines the brain as brain. Buszaki cannot even imagine a brain without oscillations because otherwise he would no longer talk about a brain (at least not of a human brain) which would be meaningless. He thus considers rhythms and oscillations to be what I describe as 'design features' of the brain that as such define the brain as brain. In short, rhythms and oscillations are design features of the brain that are intrinsic to the brain and do therefore define the brain as brain.

We can describe the brain's 'intrinsic design features' in further empirical detail. The brain's intrinsic activity seems to show an elaborate temporal and spatial structure as its design feature. The temporal structure seems to consist in the fluctuations of the intrinsic activity level in different frequency ranges (from 0.001 to 60Hz). Thereby the phases, e.g. their onsets and peaks, in the different frequency ranges are somehow coupled and linked together, which seems to provide the template with a quite elaborate (not yet fully understood) temporal structure (see Northoff 2014a). The spatial structure of the intrinsic activity seems to consist in the distribution of the activity levels across different regions yielding transregional balances and thus a certain spatial pattern or structure of intrinsic activity. Moreover, it seems that temporal and spatial structures are somehow related to each other, with the exact mechanisms of such spatiotemporal coupling remaining currently unclear (see Northoff 2014a and 2014b).

How is the neural activity in this spatial and temporal structure coded? Empirical data suggest that it is not the single peak at some discrete point in time and space that is coded. Instead, what are coded in neural activity in the resting state (and also the stimulus-induced state) are the differences in neural activity between two different discrete temporal and spatial points. This means that the neural activity is not based on the single stimulus or single activity change at one discrete point in time and space but rather on spatial and temporal differences. This is what can be called difference-based coding as distinguished from stimulus-based coding (see Northoff 2014a).

I have assumed difference-based coding as distinguished from stimulus-based coding to define the brain's neural code. Since the code very much defines what and how the brain can process neural activity, it also defines the brain as brain. Since difference-based coding describes a coding strategy that results in temporal and spatial sparsening of neural activity, sparse coding must also be regarded as design feature. The same holds for predictive coding that also seems to be unavoidable once one presupposes difference-based coding.

Besides the coding strategy, other more specific design features concern the high- and low-frequency fluctuations of neural activity in both resting-state and stimulus-induced activity. This mirrors Buszaki's assumption of rhythms and oscillations. Functional connectivity between different regions during both forms of neural activity is yet another design feature. Finally, most important, the brain's intrinsic activity, its resting-state activity, and its consecutive constitution of a spatiotemporal structure must also be regarded as a design feature of the brain without which the brain would not be a brain (at least not a human brain). 'Intrinsic feature' means here that it cannot be changed in principle by any extrinsic stimulus in the same way that the intrinsic muscle structure of the heart cannot be abolished by extrinsic blood flow Despite their differences, all these features share the idea that their absence could not even be imagined without abandoning the ground of the brain. They must therefore be assumed to define the brain as brain and are thus what I describe as the brain's design features.

We now face a serious problem. One may focus on these design features. These features may be more brain-based than other rival concepts that I regard to be more observer-based. In order to show that these concepts are brain-based, I would need to put them to experimental testing. That means that I would need to show not only that the presence of the intrinsic design features induces neuronal and phenomenal/mental effects but also that their absence makes the neuronal and phenomenal/mental effects impossible. If I were able to show the latter, I could assume that the brain's intrinsic design features are a necessary condition of possible consciousness (see Northoff 2014b).

Yet this is the point where the problems start. While I can test the effects of the presence of these design features, the experimental testing of their absence remains in principle impossible. In the same way that Buszaki cannot even imagine a brain without oscillations, let alone experimentally test its effects, we cannot imagine at all a brain without difference-based and sparse coding, a brain without functional connectivity, a brain without intrinsic activity, and a brain without spatiotemporal structure. Why? Because these are design features of the brain that are intrinsic to the brain as brain.

Let me be clear. There are principal constraints (and ultimately limits) to how far we can go experimentally. Since these principal constraints (and ultimately limits) can be traced back to the brain itself and its particular design features, I here speak of neuro-experimental constraints. These neuro-experimental constraints do constrain and limit the knowledge we can possibly acquire about the brain These epistemological constraints, i.e. the limits in our possible knowledge of the brain and its empirical function, may therefore be described as neuroepistemological constraints. Since these concern the brain's design features and their neuronal and phenomenal/mental effects, any hypothesis is very much prone to both neuro-experimental and neuroepistemological constraints.

Does that invalidate future hypotheses? Yes and No. Yes, because ultimately one remains principally unable to know whether one is right or wrong, thus being unable to overcome intrinsic observer-related intrusion. One will therefore remain principally unable to know whether the brain operates on the basis of difference-based coding independent of my concept and hypothesis of it. No, because one can at least work on minimizing the extrinsic observer-related intrusions and develop novel experimental designs in order to put my hypotheses on more secure empirical ground. Hence, empirically one may move forward while epistemologically one remains stuck in the border territory between what can and cannot possibly be known in principle about the brain. That isn't so bad after all. Or is it?

Conclusion: free will as observer-based concept and extrinsic observer-related intrusion

How does all that apply to the concept of free will? There is intense discussion in the current philosophical debate as to whether free will is compatible or incompatible with the supposed determinism of the neuronal processes in the brain. There are different versions of compatibilism and incompatibilism in response of the idea of neural determinism and various intermediate positions between them. We did not discuss any of that here. Rather, my aim was to show that the concept of free will by itself may be more related to the observer than the brain. We as outside observers of the brain experience or assume to experience free will. However, when investigating the brain we assume determinism of neuronal states as physical states which seems to be incompatible with the assumption of free will. Is there now free will in the brain or not? If so, one would assume free will to be a brain-based concept. If not, then it is an observer-based concept. We would thus make our decision based on the kind of concept free will is dependent on our results.

We may start earlier, though. The question of free will seems to presuppose the sharp and mutually exclusive distinction between free will and no free will, between indeterminism and determinism. How does that presupposition stand to the brain and its neural operations? The brain may be neither a completely deterministic nor a completely indeterministic system. Instead, it may operate on a continuum ranging between the extremes of determinism and indeterminism. But given the neuro-experimental and neuroepistemological constraints that I have described, the concept of free will may turn out to be more of an observer-than a brain-based concept.

There is yet another reason why the concept of free will may be more of an observer-based than a brain-based concept. Free will can be experienced only by persons. The brain itself cannot experience free will. Attribution of free will to the brain and specific neural mechanisms may thus lead to confusion between persons and brains implying confusion between observer and brain. The concept of free will, as person-based, is thus an observer-based concept. Characterizing free will as a brain-based concept would neglect the fact that the observer is a person, an agent who interacts with and whose actions can have an impact on the natural and social environment. Hence, it is important to consider the agent and how he experiences subjectively from the inside, in his First-Person Perspective, as well as what we as observers describe as free will from the outside in our Third-Person Perspective. We may thus need both first- and third-person approaches to properly account for free will (see also Spence 2009).

Why is all that important? By investigating such conceptual and epistemological issues, we may clear the way for subsequent experimental research into concepts that may not be suitable for inclusion in empirical investigation. Any observer-based definition of concepts that does not turn out to be brain-based has a high likelihood of not providing insight into how the brain functions and operates independently of us and our observations. In other words, by using such concepts as free will we may intrude upon the brain, yielding results that are external rather than intrinsic to the brain itself. We will produce what I described as extrinsic observer-related intrusions.

This also has important implications for claims from Libet (1985), Fried (2011), Haggard (2005 and 2008), Haynes et al. (2007) and Haynes (2010) and other neuroscientists that mechanistic processes in the brain precede our conscious intention to act and therefore rule out free will. Neuro-experimental and neuroepistemological constraints imply a gap between what we observe about the brain and what actually occurs in the brain. Because of these constraints and the difficulty of eliminating intrinsic observer-based intrusions into the brain, we can only approximate and not achieve knowledge of neural mechanisms. The argument that we lack free will and that our belief in it is an illusion appeals to recorded data about event-related potentials in motor, pre-motor and supplementary motor areas in the brain. However, if we do not have direct but only indirect access to these neural mechanisms because the data are sensitive to intrinsic observer-related intrusions, and if claims about the significance of these data are more observer-based than brain-based, then we may have good reason to be sceptical of this argument.

There is no purely brain-based concept of free will. Claims that we have or lack free will may be more reflective of observers' projections onto the organ that is being observed than of intrinsic features of the organ itself. The continuum model offers the most plausible way of discussing the neuroscience of free will. Judgments about actions being free or unfree are not absolute but fall somewhere between observer-based and brain-based concepts along the continuum. This model suggests that appeal to neural activity alone will not establish whether we have or lack free will simply because direct inference from the brain to concepts like free will is epistemologically implausible given our apparent impossibility of excluding both observer-based concepts and intrinsic observer-related intrusions.

REFERENCES

Buszaki, G. 2006. *Rhythms of the Brain*. New York: Oxford University Press.

Farah, M. 2005. Neuroethics: the practical and the philosophical. *Trends in Cognitive Sciences* 9: 34–40.

Fried, I., Mukamel, R. and Kreiman, G. 2011. Internally generated preactivation of single neurons on human medial frontal cortex predicts volition. *Neuron* 69: 548–562.

Haggard, P. 2005. Conscious intention and motor cognition. *Trends in Cognitive Sciences* 9: 290–295.

2008. Human volition: towards a neuroscience of will. *Nature Reviews Neuroscience* 9: 934–946.

Haynes, J.-D. 2010. Beyond Libet: long-term prediction of free choices from neuroimaging signals. In W. Sinnott-Armstrong and L. Nadel (eds.), *Conscious Will and Responsibility: A Tribute to Benjamin Libet*. New York: Oxford University Press, Ch. 8.

Haynes, J.-D., Sakai, K., Rees, G., Gilbert, S. Frith, C. and Passinghuam, R. 2007. Reading hidden intentions in the human brain. *Current Biology* 17: 323–328.

Libet, B. 1985. Unconscious cerebral initiative and the role of conscious will in voluntary action. *Behavioral and Brain Sciences* 8: 529–566.

Northoff, G. 2011. *Neuropsychoanalysis in Practice: Brain, Self and Objects*. New York: Oxford University Press.

2012. Immanuel Kant's mind and the brain's resting state. *Trends in Cognitive Sciences* 16 (July): 356–359.

2014a. *Unlocking the Brain*. Vol. I: *Coding*. Oxford University Press.

2014b. *Unlocking the Brain*. Vol. II: *Consciousness*. Oxford University Press.

Roskies, A. 2008. Neuroimaging and inferential distance. *Neuroethics* 1 (1): 19–30.

Spence, S. 2009. *The Actor's Brain: Exploring the Cognitive Neuroscience of Free Will*. Oxford University Press.

Walter, H. 2001. *Neurophilosophy of Free Will: From Libertarian Illusions to a Concept of Natural Autonomy*, trans. C. Klohr. Cambridge, MA: MIT Press.

3 Evolution, dissolution and the neuroscience of the will

Grant Gillett

ABSTRACT

An Aristotelian conception of the will directs us towards the efficacy of the human intellect and its deliberations and whether our reasons genuinely control the way we act in the world. It is therefore directly relevant to human adaptation rather than the mechanism by which we achieve that. The way that humankind has evolved so that our thoughts do engage with the challenges we face in the world is also the focus of John Hughlings Jackson's work on evolutionary neurology and it finesses convoluted discussions about neural mechanisms in favour of a whole organism approach to thought and action. The key role he gives to propositionising prefigures the work of the great Russian neuropsychologist A. R. Luria who is very clear about our higher control of action and our engagement in a socio-cultural world of discourse. That *potency* orientation delivers a clear and coherent view of the nature of the will as the executive function of a human being who is capable, to a degree depending on personal development, of translating the results of argument into effective action in a world where he or she is a being-among-others and who satisfies the causal requirements to be a self-governing agent.

Introduction

The will and disorders of the will are problematic concepts in current cognitive neuroscience. Some claim they are empty because our so-called acts of will are subjective illusions created by efferent copies of motor output commands. Others see the will as our ability to translate reason into action so that defects of the will (such as *akrasia*) are failures in that capacity. Aristotle noted that the human will is at its best when we consider not only how to do what we want to do but also whether our aims are truly worthwhile; so the will is truly an aspect of the intellect. He noted that the defect in *akrasia* was not a problem of movement, nor a problem in reasoning and that attempts to remedy a defect of the will through reasoning were doomed to failure because, 'If water makes a man choke, what can you give him to wash it down with?' Aristotle denied that *akrasia* is an epistemic problem, a failure to know what is really in one's best interests when one acts, and therefore departed from Plato's apparent intellectualism whereby knowledge of the Good and the True produced in the soul dispositions to act rightly. Instead he regards *akrasia* as an executive defect in the agent's adaptability to the world whereby our apprehension of what is best is given effect in our action and in turn informs a sense of what is best to do in situations like the one being responded to.

Aristotle's view helps with a key problem in understanding how reason controls action? His view is convergent with that of John Hughlings Jackson (JHJ) and focuses on the integration of knowledge and action as the key to human adaptation to the world, and it offers an entrée into cognitive neuroscience and an informed understanding of disorders of volition. Obsessive-compulsive disorder (OCD), and psychopathy, two such disorders, illustrate two very different mechanisms whereby one can fail to translate reason into action. JHJ's neurological analysis makes sense of current neuroscientific findings in these and other conditions and thus of the control of our behaviour as highly evolved beings.

John Hughlings Jackson: the evolved brain and consciousness

JHJ regarded consciousness as an amalgam of will, memory, reason and emotion, as modes of neural or sensorimotor integration that were unable to be examined through analysing functional patterns unless one considered their evolutionary significance (1887). JHJ saw neural evolution as using increasingly higher levels of representation (and re-representation) to construct a complex repertoire of responses to various environmental challenges. He believed that our coordinated activity could be understood only by considering the complexity of environmental demands and our ability to override reflex (or mechanistic) connections by using learning and interconnectedness, both with other agents (and their discourse) and with the environment, to create behavioural flexibility. A learning history uses patterns of stimuli with subjective significance, in terms of reward and avoidance, to select and moderate the exhibition of responses. For example, if a child finds that approaching the adult male most frequently in his vicinity leads to pain and distress, then normal human attachment patterns will be disrupted. Subjective significance comes from a series of dynamic interactions overlaid by explicit memories of times past and the use of reason in 'propositionising' about the events concerned. Propositionising is, as JHJ observes, largely conducted through 'structures of nervous energy organised according to word meanings'. Alexander Luria, arguably the greatest neuropsychologist of the twentieth century, agrees: 'higher mental processes are formed and take place on the basis of speech activity' (1973: 93–4). Both see the information we introduce into the control of our behaviour as a feature of a shared (intersubjective or 'objective') world where human beings construct complex inter-related courses of action in the light of 'decontextualized' truth (Mercier & Sperber, 2011).

Thus the will, for JHJ, is the highest level of evolved motor function whereby the conscious control of action factors in various present and imagined contingencies (with the aid of speech) and becomes 'the least automatic', and most integrated sensorimotor activity (1887: 41). JHJ sees increasingly more inclusive complexes of associative regularities as having a role in the structure of behaviour, and directs the study of volition towards the frontal lobes (pre-empting contemporary cognitive neuroscience). But he resists the temptation to posit a ('Frontal') Cartesian centre of subjectivity sending an impulse to motor areas 'triggering' a voluntary action (Dennett, 2003; Gillett, 2008).

Coordination and the subjective brain

JHJ notes that consciousness brings memory, emotion and reasoning to bear on action. Thus, 'acts of will' reflect a level of nervous integration that, for a neuro-scientifically minded theorist, pulls together limbic and orbito-frontal activity (the neural basis of emotive and memory functions), left hemisphere speech centres ('propositionising' or language-related activity), and on-going problem-solving and goal-related plans and strategies (mediated by dorsolateral pre-frontal areas). Trying to localize the brain areas (or centre of conscious will) underpinning voluntary action neglects this integrative and possibly distributed activity (Roskies, 2010; Zhu, 2004) and reflects misleading philosophy and poor theoretical cognitive neuroscience (Jeanerrod, 2006).

Memory (a catch-all term for a whole series of processes that include learning, autobiographical memory, source memory and semantic memory) reconstructs and consciously draws on past experience to inform present behaviour (Gillett, 2008: 84ff.). The relevant neural capacities mobilize practised schemata and allow current cognitive solutions to build on earlier successful strategies so as to enact similar problem-solving routines (adjusted if necessary for variations) and allow directed revisitation of past action contexts. In human beings the action-guiding mix uses representations combining the meanings of words (JHJ) with mnemic residues including limbic and paralimbic activity (Freud, 1986: 445–8). That integration enables intersubjective histories and experiences to either straitjacket or liberate the subject from the effects of a present set of conditions.

Emotional resonance with others, in this account, incorporates into reasoned and conscious control of behaviour strategies of coordination that, aided by 'speech', use information about the feelings and behaviour of others to inform 'centres whereby the organism as a whole is adjusted to the environment' (JHJ, 1887: 34). At that level of volitional control, the agent can take into account the intentions, plans, needs, vulnerabilities and moral demands of others (based on intersubjective resonance). Thus, for instance, I might realise that the person to whom I am talking has been deeply hurt by a friend of mine and acknowledge that in the way I speak to him.

Reasoning and its abstract propositional structure become part of volition through the pervasive influence of words and the semantically informed processing assemblies to which they contribute. JHJ notes their influence in human mental life even in those with severe aphasia. He argues that the loss of ready use of words as a tool of consciousness is such a major problem that serious damage to the left hemisphere causes a partial dissolution of our highly evolved structures of mental activity: 'The nervous arrangements for words used in speech lie chiefly in the left half of the brain; … the nervous arrangements used in understanding speech (and in other ways) lie in the right also (JHJ, 1878: 319) and, 'Words are required for thinking, for most of our thinking at least but the speechless man is not wordless; there is an automatic or unconscious service of words' (1878: 323)

The role of speech

JHJ's thinking in this area is remarkably prescient of two major twentieth-century thinkers – Luria (mentioned above) and the philosopher, Ludwig Wittgenstein. Wittgenstein is famous for the claim 'meaning is use' (1953: #43) and JHJ remarks 'an utterance is or is not a proposition according to how it is used' (1879: 210). He notes, 'superiority of speech is precision of application to new relations of things' (1879: 218) so that 'To speak is not simply to utter words, it is to propositionise' (1878: 311). In this way, the 'complex of cues and connections' arising from speech-related activity that constitute the meaning of a word (Luria, 1973: 306) relate contexts of action (whether familiar or novel) to intersubjective communication and the currency of shared social life.

The remark reinforces the view that subconscious, or relatively inarticulate, reactions and responses, based on experiences with others, become articulated by the use of words and function as neurocognitive markers – sound or graphic patterns with associated connections – unifying neural assemblies. These (possibly distributed) assemblies capture adaptive responses to regularities in our life-world and the arguments informing human responses to them (Mercier & Sperber, 2011). The integration and connection of a given moment to experiences remembered, conditions not present and trains of reasoning enabled by the cognitive role of words makes the human 'imaginary' (a domain of symbols and stories) a real element in structuring human consciousness and activity.

JHJ notes that propositionising unifies our representations (cf. Kant, [1789] 1929: B93)[1] by connecting moments of experience according to their significance to a human thinker through speech. Speech links stereotyped acoustic signals to a complex of multimodal associations enabling both a higher level of personal integration over time and discursively mediated coordination with others. Speech is therefore 'a tool for intellectual activity and . . . a method of regulating or organizing human mental processe' (Luria, 1973: 307). Speech, storying and imagination, the currencies of our mental lives, are central not only in human social cognition but also in action, intention and desire. They are associated with the posterior and anterior left hemisphere cortical areas subserving language function (Wernicke's and Broca's areas), anatomically positioned for ease of connection with both the higher levels of multimodal sensory integration (parietal) and also motor integration and patterning (frontal). JHJ realises that higher mental functions integrate information and adapt the organism as a whole to the world. This is because they make maximal use of opportunities, allow awareness of dangers likely to be encountered and combine intellect, appetite and action so that we can construct an account of strength of will.

Akrasia *(weakness of the will)*

A person who suffers from *akrasia* (weakness of the will) can 'propositionise' but not translate the result into action. Their defect is not in reasoning ability but in producing consciously controlled actions reflecting a proper engagement of the intellect such that reasoning with them does no good. As Aristotle says 'if water makes a man choke, what do you give him to wash it down?' His insight directs our attention to the lack of 'coordination' (JHJ) between emotion, reasoning and action. Effective engagement between consciousness and action – strength of will – is, for

Aristotle, a skill resting on practised attunement to the world such that the agent adaptively responds to any contingencies that arise. For instance, if a person 'descends' to passion or angry outbursts when challenged, he effectively loses the connection between bodily activation and intellect in a similar way to the condition that prevails in *akrasia* (Aristotle, 1147a14–18). For JHJ, these dissolutions, or loss of integration of activity by reason (or propositionising), link the will to social cognition.

Social and moral thought

JHJ's 'propositionising' frames and coordinates our intellect and behaviour, through the everyday associations of use (including emotive content), the imperatives (and dangers) of words, and the way that patterns of association and representation are used in reasoning and argumentation. What is more, we necessarily share the embedded reasons-responsive and propositionally integrated associations with other human beings through shared tools of cognitive adaptation constructing what we might call 'network weights' structurally disposing us to respond to reason (Spitzer, 1999).

Consciousness, for JHJ, integrates memory, emotion, reasoning and will through 'unifying centres ... whereby the organism as a whole is adjusted to its environment' (JHJ, 1887: 34) and is the basis of social and moral cognition. Thus the various 'insanities' (JHJ, 1887: 27) represent various dissolutions of this complex integrating function and the conscious self at the centre of them. The self, seen as a coordinated hierarchy of 'reservoirs of energy' and 'resisting positions' comprises both the bodily periphery, and its sensorimotor contact with the environment, and the highest centres forming 'the organ of mind' (1887: 34). Mind is, to some extent, 'independent of present experience' because it includes 'centres capable of being forced into new kinds of activity [and] centres acting in ways they have been trained to act in and resisting new ways of acting' (1887: 33). Therefore the self or subjectivity, constituted by this complex activity, does not rest on a Cartesian point of 'immaterial' (or even material) presence; rather, 'le moi est un coordination' (JHJ, quoting Ribot, 1887: 35). Moral consciousness brings to human subjectivity a sense of the lives of others, replete with needs, vulnerabilities, degrees of relatedness and separation, and everything that 'in social and personal life mean something' (Williams, 1985: 201) introducing motivations that are a proper or fitting part of a good life. We can see these more adequately through the lens of defects of volition.

Disorders of the will

Obsessive-compulsive disorder (OCD)

OCD is an anxiety-related disorder in which a pattern of inappropriate, anxiety-driven thoughts and/or rituals are used to allay the patient's subjective feelings of threat and insecurity. Recent neuroscientific research has used sophisticated neuroimaging techniques to study its dynamics and development (Whiteside et al., 2004). The empirical findings focus largely on the limbic and orbito-frontal circuits of behaviour control and attempt to forge links between the clinical features of the disorder and neural dysfunction. They show:

(i) detectable abnormalities in a range of behavioural and learning studies – in limbic and orbito-[Ventro-Medial]-frontal cortical centres and closely connected areas of the basal ganglia, such as the caudate and thalamus (Breiter and Rauch, 1996; Friedlander and Desrocher, 2006; Kwon et al., 2003; Whiteside et al., 2004);
(ii) reduced activity in dorsolateral frontal areas on tasks like reversal learning (Chamberlain et al. 2008);
(iii) increased metabolic activity in the right orbito-frontal cortex, the right hippocampus, the left putamen and the right parietal region, and decreased metabolic activity in the left parieto-occipital junction associated with the severity of OCD symptoms in patients doing tasks assessing executive function and visual memory (Kwon et al., 2003, 37).

These and other studies suggest: 'that such brain regions are ... involved in OCD, [but] the designs ... do not permit one to conclude that (a) the differences represent abnormalities in functioning or (b) the differences are related to the cause of OCD' (Whiteside et al., 2004: 76). JHJ's analysis predicts this evidence of imbalance and lack of integration between functions coordinating the excitation (vs inhibition) of responding (VM and fronto-basal ganglia circuits), problem-solving and flexibility of response (dorsolateral frontal), and the detection and creative use of anomalies and cognitive conflicts (right parietal and limbic areas).

The findings are discussed in terms of: (i) executive dysfunction, whereby the patient is thought to have poor impulse control or response inhibition and (ii) modulatory control where behaviour is thought to be maladjusted to its context (Friedlander and Desrocher, 2006: 34, 40). JHJ speaks of 'positions of resistance' (selective inhibition) and 'reservoirs of energy' (directed excitation) attuned to demands that 'ought' (adaptively) to shape the organism's behaviour such that higher levels of integration using widely interconnected and 'less automatic' processes, coordinate lower-order centres of attention and action. His view therefore accommodates both executive dysfunction and modulatory control models. It analyses the defects of will seen in impulsive and OC behaviour (both 'positive' manifestations) as forms of dissolution (negation) of higher control causing loss of conscious or reasoned coordination of action in the light of maximally informed representations of contingencies and situational constraints.

In OCD, the 'self' (*le moi est une coordination*) is dominated by emotive drivers such as anxiety and fear. OC rituals are, perhaps secondarily, associated with the alleviation of anxiety-producing states of mind (e.g. hand-washing because one feels dirty or tainted; repeatedly checking locks because one feels vulnerable) and become entrenched in a person's behavioural repertoire through the immediate reward they bring (the lessening of an aversive state).

Psychopathy (and ASPD)

In OCD the dissolution of higher-order integration and coordination of behaviour allows anxiety-driven thoughts and behaviour to disrupt a person's daily activity. But in psychopathy a different kind of insanity (sometimes called 'moral insanity') occurs. The psychopath seems to have lost rational touch with moral life such that the integrative activity of the 'highest motor centres (pre-frontal lobes)' forming 'the physical bases of volition' (JHJ, 1887: 35, 48) become disconnected from the interpersonal emotion- and memory-based resonances of acts and consequences that usually inform moral cognition and self-control (Lynam and Gudonis, 2005; Kiehl et al. 2001). Social and moral cognition both depend on inhibition of inappropriate behaviour (resistances) and an understanding of what matters to others. However, in psychopaths (and some of those with anti-social personality disorder (ASPD)) there is a 'local dissolution' that is quite specific to 'moral insanity'. Machiavellian intelligence may be intact but empathy seems to be lacking. Thus, a psychopath successfully coordinates higher mental function to do with self-serving desires and strategies and, in that respect, 'the organism as a whole is adjusted to the environment' (JHJ, 1887, 34). But, in areas of consciousness that factor into self-coordination a regard for the distress of others, higher-level integration fails, and a degenerate or lesser structure lacking an emotive, or other-regarding, element presides. Thus, we note 'affective abnormalities' in decision-making (Kiehl et al., 2001), or 'reduced ... responses to distress cues and threatening stimuli' (Blair, 2003) so that psychopaths cannot follow 'the painful path to virtue' our principal mode of 'ethical formation (Gillett, 2010). The pre-frontal areas – JHJ's 'highest centres of motor control . . . in which evolution is most actively going on' (1887: 34) draw on 'will, memory, reason, and emotion' (the elements of consciousness for JHJ) and enable a subject to learn through ontogeny 'what in social and personal life means something'. The psychopath's brain, hampered by a partial "dissolution" of this capacity, therefore falls short of the ongoing neurocognitive evolution that is moral consciousness.

Impulse disorders and addiction

JHJ sees the 'different insanities' as different 'local dissolutions of the highest centres' whereby levels of 'energizing' and 'resistance' make possible 'new adjustments of the organism, as a whole, to the environment' (1887: 34). Simple impulse control disorders show poorly inhibited or 'resisted' behaviour, energised by either environmental or internal stimuli. Addiction and more complex disorders show 'dissolution' of more widespread connections and the behavioural constraints that arise from them submerged in the workings of a mind focused on a psycho-active substance (with its associated subcultural context). Such complex disorders are maladaptive through loss of the nuanced and non-automatic balances required for proper function as beings-in-the-world-with-others. The resulting failure of the highest and most actively evolving centres of the brain, normally shaped through 'survival of the fittest' evolution in the human life world, renders the life of the individual concerned ultimately unsustainable in that world.

We can now address attacks on the very idea of the will from arguments that build on scholarship about these disorders to construct an increasingly strident version of 'neurodeterminism'.

Neurodeterminism and the will

For Aristotle, self-control is a skill trained through learning to act on the basis of reason and 'all things considered' best judgments, and it results in strength of will. His view can be illustrated through thinking about a skilled striker scoring a goal. If we ask 'How did that happen?' we could answer by detailing a complex chain of neuromuscular events, but that would illuminate neither how the neural connections enabling them occurred nor why they were triggered 'right here, right now'. The knowledge, training and imagination of the player explain the act. The neuromuscular account gets as far as the brain and no further. To understand the act as the voluntary action of an intelligent agent 'in our judgments in regard to the causality of free actions, we can get as far as the intelligible cause but no further' (Kant, CPR: B585). In essence we are asking: how did the 'unconscious neuromuscular events' get configured so as to allow the action and why were they set into motion at this time? And here Kant remarks, 'No action begins in this active being itself; but we may yet quite correctly say that the active being of itself begins its effects in the sensible world' (CPR: B569). Notice that the 'internal events' are here a subplot in a 'whole agent' story about an act in a human life. So, how was the footballer able to say: 'Know how, can do!' (This becomes automatic and almost unconscious, though still very much within his control.)

Nietzsche argues a *potency* conception of the will when he remarks, 'Unfree will is mythology; in real life it is only a question of strong and weak wills' (1886 [1975]: #21).[2] He rails against 'the prevailing mechanistic stupidity' whereby people are machines driven by biology and forces within them and argues that all creatures develop a *will to power*, usefully interpreted as the ability to take dynamic control over their activity. The will to power cultivates discernment, informed action and effective intervention to produce conditions favourable to success in life through reason, personal creativity and aspiration so as to free an agent from subjection to contextual contingencies. The agent becomes a 'dynamic system' in a relation of Continuous Reciprocal Causation (CRC) with the world so that its actions are self-determined rather than being determined by events that befall it (Clark, 2008). Such an agent in effect, transcends the metaphysics of 'stupid mechanistic systems'.

Human beings are therefore unlike causally driven creatures in that they are not dependent on the ability to learn from trial and error (or imitation).They can also formulate projections about what is not (yet) the case and pre-empt environmental contingencies by taking control, intentionally copying the strategies of others and using stories to expand their repertoires of tricks. Thus human beings can change the world through will and imagination in ways not apparent to many 'labourers in physiology' following the principle of 'the smallest possible effort' causally evoked by current conditions (BGE: #14).

> It is almost always a symptom of what is lacking in himself when a thinker detects in every 'causal connection' and 'psychological necessity' something of compulsion, exigency, constraint, pressure, unfreedom; such feelings are traitors, the person who has them gives himself away. (BGE: #21)

Monitoring and using patterns in events (including brain events) to become more potent and effect changes in the world (with potential impacts on the lives of others) connects what an agent does to two contexts of meaning:

(i) the individual's self-narrative(s);
(ii) the shared actual world in which those narratives are played out through actions.

Those connections are through stimulus arrays and structures of meaning built on a scaffolding of relationships and life-skills. They target states of affairs that do not exist except in the imagination of the agent (they are what he or she aims to bring about), and they inform motives, mistakes and purposes, shaping and making sense of what is happening to capture what is of interest to us. Thus the will, as the ability to translate reason into action (Aristotle, 1925; Wolf, 1993), rests on two major preconditions (as does the striker's goal-scoring ability).

(i) *The precondition of reason*: Reason enables the agent to discern and incorporate meaning into thought and action so as to inform his or her action (cf. seeing the opportunity to score);
(ii) *The precondition of skill*: Training enables the agent to respond to reason through self-control and a fitting range of responses to various life situations (cf. 'netting the ball').

The skills and capacities involved are often overlooked in arguments focusing on (mechanistic) causal or neural accounts of human action such as the following.

A causal argument: the acts and intentions syllogism

1. An agent is responsible for any act done with the relevant intent.
2. The relevant intent must cause the act.
3. Human actions are caused by brain processes that precede conscious acts.
4. The relevant brain processes precede the agent's conscious awareness of them.
5. An agent does not consciously cause his or her own acts.
6. Agents are not responsible for their acts.

The model implicit here underpins most writing on neuroscience and voluntary action (Haggard 2005; Libet, 1985; Zhu, 2004). It assumes that the intent is a mental (read: brain) state causally producing a bodily movement – the act. The crucial premises (2 and 3), combined with 4, then, seem to undermine our common-sense idea of voluntary or conscious action. They also raise profound metaphysical questions about causation, action and the will.

Does reason cause a decision to act?

Is an act caused by a mental event – the intention (I_A) – which, assuming that the mind *is* just a way of talking about the workings of the brain, is actually a brain event/s (BE)?

The metaphysics of causation allows for two main possibilities to fill out this model:

(i) a singular causal relation such that a preceding event brings about a later event by some plausible mechanism (i.e. two *independently existing events*);
(ii) a law-like system of mechanistic events, at time 1, produces a state at time 2 – the effect (i.e. a *closed causal nexus*).

There are many examples illustrating the two possibilities.

A singular causal relation: *That smoke was caused by that fire.*

Here a process of combustion, at a certain place and time, produces a column of hot gas and carbon-containing particles. The two are closely related and are distinct phenomena related by a well-known mechanism. They are like action explanation in that both fire and voluntary action are difficult to precisely localise in space and time (the one in the air, the other in the brain and body).

A law-like domain or *closed causal nexus* where WT_2 (the Whole state at Time 2) is determined by WT_1:

The Goldberg Variations by George Rhoads. This kinetic ball sculpture has various balls dropping into various positions at varying intervals causing a constant stream of events, each explicable by what goes before. It is not as complex as the approximately 100 billion neurons and their 100 trillion interconnections in the human brain and the infinitely varying patterns of activity possible there. But in each system results (ball movements or bodily actions) are ('in principle') explicable by what has gone before. A further example is similar.

The butterfly effect. Edward Lorenz (1963), discussing meteorology, proved that a monsoon in India could be caused by the flapping wings of a butterfly in Kansas. In the human nervous system, we could similarly posit that a micro-change, e.g. *Joe thinking that he should act selflessly* might cause him to act in a novel and distinctive way (a 'butterfly effect' in the human neurocognitive system). Now the result – his writing a cheque for Oxfam – might be traceable, in a *closed causal nexus* way (as discerned by an unlimited intellect), through the distributed neural events to the moment of his altruistic thought so that the subtle shift of a (micro-neural) brain state that could then be said to have 'caused the act'. And if his thought could do it, so could any other random unconscious event in the brain.

These analogies could underpin an attack on free will and moral responsibility through cognitive neuroscience. But clearly more philosophical work needs to be done to clinch the argument because the responsible agent only gets 'off the hook' if the mechanistic chain of events links the action – a pattern of bodily movement – to events in the unconscious recesses of the brain so that a conscious decision is not the cause. However, does that claim follow from either the *independently existing events* (singular causal) account or the *closed causal nexus* account? We can begin with the latter.

The *closed causal nexus* account of brain function is problematic because of the following:

(i) 'the explanatory gap' between 'the non-linear, non-equilibrium, non-mechanistic dynamics of self-organizing living organismic thermodynamic systems on the one hand, and the classical linear, equilibrium, mechanistic dynamics of inertial non-living systems on the other' (Hanna, 2009: 120);
(ii) the openness of the human mind/brain to the world and what constitutes explanation in meaningful terms.

Either of the above would undermine the neurodeterminism rife in the neuroscience of human action.

(i) Hanna's 'explanatory gap' allows us to concede that the reflection explored above – Joe's selfless thought – might, through a shift in the firing patterns of the brain, bring about an otherwise improbable action given his personality. It would be like what we see when a human subject, under instruction, shifts the processing pattern in the brain to perceive a stimulus array in a new way (as in the Necker's cube or other ambiguous perceptual figures). This ability to voluntarily switch 'gestalts' or undergo perceptual learning shows the conscious will, on the basis of some kind of top-down, whole-person control, changing one's own brain states (Wittgenstein, 1953: #213e).
(ii) Human beings obey the conception of laws (ideas of what it would be best to do or they ought to do) and not just laws of nature (Kant, 1948: 76). Laws of nature cause inclinations, reactions and

responses dictated by animal nature (*arbitrium brutum*), but a conception of a law that one ought to obey creates an imperative (not a disposition) and the imperative is an idea not a causal function explained by laws of nature. A rule and its prescriptive imperative do not cause obedience, but rather depend on the agent framing, endorsing and acting on certain thoughts (Gillett, 1993). Producing an action in that way does not just go on in me. Rather, framing the thought and doing what it recommends is something that I do as a whole person, open and responsive to logic or rhetoric and not just causal processes that I do not direct and which do not completely direct me in a comprehensive way. Kant's formulation of the principle scrupulously observes a distinction between obeying prescriptions and being moved by the inclinations of inner nature (Gillett, 1992), and he concludes that an intentional act may be able to be traced back to a decision and the agent's reasons but no further. The crux of the act is a verdict on the reasons delivered, in effect, by the agent's acting thus or so (Hampshire 1969).

Kant's intuition is famously captured by Davidson's 'nervous mountaineer' argument for the autonomy of the mental (1980). Given these thoughts, *the closed causal nexus* account of action explanation fails as a mechanistic causal story.

The singular causal relation account requires that we satisfy two metaphysical requirements (Morris, 1986): the *independent existence requirement* (IE) and the *non-a priori* (NAP) condition.

IE (independent existence)

This condition requires two separate identifiable events or entities in the causal relationship; just as the smoke existed separately from the fire, so they could be meaningfully related to each other. In general form this condition is:

> *There are two existents A and B such that A could exist without B but in conditions C', C", . . . causally produces/results in B.*

Further examples are: The butterfly flapping its wings in Kansas causes the monsoon in India; striking a match causes it to light; genetic behavioural programmes cause birds to migrate at certain times of the year; a flashing light in a person's visual field produces a K-complex in his brain, and so on. Other examples are illicit: oxidation of cellulose causes the flame; the pattern of bird movements causes seasonal migrations; the pattern of neuromuscular movements caused his action. In fact these examples often violate the non-a priori (NAP) condition. This says that metaphysics can deliver truths about identifies that are *a posteriori* but once discovered become *a priori*. They enter into an understanding of the concepts concerned. We can see why the burning of the match just is the (very same metaphysical event as) the oxidation of phosphorous and cellulose and other substances at a given point in time and place. Perhaps the thought/action/brain activity complex at the heart of human agency is similar so that it is problematic to say which bits of the activity going on in a brain and neuromuscular system constitute the action of, say, leaving your lover – why, there must be fifty ways. You could do it with a shrug of your shoulders in response to a question, delete his number from your cell phone directory, or block him from your Facebook page. But none of these, on any plausible mapping of your brain function, would be picked out as an act of leaving your lover.

We must now address the question about singular causes as in *the acts and intentions syllogism* which implies that the cause of any voluntary action is an unconscious event in the brain.

Action explanation and the brain

A large number of experiments in cognitive neuroscience are focused on precisely timed events at either the mental level or the neural level. To do that we have to identify:

(a) the mental event or intention causing the action (perhaps comprising a decision to act and then an initiation of the action – a 'covert action' [Jeanerrod, 2006] or a 'trying') and
(b) the act that is caused by that intention.

This schema assumes that people know the moment they decide to act and also the moment they act even if they do not know the mechanism translating the thought or intent into action.

This schema forms what we might call *The Libet model* (Lm) of intention and action (Libet, 1985):

Lm1. You decide/intend to A at T_1 and are simultaneously conscious of doing so – the event, I_A;
Lm2. You initiate action at T_2 by sending a message/motor pattern (BE_2) to your muscles arising from your brain (perhaps unconsciously) – a second event;
Lm3. You act at T3 by making a bodily movement (M_b) according to a motor pattern (A) – the effect.

However, there are certain objections to this model whereby an intention (I_A) as a brain event (BE_1) in the agent, perhaps through an/other event/s (BE_2) causes action, A, the bodily movement M_b.

Objection to Lm1

The model requires that I_A is an Independent Event with respect to the pattern of brain activity that actually produces the bodily movement (M_b or A) and is prior to it. Thus I_A is not part of, caused by or dependent on the brain events actually producing the action. In fact most of our actions are not as pictured but interactive and dynamic, effecting an outcome in the world (Luria, 1973) by aiming at and making the adjustments required to perform the operant (e.g. a button press or a shot). If that is so, then the action itself is an unfolding tract of possibly distributed brain and neuromuscular activity in which monitoring of the effect in the world is part of the Continuous Reciprocal Causation (CRC) shaping the act (Haggard, 2005). That does not look at all like the singular causal model we have outlined, and it does not have the form of a relation between two independently existing events (like the fire and the smoke). Instead, it looks a bit more like descriptions of the one complex (extended) event.

What is more, there is a problem with the second clause in the premise (simultaneous consciousness of willing or intending). The evidence seems to show that a human being does not accurately and simultaneously monitor basic neural events as they happen but rather reconstructs an account of what he or she is doing by 'interpreting' the stream of brain world activity going on (Banks and Isham, 2009) and fitting it to recognizable patterns of events (that are like what tends to happen in the agent's usual environment). This is evident not only from Libet's own experiments using his timing method to try and fix the time of the intention (2002) and work by other authors (Danquah et al, 2008) but also from the colour phi phenomenon as analysed by Dennett (1991). The colour phi phenomenon is a particularly striking example of the brain 'filling in' a conscious perception where there is no stimulus object corresponding to it in order to reconstruct a more ecologically plausible tract of experience. The conclusion emerging from the evidence is that we do not 'read off' conscious mental events from our own brain activity but rather reconstruct conscious contents from tracts of brain activity underpinning patterns of perception and action that we use to deal with the challenges of our life-world.

Therefore the moment of an intention or decision does not exist as a discrete event in time, in the brain or anywhere else. And the forced 'awareness of the time of the conscious decision to act' is a 'read-back' into, or inference from, what went on that articulates my activity in the world. Think of Looney Tunes where Tweety's trademark 'I tawt I saw a puddytat' is ecological awareness of the kind in question (i.e. 'something familiar has happened that I have a glimpse of from happenings in my brain and, going by what normally happens around here and the fact that I, as a whole agent, know how to enact my own agenda, they betoken my voluntarily acting thus and so'). The fact that there is (from the evidence) no timeable event corresponding to the decision to act implies that the readiness potential and the neural timing of events in the brain is not relevant to questions about the conscious control of action, and we must find another neuro-philosophical account.

The interim conclusion at this stage is that there is no independently existing Brain Event preceding a human action but that an agent makes a self-judgments of the form: 'I (must have) intended to Act', which can be sound or shaky depending on his or her self-knowledge and self-control. The agent has and exercises self-control on the basis of skills that translate reason (or thought) into action and that are lacking in *akrasia*.

Objection to Lm2

When we take seriously the dynamic, unfolding and interactive nature of most actions and the fact that holistic patterns of brain activity embody integrated informational complexes used to control and direct bodily activity (JHJ, 1884; Luria, 1973), it is evident that Libet's model, despite widespread acceptance in the cognitive neuroscience literature, embeds a serious mistake. The brain events intrinsic to voluntary action (BE_A comprising $I_A + BE_2$) are to A as combustion is to fire: the combustion of cellulose to form carbon-based residues is not the cause of fire; it is the fire. Similarly, describing the total complex of distributed brain activity associated with an action (Haggard, 2005) is an alternate (neuroscientific) description of human volitional action, not the cause of it. Voluntary acts are part of a complex world-directed stream of dynamic activity that is an unfolding perception-action cycle whereby the agent achieves an effect on the world (Neisser, 1976). That activity includes *everything* prior to a bodily movement: premotor processing, motor intentions and commands, *and* the prediction of the re-afferent consequences of motor processing (Jeanerrod, 2006). Thus to think of human action as comprising a series of punctate events resulting from causal chains producing discrete voluntary movements is completely unrealistic. A further objection makes that plain.

Objection to Lm3

A crucial part of the neurodeterminist account is that there is a physically describable pattern of bodily movement – the effect – that is the action. But think of 'fifty ways' mentioned above and the fact that no distinctive pattern of bodily movement, and its related motor events, is the action in question.

(i) *The wineglass at the party.* In this case I am talking to an attractive person at a party with my friend. At a certain point a rapid jerk of my hand spills red wine over his shirt and he has to go and change. I say 'Sorry mate. Damn that tic, I wish I could be rid of it!' Now the question is not whether the *bodily movement* was mine but whether it was in fact intentional. To ask that question is to ask about the context and meaning of the movement in question. Is it a random neuromuscular event or a deliberate ploy? The question concerns the fit between the bodily movement and my story as an individual in relationships with others, and that goes way beyond neuroscience. A wider description, sufficient to account for the physically indistinguishable tic includes not just motor events but diverse brain areas implicated in volition (Zhu, 2004) that are only important because they are neuroscientifically required to get conscious acts into the frame. Thus a narrow, physical or bodily movement event does not identify the act as a voluntary act

(ii) *The brain-damaged mobster case.* In this example Sean sets up a trap for his wife so that when she comes home and opens the door she will trigger a shotgun aimed at the doorway. That duly happens and we, having not been fooled by the argument that he left a note to warn her (inside the door), accuse him of killing his wife. Sean, however, is a neurodeterminist who believes the Libet model and says 'I can't have killed her because I was asleep at the time and had no readiness potential or brain events that caused the event that killed her.' A moment's thought disposes of his disclaimer because the question of the intent that informed the act is not settled by events in the brain at the time of the fatal event.

However, at this point we have the right to ask of the objector, 'How can you give me a story of reason causing a voluntary human action if you are going to disallow the normal patterns and principles of antecedent causation in the way that you have?' (in legal terms, 'What is the connection between *mens rea* and *actus reus*?')

Action, neuroscience and the will

A naturalistic analysis of human action that does not falter on the dodgy metaphysics already critiqued nor require a Cartesian or extensionless point of willing at the heart of the existential individual draws on Aristotle and Nietzsche, an implacable opponent of pretentious philosophy.

I have noted that Aristotle's account of the will focuses on the translation of reason into action such that the agent who has self-control is skilled or trained in putting his or her thoughts into practice. The outcome of reasoning or argument is not an 'all things considered' best judgment but the agent acting on an 'all things considered' best judgment. That is why Kant remarks 'the active being of itself begins its effects in the sensible world' (CPR: B569). The active being concerned here is a 'being in the world with others' engaged in discourse, propositionising and doing things to others that are potentially informed by goodness and truth.

We can, for the moment gloss this account by noting that an action is a pattern of events (including brain events) connecting the subject/agent to the world through the meaning of what is going on in the world. Through its meaningful content, this pattern maps the agent onto a human life-world clothed with meaning. As such, action is our translation of the significance we see in the world, for reasons that we accept, into effects on the lives of others (with all their moral overtones). Intentional action is therefore a manifestation of the evolution of the nervous system to the point where, in the words of Hughlings Jackson, we have progressed 'in evolution ... from the most to the least automatic, and thus the highest centres are the least automatic' (1884: 704–5). The skills to surmount environmental challenges, so as to enact a life plan, disrupt mechanistic stereotyped responses and inform the actions of human agents by deploying imagination, reason, and argument. The only question is whether the agent has the strength of will to enact his or her thought. Nietzsche regards 'free will' and 'unfree will' as myths created by philosophers and the will to power as the ability not to be 'unfree in the face of environmental contingencies'. This implies that the whole determinist conception that undercuts agency is a mistake.

The agent becomes free through the development of skills that translate the results of discourse or argument into intervention in the world. Being good at that – enacting one's story – is having a strong will, and people suffer the various impairments already discussed in developing that highly evolved capacity. The necessary skills are learned through experience and subject to various impairments so that understanding them and how they come about is far more important than pondering about brain function to illuminate intent and moral responsibility.

We are all used to coming to intuitive assessments of the extent to which a person does or does not have the life skills required to act well in this or that situation, and we have all our lives been negotiating the world of excuses. Thus what we need is 'a plea for excuses' and an educated understanding of the 'development theory of the will to power' (Nietzsche, BGE: #23) to understand human freedom and responsibility. But it is hard to see anything meaningful about that story – why people do what they do and their impairments in doing so – unless our findings in neuroscience are closely married to a sophisticated philosophical and psychological understanding of the fact that human beings are beings-in-the-world-with-others and subject to all the influences that can arise in that complex situation. That is a story of existence, the phenomena we encounter and our moral responsiveness to the true and the good, and these go way beyond the facts of science as Plato (through his primary focus on goodness and truth as related non-natural realities), and Kant and Wittgenstein (in a more naturalistic way) all realised and argued in their own ways.

NOTES

1 Hereinafter, CPR, with pagination used in this edition, e.g. B562.
2 Hereinafter, BGE, with sections referred to as #NN.

REFERENCES

Aristotle (1925) *Nichomachean Ethics* (trans. D. Ross). Oxford University Press, (pagination is standard).

Banks W. and Isham E. (2009) We infer rather than perceive the moment when we decided to act. *Psychological Science* 20.1: 17–21.

Blair, J. (2003) Neurobiological basis of psychopathy. *British Journal of Psychiatry* 182: 5–7.

Breiter, H. and Rauch, S. (1996) Functional MRI and the study of OCD: from symptom provocation to cognitive-behavioral Probes of cortico-striatal systems and the amygdala. *Neuroimage* 4: s127–38.

Chamberlain S., Menzies, L., Hampshire, A., Suckling, J., Fineberg, N. et al. (2008) Orbitofrontal dysfunction in patients with obsessive compulsive disorder *Science* 321: 421–2.

Clark, A. (2008) *Supersizing the Mind: Embodiment, Action and Cognitive Extension*. Oxford University Press.

Danquah, A., Farrell, M. and O'Boyle, D. (2008) Biases in the subjective timing of perceptual events: Libet et al. (1983) revisited. *Consciousness and Cognition* 17: 616–27.

Davidson, D. (1980) *Essays on Actions and Events*. Oxford: Clarendon.

Dennett, D. (1991). *Consciousness Explained.* London: Penguin.

(2003) The self as responding – and responsible – artefact. *Annals of the New York Academy of Sciences* 1001: 39–50.

Freud, S. (1986) *The Essentials of Psychoanalysis* (ed. A. Freud). London: Penguin.

Friedlander, L. and Desrocher, M. (2006) Neuroimaging studies of obsessive-compulsive disorder in adults and children *Clinical Psychology Review* 26: 32–49.

Gillett, G. (1992) Actions, causes and mental ascriptions, in *Objections to physicalism* (ed. H Robinson). Oxford University Press, pp. 81–100.

(1993) Freedom of the will and mental content. *Ratio* 6: 89–107.

(2008) *Subjectivity and Being Somebody: Human Identity, and Neuroethics.* Exeter: Imprint Academic.

(2010) Intentional action, moral responsibility and psychopaths, in *Responsibility and Psychopathy: Interfacing Law, Psychiatry and Philosophy* (ed. Luca Malatesti & John McMillan). Oxford University Press, pp. 283–98.

Gillett, G. and Liu, S. (2012) Free will and Necker's cube: reason, language and top-down control in cognitive neuroscience. *Philosophy* 87.1: 29–50.

Haggard, P. (2005) Conscious intention and motor control. *Trends in Cognitive Science* 9.6: 290–5.

Hampshire, S. (1969) Some difficulties in knowing, in *Philosophy, Science and Method: Essays in Honor of Ernest Nagel* (ed. S. Morgenbesser, P. Suppes & M. White). New York: St Martin's Press.

Hanna, R. (2009) Freedom teleology and rational causation. *Kant Yearbook* 1: 99–142.

Hughlings Jackson, J. (1878) On affectations of speech from disease of the brain (1). *Brain* 1: 304–30.

(1879) On affectations of speech from disease of the brain (2). *Brain* 1: 203–22.

(1884) On affectations of speech from disease of the brain (2). *British Medical Journal* 12 April: 703–7.

(1887) Remarks on the evolution and dissolution of the nervous system. *British Journal of Psychiatry* 33: 25–48.

Jeannerod, M. 2006: *Motor Cognition: What Actions Tell the Self.* New York: Oxford University Press.

Kant, I. (1789 [1929]) *The Critique of Pure Reason* (trans. N. Kemp Smith). London: Macmillan

Kant, I. (1948) *The Moral Law* (trans. H. J. Paton) London: Hutchinson, p. 76.

Kiehl, K., Smith, A. M., Hare, R. D., Mendrek, A., Forster, B. B., et al. (2001) Limbic abnormalities in affective processing by criminal psychopaths as revealed by functional Magnetic Resonance Imaging. *Biological Psychiatry* 50: 677–84.

Kwon J. S., Kim, J., Lee, D., Lee, J., Kim, M. et al. (2003) Neural correlates of clinical symptoms and cognitive dysfunctions in obsessive-compulsive disorder. *Psychiatric Research: Neuroimaging* 122: 37–47.

Libet B. (1985) Unconscious cerebral initiative and the role of conscious will in voluntary action. *The Behavioural and Brain Sciences* 8: 529–66.

(2002) The timing of mental events: Libet's experimental findings and their implications. *Consciousness and cognition* 11: 291–9.

Lorenz, E. (1963) Deterministic nonperiodic flow. *Journal of the Atmospheric Sciences* 20: 130–41.
Luria, A. R. (I 973) *The Working Brain*. Harmondsworth: Penguin.
Lynam, D. and Gudonis, L. (2005) The development of psychopathy. *Annual Review of Clinical Psychology* 1: 381–407.
Mercier, H. and Sperber, D. (2011) Why do humans reason? Arguments for an argumentative theory. *Behavioral and Brain Sciences* 34: 94–111.
Morris, M. (1986) Causes of behaviour. *Philosophical Quarterly* 36.143: 123–44.
Neisser, U. (1976) *Cognition and Reality*. San Francisco: Freeman.
Nietzsche, F. (1886 [1975]) *Beyond Good and Evil* (trans. R. J. Hollingdale) London: Penguin.
Roskies, A. (2010) How does neuroscience affect our conception of volition? *Annual Review of Neuroscience* 33: 109–30.
Spitzer, M. (1999) The Mind within the Net. *Cambridge*, Mass.: MIT Press.
Whiteside, S., Port, J. and Abramowitz, J. (2004) A meta-analysis of finctional neuroimaging in obsessive-compulsive disorder. *Psychiatry Research: Neuroimaging* 132: 69–79.
Williams B. (1985) *Ethics and the Limits of Philosophy*. London: Fontana.
Wittgenstein, L. (1953) *Philosophical Investigations* (PI) (trans. G. E. M. Anscombe). Oxford: Blackwell.
Wolf, S. (1993) *Freedom within Reason*. Oxford University Press.
Zhu, J. (2004) Locating volition. *Consciousness and Cognition* 13: 302–22.

4 The experience of free will and the experience of agency: an error-prone, reconstructive process

Matthis Synofzik, Gottfried Vosgerau, and Axel Lindner

ABSTRACT

The notion of free will largely results from one's own *experience* of free will with respect to many of our actions in daily life. But how does this experience arise? Is it grounded in brain processes? And would this imply that free will – or at least the experience of it – is exclusively a biological phenomenon? We will here analyze these questions by linking philosophical and psychological accounts with neurocognitive mechanisms and neuropsychiatric disturbances. Our thesis is that *self-attributions of free will* are tightly connected to *self-attributions of responsibility*, which in turn are rooted in *self-attributions of actions*, i.e., in the experience of being the agent of one's actions. This experience of agency results from a reconstructive process weighting different agency cues. Disorders of agency, as in schizophrenia, reveal that this process is prone to errors. Despite these neurocognitive underpinnings, free will (and the experience of it) cannot be fully reduced to the biological make-up of individuals. Rather, free will is foremost a social phenomenon, and self-attributions of free will largely result from an "internalization" of social perspectives and norms on what counts as the exercise of free will. They are essentially a personal-level "reflex" of the social phenomenon of free will.

The experience of free will: grounded in neural mechanisms, but a social phenomenon

The notion of free will largely results from the *experience* of free will with respect to many of our actions in daily life. But how does this experience arise, and is it grounded in brain processes? And, if it is grounded in

MS and GV work jointly on the research project "ThinkAct – Grounding Thoughts in Actions," which is generously founded by the Volkswagen Stiftung (VW II/85 158 awarded to MS; and VW II/85 068 awarded to GV). This work was also supported by the DFG (Werner Reichardt Centre for Integrative Neuroscience; support to AL and MS).

brain processes, how could these processes account for this complex and inherently subjective phenomenon? And: Would it imply that free will – or at least the experience of it – is exclusively a *biological* phenomenon?

Rather than starting off by searching for material facts that constitute free will, we here propose to analyze how *self-attributions* of free will are generated in everyday contexts and how and to what extent they are grounded in neurocognitive mechanisms. This approach allows us not only to link philosophical and psychological accounts of free will with neurocognitive approaches but also to learn about the experience of free will and its neurocognitive underpinnings from neuropsychiatric disorders in which this experience goes astray.

Our thesis is that *self-attributions of free will* are tightly connected to *self-attributions of responsibility*. These in turn are rooted in *self-attributions of actions*, in the experience of being the agent of one's actions. The self-attribution of an action results from a reconstructive process integrating and weighting different agency cues which precede, accompany, and follow the particular action. Disorders of agency, such as, for example, in schizophrenia patients with delusions of control, reveal that this process is prone to errors: a disturbance in the self-attribution of action can be triggered by a disturbance on a very basic sensorimotor level, and this basic disturbance – if complemented by additional deficits on affective or cognitive levels – can lead to the rejection of agency, of responsibility, and of free will for a particular action.

Although we will show that this account and the study of neuropsychiatric patients open a window to understand the basic neurocognitive underpinnings of the experience and the self-attribution of action and responsibility, we will at the same time show that this does not imply that free will (and the experience of it) is a phenomenon that can be fully reduced to the biological make-up of individuals. Rather, we will argue that free will is foremost a social phenomenon, and that self-attributions of free will largely result from an "internalization" of social perspectives and norms on what counts as the exercise of free will and what does not. This means that the experience of free will is essentially a personal-level "reflex" of the social phenomenon of free will. This experience is highly formed by the personal representations of social norms and expectations.

Self-attribution of action and the underlying neurocognitive mechanisms

One basic hallmark that is necessary for the experience of free will is the registration that I am the agent of the actions I perform, i.e., the sense of agency (Gallagher, 2000; Synofzik et al., 2008; Synofzik and Vosgerau,

2012). Importantly, two distinct levels of the sense of agency should be distinguished: the *feeling of agency*, which consists of a non-conceptual, automatic registration of whether I am the initiator or not, and the *judgment of agency*, which is the formation of a belief about who the initiator of the movement was (Synofzik et al., 2008).The automatic registration on the level of feeling does not necessarily have to go along with an experiential quality; that means it does not necessarily need to be an actual *experience* in itself, but can also be, for example, an *unconscious registration* process. This registration process can lead to the perception of a particular action or sensory event as self-caused. Subsequently and based on this feeling, a judgment might be established (depending on the demands of the context) which takes into account not only the feeling itself but also context information, background beliefs, general social norms, etc.

A *sense of feeling in control* about one's actions is not identical and should thus not be confused with the *feeling of agency*: while patients with Parkinson's disease or cerebellar ataxia have often a strongly diminished feeling of control about their actions – since the movement trajectories do not match what they aim to do – they do not have a disturbed feeling of agency, that is, they do not falsely register their movements as not being caused by themselves. Accordingly, these patients always attribute their own actions to their own agency on the judgment level. Moreover, the feeling of agency should not be confused with any kind of *awareness of preparing or wanting to move*. A famous example for this awareness is the widely discussed Libetian "urge to move" (Libet et al., 1983). The latter is just one form of an attitude. Just like the awareness of having a certain thought, this is simply the awareness of wanting to move, but not yet an authorship registration, an agency attribution, or let alone an experience of free will.

The comparator model as one cue for the self-attribution of actions

But how do we "know" whether a certain action X – or any other sensory event – is self-caused or not? The problem here is that self-produced and externally produced sensory information do not differ intrinsically. Thus, to draw a distinction on a feeling level, an efferent mechanism is necessary which differs from purely afferent registration. One possible mechanism is proposed by the so-called comparator model (Frith, 1992; Frith et al., 2000a). According to this model, the nervous system predicts the sensory consequences of an action on the basis of internal action-related information, such as efference copies (von Holst and Mittelstaedt, 1950) or corollary discharge (Sperry, 1950) of motor commands. These *internal sensory predictions* are likely issued by forward models which account for the current state of the motor and the sensory system (Wolpert et al., 1995; Wolpert et al., 1998). By comparing the actual and the predicted afference, the cause of the sensory input can be established. In case of a match, the afference is experienced as a result of our own actions. In case of a mismatch, the difference is registered as externally caused.

This idea of a comparator as a subpersonal mechanism underlying a subject's registration of self-agency has manifold theoretical advantages: (1) The information necessary for agency is not added to the perception of an action, e.g., by a higher-order cognitive reasoning process but is an integral part of the perceptual registration and action generation itself and thus directly frames our phenomenal content. (2) The experience of agency is not dependent on conceptual capacities but functions on a pre-conceptual, subpersonal level. (3) Correspondingly, the self-relation involved in agency is not assumed to be represented as independent of action processing, as suggested by many philosophical conceptions (e.g., Descartes' dualism which presupposes an independent self that is able to initiate an act of will unrelated and prior to any bodily movement, or Kant's transcendental philosophy which presupposes a transcendental I as an independent entity which constitutes the experience of agency by unifying all our sense-experiences), but is an intrinsic property of the action processing itself. (4) The comparator mechanism can nicely be experimentally tested in various behavioral and imaging paradigms, throughout healthy and neuropsychiatric subjects, and even across different species (Frith et al., 2000b; Frith, 2005; Synofzik et al., 2008). And, indeed, a magnitude of behavioral, electrophysiological, and imaging studies has provided evidence that a constant comparison between internal predictions and external sensory information ensures that we correctly attribute self-produced sensations to our own agency rather than to external causal forces (Blakemore et al., 1999; Bell, 2001; Bays et al., 2005; Crapse and Sommer, 2008; Dicke et al., 2008) and that, in turn, it is this mechanism which goes astray in neuropsychiatric patients exhibiting disorders of agency (Lindner et al., 2005; Shergill et al., 2005; Synofzik et al., 2010).

Optimal integration of agency cues might underlie self-attribution of actions

Although the output of an underlying comparator process is a major cue informing our feeling of agency, it is neither a sufficient condition nor, seemingly, a necessary condition for this registration process (for details, see Synofzik et al., 2008).[1] For example, we have recently investigated whether the perception of one's own actions is fully determined by efferent processes directly related to one's action itself (such as internal predictions/the comparator model) – or, alternatively, whether even the very immediate perception of one's action trajectories also draws on *post hoc* information, such as the valence of an affective action outcome (Wilke et al., 2012). The results indicate that – although self-action perception is constrained by signals related directly to the action itself – it can nevertheless also be modulated by unpredictable *post hoc* action outcomes that are not part of the intentions or any other prospective representation preceding or guiding one's actions. This study provides evidence for the fact that the perception of one's actions – and thus the feeling of agency – builds not only on *one* signal, such as the comparator output, but also on *multiple* cues that precede, accompany, or follow one's action (the modifying cue here: the affective valence of action outcomes).

A study by Moore, Wegner, and Haggard (Moore et al., 2009) showed that, if consistent primes were available, a temporal binding (also referred to as "intentional binding"; compare Haggard et al., 2002) of a movement and its effects occurs even in case of passive movements. If in their study such temporal binding is indeed seen as a signature of the feeling of agency (which not all authors do, cf. Synofzik et al., 2009), and if this binding cannot simply be explained by purely sensory priming (Synofzik et al., 2009), the aforementioned finding could be taken as evidence for the fact that internal predictions (issued in case of active movements) and a subsequent comparator process are not even *necessary* to induce a sense of agency. Rather, as suggested by the study of Moore and colleagues, external cues (here: primes) could substitute them.

But how can the brain integrate multiple agency cues to form a nevertheless valid and reliable sense of agency for a given sensory event in a particular situation? A proposal of *optimal integration of agency cues* has recently emerged: the brain could constantly integrate several different agency cues and weight each cue according to its relative reliability in a given situation (on both the feeling and the judgment level, respectively) (Synofzik et al., 2009; Synofzik et al., 2010; Synofzik and Voss, 2010). This notion follows the framework of optimal cue integration established in the field of object perception: according to this framework, we are not using just a single information signal to convey an adequate representation of a certain perceptual entity under all everyday conditions. Instead, all available information cues are integrated according to their relative reliability. As already mentioned above, such an optimal integration strategy could also be used to frame the weighting of sensory and motor signals. For example, if internal sensory predictions are imprecise or absent, external cues (like, e.g., primes) should receive a higher relative weight in determining one's sense of agency.

Thus, optimal cue integration might not only allow robust perception of objects and the world (Ernst and Banks, 2002; Ernst and Bulthoff, 2004) and efficient sensorimotor learning (Kording and Wolpert, 2004) but also provide the basis for subjects' robust and, at the same time, flexible agency experience in variable contexts (Moore and Fletcher, 2012).

Self-attribution of actions in schizophrenia

Schizophrenia patients suffering from *delusions of influence* can be seen as a pathophysiology model for agency processing, that is, they provide a window into the processes underlying one's self-attribution of actions: patients experiencing this first-rank symptom and hallmark of schizophrenia feel that their actions are no longer controlled by themselves. Sometimes they not only experience their actions as not self-caused, leading only to a "vague" or "strange" feeling of agency, but also attribute them to some specific other agent on the judgment level (e.g., to a friend, neighbor or the devil) (Frith, 1992).

How can this experience be explained by the comparator model and the – more comprehensive – approach of optimal integration of authorship cues? Several recent studies using very different paradigms – namely a visual distortion paradigm for eye movements (Lindner et al., 2005) and for hand movements (Synofzik et al., 2010), an "intentional binding" paradigm (Voss et al., 2010), and a force matching paradigm (Shergill et al., 2005) – demonstrated that schizophrenia patients indeed show imprecise internal predictions about the sensory consequences of their own actions. Two of these studies were actually also able to show that this deficit correlated with the severity of the psychopathology: the higher the imprecision in predicting the sensory consequences of one's own actions, the higher the score for delusions of influence (Lindner et al., 2005; Synofzik et al., 2010). Following the suggestion of an optimal integration of agency cues (and extending the classical comparator model), imprecise predictions should prompt the perceptual system to rely more strongly on external action-related information in order to receive a more reliable account of one's own actions. And indeed, the study by Synofzik and colleagues found that schizophrenia patients relied more heavily on external information about their actions (in this study: vision) (Synofzik et al., 2010).

An optimal integration of agency cues might provide a common basis for the various misattributions of agency in schizophrenia patients, including their episodic nature (Synofzik et al., 2010; Synofzik and Voss, 2010). In schizophrenia, and even more so in an acute psychotic state, internal predictions about the sensory consequences of one's actions could be frequently imprecise and unreliable. Patients should therefore be prompted – at least in certain situations – to rely more on (seemingly more reliable) alternative cues about self-action, such as vision, auditory input, prior expectations, or *post hoc* thoughts. The stronger weighting of these alternative cues could help patients to avoid a misattribution of agency for self-produced sensory events that was due to imprecise internal predictions. However, as a consequence of giving up the usually most robust and reliable internal action information source, i.e., internal predictions, the sense of agency in psychotic patients is at constant risk of being misled by contingent events, invading beliefs, and confusing emotions and evaluations. In other words: schizophrenia patients would be at constant risk of becoming "a slave to every environmental influence" (Frith, 1994: 151) – and to every affective and moral ad hoc evaluation. Different agency judgment errors may result: patients might over-attribute external events to their own agency whenever these more strongly weighted alternative agency cues are not veridical and misleading, as is the case in delusions of reference (also referred to as "megalomania"). Conversely, if alternative cues are temporarily not attended or unavailable, patients might fail to attribute self-produced sensory events to their own agency and instead assume external causal forces (as is the case in delusions of influence). A context-dependent weighted integration of imprecise internal predictions and alternative agency cues may therefore reflect the basis of agency attribution errors in both directions: over-attribution, as in delusions of reference/megalomania, and under-attribution, as in delusions of influence.

The approach of cue integration holds also another explanatory advantage: it might be able to explain why such basic impairments – such as in sensorimotor predictions – might trigger specific delusional beliefs. If only deficits in basic sensorimotor mechanisms would be assumed, it would be difficult to explain how a deficit in internal predictions could be sufficient to cause the (wrong) judgment of agency observed in schizophrenia. In order to transit from an abnormal experience to a delusional belief, a distorted belief-formation processing must be postulated. Only such an idiosyncrasy in the belief-formation process could explain why schizophrenia subjects (1) do not accept an alien experience as a strange experience (as, for example, healthy subjects or most neurological patients with alien motor phenomena would do) but (2) devise a delusional agency hypothesis about this experience, and (3) maintain it despite different stored encyclopedic knowledge about their behavior and despite the testimony of others (Davies et al., 2001). Thus, an explanation of delusions of agency also needs to account for the abnormalities in the belief-formation system with respect to a person's method of action rationalization and self-theorizing. A deficit in internal predictions per se can also not provide any explanation for the semantic context of the delusional belief: Why is it that agency attribution fails only in certain semantic contexts that are often highly specific to the history of the delusional individual? And why does it have its specific semantic content (e.g., an action is caused by a neighbor or by the devil)? To explain this, one would have to integrate information from a person's broader belief and evaluation system.

The cue integration framework allows combining deficits in sensorimotor mechanisms with alterations in thought and affective processes: (1) an imprecision in efferent action-related information leads to a fluctuating, unreliable feeling of agency, prompting these patients to rely more on other agency cues. (2) An altered weighting of affective cues and the well-established disturbances in formal thinking in schizophrenia will then lead to an unbalanced and disturbed integration of the feeling of agency into the belief-formation process on the level of the judgment of agency. (3) This leads to the formation of a delusional belief, which is formed according to the weighting of cognitive and affective cues given a particular situation and according to the person's individual background beliefs and history.

This would also explain the impression that delusions of control mostly refer *not* to trivial, non-emotional actions in daily life (e.g., brushing teeth), but to very specific, singular actions with a high affective and/or moral value, which are usually morally and socially not acceptable or at least negatively connoted (e.g., causing an accident, hurting someone, behaving inappropriately in the presence of one's peers). Although proper empirical evidence is still warranted for this clinical observation, we here speculate that in this case negative cues, which arise from affective processing or moral evaluation, are given high weight in the integration of agency cues, and that agency for one's action is consequently rejected on the judgment level.

The nature of free will and the self-attribution of free will

If schizophrenia patients suffering from delusions of influence gave a higher weight to the affective and moral outcome of one's action (in particular if it is negative), as was suggested above, this could subsequently lead to a lack of agency experience for this action if the affective and moral outcome is not compatible with the patient's evaluative and belief system. Accordingly, patients might also not experience responsibility and free will with respect to this action.

This idea illustrates two essential general aspects of the self-attribution of responsibility:

1. The registration (feeling) and self-attribution (judgment) of agency with respect to a particular action lead to the experience and the self-attribution of responsibility and of free will. If subjects experience and claim agency for an action (even with negative outcomes), they also have to assume responsibility for it. In turn, if they reject agency, they can also reject responsibility and free will control. Since the experience and self-attribution of agency integrates and weights various cues, also the experience and self-attribution of responsibility and free will cannot be seen as immediate, monolithic processes, but rather as reconstructive processes that draw on sensorimotor cues, action beliefs, context evaluations, and background beliefs (including social norms assumed by the subject).
2. Cues like affective, normative, and social evaluations and background beliefs, which – in addition to sensorimotor cues – construe the feeling and judgment of agency (Synofzik et al., 2008; Wilke et al., 2012), might in fact receive even more weight in the experience and self-attribution of *responsibility* and of *free will*. Persons could "internalize" social perspectives and moral norms conveyed by society and integrate them as strong cues in their weighting process underlying the experience and self-attribution of responsibility: depending on one's personality traits and individual attribution style (as well as on one's agency registration process), somebody could be more or less prone to experience and self-attribute responsibility also for those actions with socially and/or morally negative outcomes.

In order to assess the principles behind the attribution of responsibility and free will beyond their dependence on the sense of agency, it is useful to have a closer look at the role of free will and responsibility in everyday life. The basic assumption is that (moral) responsibility and free will are deeply interconnected (a position generally acknowledged in philosophical discussions; cf. Pereboom, 2005; Fischer et al., 2007; O'Connor, 2009). The idea that we are free in executing an action is a necessary prerequisite for the ascription of moral responsibility[2] for this action, which in turn gives rise to praise and blame. In other words: if we would not assume that we are free in doing this or that, we could not blame or praise anybody for doing this and that.

But what are the reasons for praising and blaming each other in the first place? We propose to consider the evolution of man to answer this question. Human beings are special in the animal world foremost because of their vast involvement in cooperative behavior (Tomasello, 2008, 2009). In order to cooperate, it is necessary to rely on the other in general, because the advantage of cooperation for me depends also on the commitment of the other to the shared goal. Thus, it is a prerequisite for cooperative behavior that we know our cooperation partners to be good cooperation partners beforehand. Since human social groups became too large for every individual to know each other (often we have to cooperate with people we have never met before), social mechanisms evolved to secure the in-principle commitment to cooperative behavior for each member. This mechanism is often called "social control," and its basic "tools" are praise and blame. Members of the society that have proved to be good cooperators are praised by the community and known as good members of it. On the contrary, cheaters and "free riders" are blamed by the community and known as bad cooperators. In this way, social communities developed a social tool, namely moral responsibility, that enables them to ensure enduring cooperative behavior among their members (at least on a large scale). Since free will is a presupposition for moral responsibility, it also rests on the same mechanisms described for moral responsibility. In particular, its ascription is based on the same evolutionary and social grounds.

But how can moral responsibility and free will be represented by the brain, but nevertheless essentially be social phenomena? Social phenomena are phenomena that are essentially constituted by social norms. One example is the monetary value of a coin: there is no physical property of a coin that determines (or even has an influence) on its monetary value. The monetary value is exclusively determined by the social norms (or social practices) that govern the use of coins – i.e., by the norms that make us accept/pay certain coins for certain goods. Free will, so the hypothesis here, is equally constituted by the social norms of responsibility ascription (which presuppose free will ascriptions). These norms are essentially conventions of a social community, i.e., nothing that an individual invents or rules above, but something which emerges from the interactions within a social community.

Moral responsibility, and hence free will, is thus not something found on the level of individuals. It is essentially a social phenomenon grounded in our social nature, supporting the highly differentiated cooperative behavior that probably constitutes one of the biggest evolutionary advantages of human beings. Like every social norm, the norms that govern the ascription of free will and the ascription of responsibility are learned during childhood and "internalized" by each individual. This means that the individual will acquire a set of background beliefs about free will and responsibility ascriptions, which are ultimately reflexes of the norms in their surrounding society. These "internalized" social norms, in turn, heavily influence the sense of agency on the judgment level, such that social norms have an indirect, yet substantial influence on our experience of agency and our experience of free will. This means that the experience and self-attribution of free will is essentially a personal "reflex" of the social phenomenon of free will. This experience is highly formed and constrained by the personal representations of social norms and expectations.

Conclusions

Many lines of research in the last few years have focused on the question of whether and how free will might be implemented in the brain. This quest for brain processes might be misleading in that it assumes that "free will" is an inherently biological phenomenon. Here we suggested that it might be more productive to head in a different direction: rather than mainly searching for biological facts that constitute free will, we propose to analyze how self-attributions of free will are generated in everyday contexts and how they are grounded in neurocognitive mechanisms.

A necessary condition and key element of self-attributions of *free will* are self-attributions of *actions*. These are not monolithic processes but result from a reconstructive process that draws on sensorimotor cues, internal action beliefs, context evaluations, and background beliefs (including social norms assumed by the subject) which both precede and follow an action. These cues might be integrated and weighted according to their availability and reliability in a given situation. Within each cue and at each stage of this reconstructive process, disruptions and errors can occur and diminish the experience of agency. A resulting attribution of agency is also the necessary basis for an experience of free will and for assuming responsibility for this action and its outcomes. (This does not, of course, mean that – in turn – *any* attribution of agency will lead to an experience of free will and responsibility.)

Based on the argumentation proposed here, the self-attribution of actions results from a multi-cue process and, consequently, so too do the self-attribution of responsibility and free will. Individuals hereby also integrate an "internalized" notion of their respective society on what counts as the exercise of free will and what does not. This means, that the experience of free will is essentially a personal "reflex" of the social phenomenon of free will. Thus, although to a great extent formed by the personal representations of social norms and expectations, free will is essentially a social phenomenon. Therefore, the quest for brain processes underlying "free will" is heading in the wrong direction: social phenomena are not in the brain – just as monetary value is not in the coin. Nevertheless, the investigation of brain processes is very important for our understanding of the *representation and experience* of free will – namely for the understanding of the sense of agency, which is an important (although by far not the only) factor contributing to our experience of free will.

NOTES

1 Moreover, the comparator model cannot explain the judgment of agency and is hence not suitable as a model for the sense of agency (cf. Synofzik et al., 2008).
2 Moral responsibility is the kind of responsibility connected to praise and blame as opposed to responsibility connected to obligations, as, e.g., the responsibility of parents for their children. In this article, we are only concerned with moral responsibility.

REFERENCES

Bays, P. M., Wolpert, D. M., and Flanagan, J. R. (2005) Perception of the consequences of self-action is temporally tuned and event driven. *Current Biology* 15:1125–1128.

Bell, C. C. (2001) Memory-based expectations in electrosensory systems. *Current Opinion in Neurobiology* 11:481–487.

Blakemore, S. J., Frith, C. D., Wolpert, D. M. (1999) Spatio-temporal prediction modulates the perception of self-produced stimuli. *Journal of Cognitive Neuroscience* 11:551–559.

Crapse, T. B. and Sommer, M. A. (2008) Corollary discharge across the animal kingdom. *Nature Reviews Neuroscience* 9:587–600.

Davies, M., Coltheart, M., Langdon, R., and Breen, N. (2001) Monothematic delusions: towards a two-factor account. *Philosophy, Psychiatry & Psychology* 8:133–158.

Dicke, P. W., Chakraborty, S., and Thier, P. (2008) Neuronal correlates of perceptual stability during eye movements. *European Journal of Neuroscience* 27:991–1002.

Ernst, M. O. and Banks, M. S. (2002) Humans integrate visual and haptic information in a statistically optimal fashion. *Nature* 415:429–433.

Ernst, M. O. and Bulthoff, H. H. (2004) Merging the senses into a robust percept. *Trends in Cognitive Sciences* 8:162–169.

Fischer, J. M., Kane, R., Pereboom, D., and Vargas, M., eds. (2007) *Four Views on Free Will*. Walden, MA: Blackwell Publishing.

Frith, C. (1992) *The Cognitive Neuropsychology of Schizophrenia*. Hillsdale, NJ: Lawrence Erlbaum Associates.

(1994) Theory of mind in schizophrenia. In *The Neuropsychology of Schizophrenia* (A. S. David & J. C. Cutting, eds.), pp. 147–161. Hillsdale, NJ: Lawrence Erlbaum Associates.

(2005) The self in action: lessons from delusions of control. *Consciousness and Cognition* 14:752–770.

Frith, C. D., Blakemore, S., and Wolpert, D. M. (2000a) Explaining the symptoms of schizophrenia: abnormalities in the awareness of action. *Brain Research Reviews* 31:357–363.

Frith, C. D. (2000b) Abnormalities in the awareness and control of action. *Philosophical Transactions of the Royal Society of London, B: Biological Sciences* 355:1771–1788.

Gallagher, S. (2000) Philosophical conceptions of the self: implications for cognitive science. *Trends in Cognitive Sciences* 4:14–21.

Haggard, P., Clark, S., and Kalogeras, J. (2002). Voluntary action and conscious awareness. *Nature Neuroscience* 5: 382–385.

Kording, K. P. and Wolpert, D. M. (2004) Bayesian integration in sensorimotor learning. *Nature* 427:244–247.

Libet B., Gleason, C. A., Wright, E. W., and Pearl, D. K. (1983) Time of conscious intention to act in relation to onset of cerebral activity (readiness-potential): the unconscious initiation of a freely voluntary act. *Brain* 106 (Pt 3):623–642.

Lindner, A., Thier, P., Kircher, T. T., Haarmeier, T., and Leube, D. T. (2005) Disorders of agency in schizophrenia correlate with an inability to compensate for the sensory consequences of actions. *Current Biology* 15:1119–1124.

Moore, J. W. and Fletcher, P. C. (2012) Sense of agency in health and disease: a review of cue integration approaches. *Consciousness and Cognition* 21:59–68.

Moore, J. W., Wegner, D. M., and Haggard, P. (2009) Modulating the sense of agency with external cues. *Consciousness and Cognition* 18:1056–1064.

O'Connor, T. (2009) Conscious willing and the emerging sciences of brain and behavior. In *Downward Causation and the Neurobiology of Free Will* (G. F. R. Ellis, N. Murphy, and T. O'Connor, eds.), pp. 173–186. New York: Springer Publications.

Pereboom, D. (2005) Defending hard incompatibilism. *Midwest Studies in Philosophy* 29:228–247.

Shergill, S. S., Samson, G., Bays, P. M., Frith, C. D., and Wolpert, D. M. (2005) Evidence for sensory prediction deficits in schizophrenia. *American Journal of Psychiatry* 162:2384–2386.

Sperry, R. W. (1950) Neural basis of the spontaneous optokinetic response produced by visual inversion. *Journal of Comparative Physiology and Psychology* 43:482–489.

Synofzik, M. and Voss, M. (2010) Disturbances of the sense of agency in schizophrenia. In *Neuropsychology of the Sense of Agency* (M. Balconi, ed.), pp. 145–156. New York/Heidelberg: Springer.

Synofzik, M. and Vosgerau, G. (2012) Beyond the comparator model. *Consciousness and Cognition* 21:1–3.

Synofzik, M., Vosgerau, G., and Newen, A. (2008) Beyond the comparator model: a multifactorial two-step account of agency. *Consciousness and Cognition* 17:219–239.

Synofzik, M., Vosgerau, G., and Lindner, A. (2009) Me or not me: an optimal integration of agency cues? *Consciousness and Cognition* 18:1065–1068.

Synofzik, M., Thier, P., Leube, D. T., Schlotterbeck, P., and Lindner, A. (2010) Misattributions of agency in schizophrenia are based on imprecise predictions about the sensory consequences of one's actions. *Brain* 133:262–271.

Tomasello, M. (2008) *Origins of Human Communication*. Cambridge, MA: MIT Press.

(2009) *Why We Cooperate*: Cambridge, MA: MIT Press.

von Holst, E. and Mittelstaedt, H. (1950) Das Reafferenzprinzip. *Naturwissenschaften* 37:464–476.

Voss M., Moore, J., Hauser, M., Gallinat, J., Heinz, A., and Haggard, P. (2010) Altered awareness of action in schizophrenia: a specific deficit in predicting action consequences. *Brain* 133:3104–3112.

Wilke, C., Synofzik, M., and Lindner, A. (2012) The valence of action outcomes modulates the perception of one's actions. *Consciousness and Cognition* 21:18–29.

Wolpert, D. M., Ghahramani, Z., and Jordan, M. I. (1995) An internal model for sensorimotor integration. *Science* 269:1880–1882.

Wolpert, D. M., Miall, R. C., and Kawato, M. (1998) Internal models in the cerebellum. *Trends in Cognitive Sciences* 2:338–347.

Part III

Mental capacities and disorders of the will

5 Being free by losing control: what obsessive-compulsive disorder can tell us about free will

Sanneke de Haan, Erik Rietveld and Damiaan Denys

ABSTRACT

It is often assumed that the exercise of free will depends on the ability to consciously decide between available options. Consequently, the more *conscious control* one has over one's actions, the freer one is. Since neuroscientific research shows the limitations of what we in fact consciously control, it seems that our free will is in trouble. A closer look at the phenomenology of obsessive-compulsive disorder (OCD) gives us reason to doubt this concept of freedom. OCD patients feel unfree. They do things they do not want to do, or think things they do not want to think. In order to regain control, they deliberate or pay extra conscious attention to what they do. Paradoxically, their recourse to conscious control often makes matters worse, resulting in a *diminishment* of the experience of freedom. Here, we combine Arendt's conception of *freedom in terms of action* with phenomenological insights into skilled action to get a better understanding of the role of deliberation in the experience of freedom. We argue that this experience depends on the ability to rely on our skills as much as on the ability to deliberate. This implies that the dichotomy between unreflective action and freedom in the current debate is a false one.

> If men wish to be free, it is precisely sovereignty they must denounce.
>
> Hannah Arendt (1954/2006: 163)

Introduction

According to the traditional Western concept of freedom, the ability to exercise free will depends on the availability of options and the possibility to consciously decide which one to choose.[1] Given that there are different options, the consequence of this view is that the more *conscious control* one has over one's actions (as opposed to merely impulsive responses), the freer one is. Since neuroscientific research increasingly shows the limits of what we in fact consciously control, it seems that our belief in free will and hence in personal autonomy is in trouble. If the free will sceptics are right, the consequences would be far-reaching, not only with regard to our self-understanding but also with regard to ethical and legal matters.

A closer look at the phenomenology of obsessive-compulsive disorder (OCD) gives us reason to doubt the traditional concept of freedom in terms of conscious control. Patients suffering from OCD experience themselves as unfree. They feel trapped in their fears, in their obsessions and compulsions, and in fact their daily life is often severely hindered by the imprisonment of their disorders. The question is whether their lack of freedom is due to a lack of will power. Do they have too little conscious control over their thoughts and actions? Or could it be the opposite: are they exerting *too much* conscious control over their thoughts and actions?

In this chapter, we will argue that OCD patients testify to the general condition that exercising an increased conscious control over actions can in fact *diminish* the sense of agency rather than increase the experience of freedom. Referring to Heidegger (1927/2001) and Merleau-Ponty (1945/2002), we argue that conscious control and deliberation may be useful when the natural flow of action is disturbed: for instance when a necessary tool is broken or missing (Heidegger 1927/2001) or when one learns a new skill (Dreyfus 2002). However, deliberation itself may also disturb the flow of unreflective action. Too much deliberation on and analysis of one's unreflective, habitual actions may cause insecurity and even a breakdown of what was once 'second nature'. We introduce three different ways in which too much deliberation can have negative effects on patients with OCD, rendering them even more unfree.

The experiences of these patients show that the traditional conception of freedom in terms of 'free will' has major shortcomings. There is an alternative, however, to be found in the work of Hannah Arendt. She advocates a conception of freedom as *freedom in action*. Combined with phenomenological insights on action, Arendt's account of freedom helps us to get a more adequate understanding of the role of deliberation in the experience of freedom. We argue that the experience of freedom depends on the right balance between deliberate control *and* unreflective actions.

Our alternative conception also has important implications for the debate on free will in cognitive neuroscience. In particular, a phenomenological perspective on the balance between deliberation and unreflective action can correct the false dichotomy that plagues the neuroscientific debate on free will: it is generally assumed that *either* one has conscious control over one's actions and thus counts as a free agent *or* automatic processes are at work that have nothing to do with the agent. Phenomenological investigation of unreflective action shows that this latter assumption is a crude misconception of what it means to be an autonomous agent. We are our habits as much as we are our conscious control.

The lack of freedom in OCD

Patients suffering from OCD are plagued by persistent, intrusive thoughts or images that they feel are inappropriate and which cause anxiety or distress (obsessions). They try either to ignore or suppress these thoughts or images, or to neutralize them with some other thought or action (compulsions) (American Psychiatric Association 2000). OCD patients recognize that their fears are irrational or at least excessive. However, this does not help them. They still fail in their attempts to keep control over their upsetting thoughts and images, and they still feel compelled to perform their neutralizing compulsions.

OCD patients are thus compelled to think or do things they do not want to think or do. They experience themselves as unfree. Their disorder forces them to behave in ways that they can themselves acknowledge to be disproportional. They admit and realize that their compulsive behaviours, hours of cleaning, checking, washing on a daily basis are inadequate and inefficient. This recognition of the irrational character of their deeds adds to their suffering and their feeling unfree.

> I am constantly worried that I might say something that would hurt other people. When I talk to someone, I pay close attention to what I say, but afterwards I am never sure whether I did not unintentionally say something offensive. I am constantly aware of all the possibilities for being offensive or insulting. Therefore I avoid people as much as I can. I hate it: I feel trapped inside my own head. (OCD patient, personal communication with SdH)

OCD patients feel trapped: they want to free themselves of their obsessions and compulsions. But when the tension they experience gets too high, they feel they *have to* wash their hands, check the oven, or order their furniture – just to make the tension bearable. The daily lives of people with OCD are severely limited by their disorder. When the symptoms are severe, patients hardly venture outside of their houses anymore.

To get a feel for these limitations, imagine that the things you do between waking up in the morning and going to work would take you not just an hour, but rather all day. Imagine you have to take a shower for three hours, wash your hands five hundred times, or clean the house for twelve hours a day. Imagine that it would take you four hours to get prepared for going to a party, so that it might already be over by the time you get there. Probably next time, you would not even bother to go – also because the party itself will need to be followed again by hours and hours of cleaning rituals. Since repetitive rituals are not just time-consuming, but are also accompanied by extreme tension and concentration, the compulsive behaviour is extremely tiring. Moreover, as a patient explained, this is not the kind of tiredness you experience after a day of hard work, because 'you have not been doing anything *real*'. It is not a satisfied form of tiredness after completing or establishing something.

Instead of going out in the world and doing things, OCD patients spend much of their time worrying about what might go wrong, or in other ways exhaustingly preparing themselves for all possible scenarios. Patients explain their situation as being 'locked inside' of their head. Often, patients also have 'meta-anxieties': they worry about worrying too much, or they are afraid that they might act out their obsessions, or afraid of losing even more control and going mad.

The paradoxical role of conscious control

Our focus here is on these patients' failing attempts to gain control. How can we explain this? Is their failure due to a lack of will power? Do they have too little conscious control over their thoughts and actions? Indeed, patients report that they cannot keep control over their thoughts and worries *and* that they feel unfree. Do these patients perhaps lack a free will? That would fit the traditional idea that the experience of being a free, autonomous agent, depends first and foremost on the level of conscious control that one is able to exert over one's actions. Esquirol, the first psychiatrist who described a patient with what we now call OCD, indeed thought it was a disease of the will (Esquirol 1838). However, since then, many other conceptions of the nature of OCD have been formulated, focusing on either the emotional dimension, or the will, or the intellect (De Haan et al. 2013).

But is a lack of conscious control really what the problem amounts to? What speak against the conception of OCD in terms of a lack of conscious control are the experiences of the patients themselves. Patients rather exert much *more* conscious control over their actions and thoughts than people ordinarily do. In fact, normally we do not deliberate about our thinking or our behaviour so often at all. Compared to OCD, normal behaviour appears to be very naïve, trustful and perhaps even a bit superficial. Are you actually sure you locked your door this morning? You probably did not pay any conscious attention to your movements.

Are you actually aware of the possibility that your food may contain too much pesticide, or that there could be pieces of glass in your peanut butter? Did you check that before taking a bite? And did you ever think about all the germs you may get from using a public toilet? And how these germs may spread on everything you touch – including other people?

All in all, in everyday life, we do so many things without thinking, without paying conscious attention, just relying on our habits and trusting that everything will be fine. We do not question and doubt everything, but we rather exhibit a *basic trust* in both the world and our own abilities (De Haan et al. 2013). Patients with OCD *do* worry about these things and *do* pay conscious attention to their actions. On the one hand, these patients report that they feel unfree and may even point to their failure to exercise control to explain their lack of freedom. On the other hand, it appears that they exercise much more conscious control over their thoughts and actions than people normally do. On the account of freedom in terms of free will, the degree of conscious control is the measure for the degree of freedom. This traditional conception thus cannot account for the experiences of these patients. How can we explain this paradox of feeling unfree whilst exerting a high degree of conscious control?

Freedom of will versus freedom in action

This paradox brings us right to the heart of a philosophical debate on how to understand freedom – or more specifically, how to understand the role that conscious deliberation plays in our experience of freedom. In her important essay 'What Is Freedom?', Arendt (1954/2006) sketches the historical shift in the conception of freedom as *freedom to act* to freedom in the sense of *inner freedom*. Initially, in Greek and Roman culture, men were regarded as free to the extent that they could be politically active. Arendt generalizes this idea as 'freedom to act', which refers to the capacity to start something new; to participate in a community or a political realm. Being free means to be able to act and take part in the (social) world. Interestingly, this implies that individuals in fact need other people and social practices to be free. By contrast, freedom is nowadays usually regarded as 'inner freedom', that is, the subject's freedom of thought or freedom of the will. On this account, the inner realm in which no other can interfere is taken to be the instantiation par excellence of freedom. Given its domain of the inner realm, the degree of inner freedom is measured by the amount of control one exerts over oneself, as opposed to the amount of influence one has in the outer world.

Arendt points to the political and religious motivations for this shift, and she heavily critiques the impotence of such an inner freedom as compared to the freedom to act out in the world. Inner freedom is the diluted derivative of freedom to act: 'The experiences of inner freedom are derivative in that they always presuppose a retreat from the world, where freedom was denied, into an inwardness to which no other has access. The inward space where the self is sheltered against the world must not be mistaken for the heart or the mind, both of which exist and function only in interrelationship with the world' (1954/2006: 145). According to Arendt, freedom is first of all at stake in our intercourse with others, not with ourselves.

But it was not only political and religious developments that fostered this shift. There is also an influential philosophical background for this way of thinking. For in the mainstream philosophical tradition, contemplation and reflection have been celebrated for ages as the most important and most valuable of human capacities. Thinking about things is valued more than doing things. Arendt challenges this view and argues for the importance of the active life instead.

A phenomenological account of action

Arendt has clearly been influenced by Heidegger. Heidegger (1927/2001) pointed to the primacy of our practical engagement with the world over deliberation. First of all we go out and do things in the world: we have our projects, we want to achieve something. And in doing so, we are immersed in our actions, which is rather the opposite experience of deliberation. In fact, Heidegger argues, we only deliberate when something goes wrong: for instance, when a tool we want to use is broken or missing; or when there are other tasks waiting for us that distract us from our present job. In such cases, we need to interrupt the flow of our actions, take a step back and reflect on what to do. Once we have figured this out, we will again return to our unreflective flow of action.

Conscious deliberation also plays an important role in learning new skills. Drawing on the work of Merleau-Ponty, Dreyfus (2002) argues that we can distinguish several stages in the acquisition of a skill and that the more proficient one becomes, the less one needs to rely on rules and theories, and conscious deliberation of what to do. Expertise is rather characterized by an 'immediate intuitive situational response' (p. 6). For example, when we learn to drive, we at first need to pay conscious attention to when and how to shift gears. The more proficient we get, the more we can rely on our habitual responses. In fact, once we are skilled, deliberation can even disturb our flow of action. Exerting conscious control is thus a necessary step on the way. But the hallmark of skill acquisition is the transfer from consciously controlled to intuitive habitual actions, with particular aspects such as timing and attunement to the situation, none of which is under our conscious control. Thus, once we have acquired a skill explicit deliberation is no longer needed: the skill has become our second nature. Or, as William James (1890/1950) put it over a century ago: 'It is a general principle in psychology that consciousness deserts all processes where it can no longer be of use' (p. 496)

This brings us to another important characteristic of our way of 'being-in-the-world' – as phenomenologists call it. The French phenomenologist Merleau-Ponty (1945/2002) pointed out that our practical engagement in the world is first and foremost a *bodily* engagement. We generally rely on our habits that have become our second nature. That is, we have incorporated these skills in our bodies. Our spontaneous, intuitive interaction with the environment and with others relies to a large extent on our bodily skills. Accordingly, Merleau-Ponty (1945/2002) argues that 'consciousness is in the first place not a matter of "I think that", but of "I can"' (p. 159).

It is important to note that these spontaneous, intuitive responses are not mere *reflexes* or *instincts*. In many situations in ordinary life, I respond appropriately without the need to first deliberate. I behave appropriately in the bakery, waiting for my turn; I talk to my colleagues over lunch; I can cycle through Amsterdam while thinking about theories of freedom. In many cases I act without conscious deliberation because I can rely on my spontaneous inclinations. In contrast to mere reflexes, which are motoric neurological closed loop systems, or instincts which are pre-programmed sets of fixed behaviours, these are skills that I have *developed,* and this development has taken time and effort. Some skills we have developed already very early in life, so that they are deeply engrained. Others we have mastered at a later age. But either way, our spontaneous, unreflective actions are informed and learned. They are the result of a cultivation, or *Bildung*, within our socio-cultural practices (Rietveld 2008a).

The role of deliberation in the experience of freedom in action

The phenomenological tradition offers a fundamentally embodied and embedded account of freedom. Phenomenologists emphasize the primacy of our practical, bodily engagement with the world. Moreover, because we are always part of social practices, we do not act in a vacuum. Our embodied and embedded nature precludes freedom in the sense of absolute sovereignty. Even the sterile version of 'inner freedom' cannot escape the fact that what we think and will is highly influenced by our socio-cultural environment. The attractive power of Arendt's notion of freedom in terms of action is that it provides an alternative in which other people and our environment are perceived not just as hindrances to freedom, but rather as the *enabling domain* in which our free actions first make sense. This fits with Merleau-Ponty's (1945/2002) explanation of freedom as 'commitment in the world' (p. 526). Of course, other people and our environment can hinder our free action, but this potential hindrance is secondary to their enabling role. That is, they can hinder us precisely *because* we first of all need them for this realm of freedom to be opened up for us.

Now, what role does conscious deliberation play in the experience of freedom on such a phenomenological, action-oriented account? If freedom is indeed 'an inherent quality of the I-can' (Arendt 1954/2006:1 58) (instead of the I-will, or I-think), and if we take into account phenomenological insights on (expert) acting, it follows that our experience of freedom will be characterized foremost by our spontaneous, bodily responsiveness to the situation at hand. However, whereas Arendt opposes contemplation and action, we saw that phenomenological accounts of action (Heidegger 1927/2001; Merleau-Ponty 1945/2002; Dreyfus 2002) are more nuanced. Deliberation does play a role, a vital role even, but it is a *serving* role. Deliberation is sometimes needed to come to the aid of the unreflective flow of action in case of disturbances or problems or when we start to learn something new. Acting freely thus requires a proper *balance* between deliberation and unreflective action.

We noted before that freedom of the will is measured by the extent of conscious control one has over one's thoughts and actions. So what determines the degree of freedom in action if it is not conscious control? According to Arendt, the extent of freedom in action depends on the extent of 'virtuosity', understood in a very specific way. She refers to Machiavelli's concept of *virtù*: 'the excellence with which man answers the opportunities the world opens up before him in the guise of *fortuna*' (Arendt 1954/2006: 151). That is, freedom lies in the virtuosity enacted in our actions, which in turn depends upon the coupling between 'fortuna' (that which the world has on offer) and 'virtù' (personal skills). In other words, the level of freedom in action depends upon two things: (a) to see the relevant opportunities for action, and (b) to act well on them.[2]

Arendt's account of virtuosity as a measure of freedom remains somewhat abstract, however. For how do we distinguish the relevant opportunities from the irrelevant ones? And what determines whether or not we act well on them? In reference to both Arendt and Merleau-Ponty, Rietveld (2008b) argues that one's commitment in the world is motivated by one's *concerns*, that is, by what one cares about. One's concerns include one's needs, preferences and interests. These are not limited to one's own well-being. For example, it is likely that what one cares about also includes the needs and interests of one's loved ones. Which opportunities the world opens up for one, and more specifically, which opportunities are *relevant*, will depend upon what one's concerns are. Reflection is not necessary for this responsiveness to relevant opportunities. As Rietveld remarks: 'even though there is no wilful choice by a deliberating subject, that which the individual cares about nevertheless motivates the way she acts freely' (2008b: 152).

This is a crucial element that remains undeveloped in Arendt's work: freedom in action is motivated by what one cares about. One's concerns determine which possibilities for action are relevant and solicit action and which are ignored. Now, when we take up the role of our motivating concerns we can specify virtuosity as the ability to act in coherence with one's concerns. That is, the freedom one experiences will increase the more one is able to act in accordance with what one cares about. If I can act according to what matters to me, I will feel free – regardless of the amount of conscious control I exert during this action. In other words, we can conclude that the experience of freedom depends on the *coherence between my concerns and my actions*.[3]

Too much control is counter-productive: three mechanisms

What does this philosophical excursion bring us with regard to understanding the lack of freedom as experienced by OCD patients? First of all, the conception of freedom in action that we have developed understands freedom as the coherence between my concerns and my actions. It is clear that patients suffering from OCD are unfree in this sense: they feel compelled to think and do things that are not in accordance with the way they would want to live. Also, when these patients recover, and we ask them about their experience of freedom, they generally report how they have taken up those activities in life that their disorder had made impossible for them. The freedom they gained is the freedom to do what matters to them.

The conception of freedom in terms of action acknowledges the importance of acting in the world, of engaging oneself in projects, together with other people. Crucially, the ability to perceive the possibilities for engaging in the world requires an attitude of acceptance: of basic trust. This attitude of trustful openness to the outside world stands in contrast with deliberation which rather entails turning one's attention inwards instead of outwards. Too much inward directedness leads to closing oneself off in one's own inner world. Now, the problem in many forms of psychopathology is precisely that patients 'live in their own world'. As Van den Berg pointed out in his book on the principles of phenomenological psychopathology *A Different Existence*: 'The psychiatric patient stands apart from the rest of the world ... he has a world of his own' (1972: 105). Patients are trapped in themselves, and their inward directedness attributes to the continuation of the pathologies.

Moreover, we are now in the position to explain the paradox that OCD patients experience themselves as unfree, even though they exert more conscious control over their thoughts and actions than people normally do. The phenomenological account of action assigns conscious deliberation a *serving* role in order to attain a spontaneous flow of action. We switch to deliberation when we encounter a problem, or when we are still in the process of learning a new skill. Too much deliberation, however, may rather disturb our flow of action. Think, for instance, of learning how to dance tango. Initially, this requires a lot of conscious attention. One has to think about one's posture, and the position of one's feet and so on. But the more skilled one becomes, the less one needs to think about these things. One just moves fluently. Imagine the dancing has become a second nature. When one would then be asked to pay conscious attention to one's feet during the dance, this will rather disturb one's fluency. But also just looking at one's feet while quickly descending the stairs can be a dangerous example of how conscious control may disrupt one's actions.

Here we will look at three counter-productive control mechanisms that are at stake in OCD: one concerning one's thoughts, and two concerning one's actions.

The pink-elephant effect

Patients suffering from OCD try very hard to control their thoughts. But how much control do we ordinarily have over our thoughts? Is it not rather part of the phenomenology of thinking that thoughts 'pop up' and that we can at best 'funnel' them? At least we never completely steer or control our thinking. There is always an element of 'emergence' of our thoughts. If having limited control over one's thoughts is normal, perhaps these patients strive for an exaggerated and impossible control.

It has long since been suggested that striving to control and particularly to suppress specific thoughts can in fact have an opposite effect. The 'pink elephant' has become the symbol of the difficulty of thought suppression: when instructed not to think of a pink elephant, this rather induces this image to come to mind. The most well-known research on thought suppression started off with white bears. In 1987, Wegner and colleagues conducted a series of experiments in which they asked participants *not* to think of a white bear for the next five minutes. If the experimenters hadn't brought up the white bear, the chances that participants would have spontaneously thought about white bears would have been next to zero. However, the assignment directed their attention to what it was now 'forbidden' to think. Wegner and colleagues showed that deliberately not wanting to think about a white bear makes it in fact much harder not to do so. They write:

> The paradoxical effect of thought suppression is that it produces a preoccupation with the suppressed thought. These findings suggest that the task of suppressing a thought is itself difficult, leading people to hold the thought in consciousness repeatedly even as they try to eliminate it. When they are then released from the suppression task and asked instead to go ahead and express the thought, they do so at an accelerated rate, mentioning it more often than if they had simply been asked to express the thought from the start. There are thus both immediate and delayed tendencies toward conscious preoccupation with the very thought that is being suppressed. (Wegner et al. 1987:8)

Such a mechanism appears also be at play in patients with OCD (Salkovskis and Campbell 1994; Rassin et al. 2001; Purdon 2004). The counter-productive effect of suppression could in their case be even more stringent, since the thoughts and images that bother them are not just neutral stimuli like white bears and pink elephants. Rather, they are depictions of what the person in question considers to be most repulsive, usually of a sexual, aggressive or blasphemous content. A mother, for instance, pictures herself murdering her baby, a father is plagued by incestuous thoughts and others worry about how they might cause fatal accidents. As Salkovskis and Campbell (1994) point out, such 'emotionally valenced and personally relevant' thoughts and images are likely to be more intrusive than emotionally neutral stimuli.

Moreover, patients tend to attribute much meaning to these images. Shafran and colleagues (1996) distinguished two biases: the likelihood bias; and the moral bias. The likelihood bias refers to the finding that OCD patients are inclined to assume that thinking about an event will make this event more likely to happen. Thus, they fear that their negative intrusions will increase the chance that their fears will indeed become reality. The moral bias refers to the idea that having a thought about something is morally equivalent to actually doing it. OCD patients tend to think that their unwanted thoughts reveal something about what they are really like or what they would be capable of doing when they lose their self-control. Taken together, these biases are referred to as 'thought–action fusion'. Naturally, this inflated meaning provides an extra motivation for trying to suppress these thoughts – unfortunately with counter-productive effects.

Apart from the propensity of OCD patients to control their thoughts by trying actively to suppress them, it has also been noted that patients tend to be 'hyper-aware' of these thoughts (Salkovskis and Campbell 1994). Salkovskis and Campbell conclude that not only thought suppression itself, but also this constant self-monitoring 'play a key role in the maintenance of obsessional thinking' (1994: 7). We would suggest that this tendency to exert control and the inward directedness of attention are parts of the same process.

The self-sustaining prophecy

With regard to the role of conscious control in action, we can distinguish two different counter-productive mechanisms: the self-sustaining prophecy and the hyper-reflectivity trap. Starting with the first, part of the problem simply comes from the fact that the time spent worrying, or thinking and performing one's compulsions, is time *not spent* engaged in meaningful actions – which implies that patients' worst-case scenario's are not corrected by real-life experiences.

In addition, there is a basic mechanism of avoidance at work. Beck and Clark (1997) point out that pathological anxiety consists of both an 'erroneous or biased interpretation of stimuli as dangerous or threatening' along with the underestimation of 'personal coping resources and the safety or rescue features in the environment' (pp. 50–51). Unfortunately, the experience of anxiety generally prompts people to *avoid* the anxiety-provoking situation – which means that they will not be in the position to correct their overestimation of the danger and the underestimation of their own skills on the basis of their own experience.[4] In other words, as long as patients do not go out and act, they do not accumulate positive, correcting experiences with regard to both the world and themselves.

The avoidance prevents patients from experiencing that their convictions are distorted. They cannot prove themselves wrong, because they do not put their convictions to the test of real-life activities – resulting in a self-sustaining prophecy.

The hyper-reflectivity trap

Not only do OCD patients engage less in meaningful activities both out of avoidance and out of sheer time pressure, but when they do, another mechanism may come into play. As we noted before, OCD patients exert much more conscious control over their actions *during* these actions. That is, they pay more conscious attention to what they do than people usually do. We suggest that here too, excessive conscious control can have a counter-productive effect.

Many OCD patients are insecure about whether they have done something, or have done something correctly. Did I really properly lock the door? Just to be sure, patients may repeat their action, whilst paying extra attention to all their movements. Now, it is completely normal to exert conscious control over one's deeds when one is insecure or when it is particularly important that one do things right. For instance, if one locks the door before leaving for a long holiday, one probably pays more attention to turning the key, than on an ordinary morning when one is going to work. Switching to conscious control can be a very helpful strategy.

However, as we noted before, too much conscious control may disturb the flow of action. Especially with those actions that we are experts at, that are already part of our second nature, thinking about these actions implies taking a step back in the stages of skill acquisition (Dreyfus 2002). You may have tied your shoes this morning. How *exactly* did you do that? If I asked you to explain, you would probably be inclined to just show how you do it. But suppose I ask you to *describe* each movement; this would probably not be easy. And if you think long enough, you may even get confused about how you in fact tie your shoes. Paying conscious attention to your habits may actually foster a feeling of estrangement or insecurity.[5]

The exaggerated reflection on and deliberate attention to what one is doing is called 'hyper-reflectivity'. Every act becomes a conscious, deliberate decision instead of just spontaneous responsiveness. What is normally taken for granted, unthinkingly relied upon, is now brought to awareness. As Fuchs (2011) points out, making such tacit processes explicit actually *disturbs* their functionality. He writes: 'Self-centeredness and hyper-reflection are … on the one hand, the result of the illness, but on the other hand, they often additionally contribute to it' (p. 239).

This process of hyper-reflection can be recognized in many different forms of psychopathology – in fact it was first described with regard to schizophrenia (Laing 1959/1990; Sass 1992). In the case of OCD patients, we can also see such a negative spiral at work. We have proposed to call this mechanism the 'hyper-reflectivity trap' (De Haan et al. 2013). It proceeds through several stages:

1. First, there is the feeling of insecurity, anxiety or tension.
2. This feeling leads to attempts to regain control through *deliberation* (e.g. what might go wrong and how could I prevent that?) and *reflective action* (e.g. trying to consciously control the performance of one's actions).
3. But too much reflection can be dangerous: analyzing and paying attention to your actions may lead to estrangement and typically *augments* insecurity.
4. As a last step, the increase of insecurity brings us back to the first step.

The initial feeling of insecurity may already be the result of a more fundamental lack of basic trust. The subsequent exercise of increased conscious control in turn *diminishes* the sense of agency rather than increasing the experience of freedom. Too much deliberation on and analysis of one's unreflective, habitual actions may cause insecurity and even a breakdown of what was once 'second nature'.

Solving the paradox: being free by losing control

Concluding, we can say that OCD patients experience themselves as unfree. Their condition is, however, not due to a *lack* of conscious control, but rather the result of *too much* conscious control. The combination of feeling unfree whilst exerting conscious control only appears to be contradictory when one understands freedom as 'inner freedom', or freedom of the will. The phenomenological alternative conception of freedom in action can very well explain this combination. Moreover, by introducing the idea of a proper balance between deliberation and unreflective action, we could better understand several of the aggravating mechanisms that can be at stake in OCD.

Interestingly, in our research on the phenomenological effects of deep-brain stimulation (DBS) we find that patients suffering from severe OCD who are treated successfully with DBS report an increase in spontaneous actions. As one patient remarked: 'my actions now go faster than my thoughts: I now do things without thinking. That is pretty scary!' (de Haan et al. 2013). Successful treatment seems to restore the balance between unthinkingly relying and deliberating. Also, over-stimulation may lead to problematically increased impulsivity (Luigjes et al. 2011). This finding is a further indication that DBS influences the balance between spontaneous action and conscious control, as well as a warning that although an increase in impulsivity is helpful, the balance should not tip to the other side either.

Our hypothesis is also in line with findings from fundamental brain research at our department. fMRI and EEG research in OCD patients stimulated at the nucleus accumbens shows changes in the *connectivity* between the nucleus accumbens and the prefrontal cortex. Stimulation restores intrinsic frontostriatal network dynamics rather than merely having inhibitory or excitatory effects at the target area (Figee et al. 2013). In particular, stimulation of the nucleus accumbens of OCD patients decreases excessive frontostriatal connectivity, which is moreover strongly correlated with OCD symptom improvement.

We suggest that the excessive frontostriatal connectivity in OCD patients may be a reflection of their excessive use of conscious control at the cost of more unreflective skill-driven behaviour or responsiveness. The fact that the diminishment of the frontostriatal connectivity correlates so strongly with the improvement of the patients' symptoms may provide a neuroscientific affirmation of our phenomenologically based hypothesis that these patients exert too much conscious control rather than too little. However, further empirical research is needed to test this hypothesis directly.

Being free by losing control: implications for the neuroscientific debate on free will

A phenomenological analysis of the experiences of OCD patients confirms a conception of freedom that requires unreflective action just as much as conscious deliberation. To feel free, one needs to find a proper balance between deliberation and conscious control on the one hand and spontaneous, unreflective actions on the other. In other words, being free also requires losing control. Moreover, our unreflective habits or abilities are just as much part of who we are as our conscious deliberation is. To appreciate the importance of our habits, one only needs to keep in mind that spontaneous actions are informed. They are not mere reflexes or instincts but are flexible and context-sensitive, and it has taken time and energy to turn them into habits. The learning of any new skill attests to the effort it takes to incorporate skills as second nature.

This alternative conception of what it means to be a free autonomous agent has some important implications for neuroscientific research on free will. Ever since Libet's landmark experiments (Libet 1985), many neuroscientific studies have shown that the role of our conscious control is limited (Wegner 2002). These findings are often taken to imply that we have no free will. We might like to think of ourselves as autonomous agents, these free will sceptics say, but all our supposed reasons for our behaviour turn out to be confabulations after the fact. That is, our reasons are not causing our behaviour but are rather rationalizations of our behaviour after it has already occurred. Hence, we are not in control of our behaviour. Everything has already been decided long before by or in our brains. After the 'masters of suspicion' (Ricoeur 1970) Marx, Freud and Nietzsche cast doubt on our traditional conception of the autonomous subject in the late nineteenth century, present-day research in cognitive neuroscience confirms the limits of our conscious control.

There are, however, two fundamentally different perspectives that we can take on the crumbling of our notion of the subject as a rational being who is only free when she or he is in conscious control. Nowadays, it is popular to interpret the limited influence of our conscious control as a *void*, as a proof of the illusory character of our autonomy, our free will and even our 'self' (Metzinger 2003; Wegner 2003). We may think that we are in control, these sceptics say, but in fact everything has already been decided for us by our brain. Now, even apart from its inherent conceptual confusions (How could an organ decide anything for us? And whose brain would it then be? (Bennett and Hacker 2003)), this interpretation unquestioningly assumes the traditional concept of autonomous agency with its emphasis on the role of conscious control that it subsequently dismisses. Moreover, this interpretation also assumes that explicit, deliberate intentions must precede actions, an assumption which is increasingly questioned.[6]

On the other hand, we could also regard the limits of conscious control as a matter of *redistribution*: perhaps our conscious control does less, whereas our skilled bodies, our second nature does more (De Haan 2012). This latter perspective acknowledges that our spontaneous, unreflective actions and our bodily skills make out a fundamental part of our personhood. Moreover, as our analysis has shown, the experience of freedom too not only resides in conscious deliberation, but just as much depends on our ability to do things *without* thinking, to rely on the flow of our know-how. Our analysis thus shows that these sceptical interpretations are based on a false dichotomy: it is assumed that *either* one has conscious control over one's actions and thus counts as a free agent *or* automatic processes are at work that 'thus' have nothing to do with the agent. As the investigation of unreflective action has shown, this latter assumption is a crude misconception of what it means to be an autonomous agent. Our unreflective skilful actions do not form a threat to our personal autonomy, but rather together with conscious deliberation co-constitute our autonomy and our experience of freedom.

Conclusion

Patients suffering from OCD feel unfree. They cannot do the things they want to do, or think the things they want to feel. Instead, they feel they are trapped inside their head. In order to regain control over their lives, they deliberate or try to pay extra conscious attention to what they do. Paradoxically, their recourse to conscious control often makes matters worse, resulting in a diminishment of the experience of freedom and agency. The traditional conception of freedom in terms of conscious control cannot do justice to this phenomenon. We have introduced Arendt's conception of freedom in terms of action as an alternative. Drawing on phenomenological insights on action, we have formulated a more adequate account of the role of deliberation in the experience of freedom. We suggest that there is an optimal level of conscious control. Beyond a certain point, the desire for and exercise of conscious control becomes pathological and results in loss of control of one's behaviour. To feel free requires first and foremost that one can act in accordance with what one cares about. Consequently, we need to be able to engage in the world, to engage with others. And this engagement requires the ability to rely on one's bodily skills as much as on our ability to reflect and deliberate. For OCD patients, the challenge lies in lessening their conscious control and learning to trust, to rely on their abilities and their surroundings instead.

NOTES

1 As Timothy O'Connor starts the entry on 'Free Will' in the *Stanford Encyclopedia of Philosophy*: '"Free will" is a philosophical term of art for a particular sort of capacity of rational agents to choose a course of action from among various alternatives' (2011).

2 Arendt's conception of virtuosity as depending upon the combination of both worldly opportunities and personal skills strongly resembles the notion of responsiveness to *affordances*. The ecological psychologist James J. Gibson, in his *The Ecological Approach to Visual Perception* (1979), introduced this notion to designate the intricate relation between the available opportunities for action and the specific biological make-up and skills of an organism – an idea that was already developed by J. Von Uexküll (1920) in his notion of the *Funktionskreis*.

3 Note that on this conception, the experience of freedom is not all or nothing, but rather a matter of degree. The more I am able to act in accordance with what I care about, the freer I am. Someone who would succeed in acting in total accordance with his or her concerns would be as free as one could be. Thanks to the editor for suggesting this point to us.

4 Meynen (2011) recently pointed out that patients who worry excessively overestimate the helpfulness of deliberation, at the cost of relying on their bodily skills. That is, they may endorse a 'metacognition that overrates the value of detached contemplation about future situations while underrating the value and resources of actual embodied-embedded engagement' (p. 1).

5 Research on memory shows that patients with OCD do not have memory impairments per se, but rather *distrust* their memory: it is thus the *attitude towards* their memory that is affected. Interestingly, the same happens to normal controls who are instructed to repeatedly check their tasks. The checking thus augments the feeling of insecurity. See Van den Hout and Kindt (2003: 301–16).

6 The interpretation of free will sceptics relies on the view of Hurley (2005). This is called 'the classical sandwich-model of the mind', that is, perception is regarded as input from the world to the mind, action is seen as the output from the mind to the world, and cognition (e.g. intentions) refers to the internal processes that take place in between. The adequacy of this linear, vertical model is increasingly under pressure from non-linear, dynamical models of both neural processes (Kelso 1995; Beer 2000: 91–9) and the relations between perception, action, and cognition (O'Regan and Noë 2001: 883–917; Noë 2004).

REFERENCES

American Psychiatric Association (2000). *Diagnostic and Statistical Manual of Mental Disorders*, 4th edn, DSM-IV-TR (text revision). Washington, DC: American Psychiatric Association.

Arendt, H. (1954/2006). *What Is Freedom? Between Past and Future*. New York: Penguin Classics.

Beck, A. T. and D. A. Clark (1997). 'An information processing model of anxiety: automatic and strategic processes'. *Behaviour Research and Therapy* **35**(1): 49–58.

Beer, R. D. (2000). 'Dynamical approaches to cognitive science'. *Trends in Cognitive Sciences* **4**: 91–9.

Bennett, M. R. and P. M. S. Hacker (2003). *Philosophical Foundations of Neuroscience*. Malden, MA: Blackwell.

De Haan, S. (2012). 'Fenomenologie van de lichaamservaring'. In *Handboek Psychiatrie en Filosofie*, ed. D. Denys and G. Meynen. Utrecht: de Tijdstroom, pp. 213–27.

De Haan, S., E. Rietveld and D. Denys (2013). 'On the nature of obsessions and compulsions'. In *Anxiety Disorders*, ed. D. S. Baldwin and B. E. Leonard. Modern Trends in Pharmacopsychiatry, Vol. 29. Basel: Karger, pp. 1–15.

De Haan, S., E. Rietveld, M. Stokhof and D. Denys (2013). 'The phenomenology of deep brain stimulation-induced changes in OCD patients: an enactive, affordance-based model'. *Frontiers in Human Neuroscience* 7: 1–14.

Dreyfus, H. L. (2002) 'A phenomenology of skill acquisition as the basis for a Merleau-Pontian non-representationalist cognitive science'. Unpublished paper. Available at http://socrates.berkeley.edu/~hdreyfus/pdf/MerleauPontySkillCogSci.pdf

Esquirol, E. (1838). *Des maladies mentales considérées sous les rapports médical, hygiénique et médico-légal.* Paris: J. B. Baillière.

Figee, M., J. Luigjes, R. Smolders, C. Valencia-Alfonso, W. Van Wingen et al. (2013). 'Regaining control: deep brain stimulation restores frontostriatal network activity in obsessive-compulsive disorder'. *Nature Neuroscience* **16**: 386–7.

Fuchs, T. (2011). 'The psychopathology of hyperreflexivity'. *The Journal of Speculative Philosophy* **24**(3): 239–55.

Gibson, J. J. (1979). *The Ecological Approach to Visual Perception.* Boston: Houghton Mifflin.

Heidegger, M. (1927/2001). *Sein und Zeit.* Tübingen, Niemeyer.

Hurley, S. (2005). 'Active perception and perceiving action: the shared circuits hypothesis'. In *Perceptual Experience*, ed. T. Gendler and J. Hawthorne. Oxford University Press, pp. 205–59.

James, W. (1890/1950). *The Principles of Psychology.* Vol. II. New York: Dover Publishers.

Kelso, J. A. S. (1995). *Dynamic Patterns: The Self-Organization of Brain and Behaviour.* Cambridge, MA: MIT Press.

Laing, R. D. (1959/1990). *The Divided Self.* London: Penguin Books.

Libet, B. (1985). 'Unconscious cerebral initiative and the role of conscious will in voluntary action'. *Behavioral and Brain Sciences* **8**(4): 529–66.

Luigjes, J., M. Mantione, W. Van den Brink, P. R. Schuurman, P. Van den Munckhof and D. Denys. (2011). 'Deep brain stimulation increases impulsivity in two patients with obsessive-compulsive disorder'. *International Clinical Psychopharmacology* **26**(6): 338–40.

Merleau-Ponty, M. (1945/2002). *Phenomenology of Perception.* London: Routledge.

Metzinger, T. (2003). *Being No One: The Self-Model Theory of Subjectivity.* Cambridge, MA: MIT Press.

Meynen, G. (2011). 'Generalized anxiety disorder and online intelligence: a phenomenological account of why worrying is unhelpful'. *Philosophy, Ethics, and Humanities in Medicine* **6**(1): 7.

Noë, A. (2004). *Action in Perception.* Cambridge, MA: MIT Press.

O'Connor, T. (2011). 'Free will'. In *The Stanford Encyclopedia of Philosophy* (Fall 2014 edn), ed. E. N. Zalta. Stanford University, available at http://plato.stanford.edu/archives/fall 2014/entries/free will/.

O'Regan, J. K. and A. Noë (2001). 'A sensorimotor account of vision and visual consciousness'. *Behavioral and Brain Sciences* **24**(5): 883–917.

Purdon, C. (2004). 'Empirical investigations of thought suppression in OCD'. *Journal of Behavior Therapy and Experimental Psychiatry* **35**(2): 121–36.

Rassin, E., P. Diepstraten, H. Merckelbach and P. Muris. (2001). 'Thought-action fusion and thought suppression in obsessive-compulsive disorder'. *Behaviour Research and Therapy* **39**(7): 757–64.

Ricoeur, P. (1970). *Freud and Philosophy: An Essay on Interpretation*. New Haven: Yale University Press.

Rietveld, E. (2008a). 'Situated normativity: the normative aspect of embodied cognition in unreflective action'. *Mind* **117**(468): 973–1001.

(2008b). *Unreflective Action: A Philosophical Contribution to Integrative Neuroscience*. University of Amsterdam: ILLC-Dissertation Series.

Salkovskis, P. M. and P. Campbell (1994). 'Thought suppression induces intrusion in naturally occurring negative intrusive thoughts'. *Behaviour Research and Therapy* **32**(1): 1–8.

Sass, L. A. (1992). *Madness and Modernism: Insanity in the Light of Modern Art, Literature and Thought*. New York: Basic Books.

Shafran, R., D. S. Thordarson and S. Rachman (1996). 'Thought-action fusion in obsessive compulsive disorder'. *Journal of Anxiety Disorders* **10**(5): 379–91.

Van den Berg, J. H. (1972). *A Different Existence: Principles of Phenomenological Psychopathology*. Pittsburgh: Duquesne University Press.

Van den Hout, M. and M. Kindt (2003). 'Repeated checking causes memory distrust'. *Behaviour Research and Therapy* **41**(3): 301–16.

Von Uexküll, J. (1920). *Theoretische Biologie*. Berlin: Paetel.

Wegner, D. M. (2002). *The Illusion of Conscious Will*. Cambridge MA: MIT Press.

(2003). 'The mind's best trick: how we experience conscious will'. *Trends in Cognitive Sciences* 7(2): 65–69.

Wegner, D. M., D. J. Schneider, S. Carter and T. L. White. (1987). 'Paradoxical effects of thought suppression'. *Journal of Personality and Social Psychology* **53**(1): 5.

6 Psychopathy and free will from a philosophical and cognitive neuroscience perspective

Farah Focquaert, Andrea L. Glenn, and Adrian Raine

ABSTRACT

In our chapter, we discuss one of the most influential compatibilist accounts of free will, Fischer and Ravizza's (1998) reasons-responsiveness theory, and review the empirical literature on psychopathy that addresses the requirements for moral responsibility that are put forward in their account. Reasons-responsive compatibilist views seem to argue for the absence of moral responsibility or at least diminished responsibility when considering psychopathy. Their view draws upon impairments in the relevant kind of reasons-responsiveness in which one is responsive to both prudential *and* moral reasons. If moral reasons as genuine reasons that may motivate behavior are somehow *alien* to individuals with psychopathy, can we argue that these individuals are fully responsible for their immoral behavior? Based on empirical findings, we argue that psychopaths have core affective and cognitive deficits that may impair moral rationality. We conclude that the hard determinist, hard incompatibilist, and reasons-responsive compatibilist view suggest that offenders with severe psychopathy should not be held criminally responsible, and that mild psychopathy should function as a mitigating factor allowing for partial criminal responsibility. We should greatly increase our emphasis on early prevention and rehabilitation while ensuring that society is adequately protected and the feelings and rights of victims are respected.

> What we fear – or at any rate a very important part of what we fear – in determinism is the prospect that determinism would rule out control, and we very definitely do not want to lose control or be out of control or be controlled by something or someone else – like a marionette or puppet.
> (Dennett, 1984: 51)

Introduction

Psychopathy is a personality disorder that is characterized by a combination of personality and behavioral features. The interpersonal and affective features encompass specific personality traits such as glibness, deceitfulness, conning, superficial charm, manipulativeness, and a lack of empathy, guilt, or remorse. In addition to reactive aggression, psychopaths also uniquely show instrumental (unprovoked) aggression. In the USA, about 20–25 percent of prisoners would be considered psychopaths as measured by the Psychopathy Checklist-Revised (PCL-R). Psychopathic traits are considered one of the strongest predictors of violent recidivism. Research studies have had little success in identifying behavioral treatment programs that work in adult psychopaths.

A growing body of evidence has begun to identify both genetic and environmental factors that appear to contribute to the development of psychopathic traits and demonstrate that regions of the brain function differently in these individuals. This research raises many questions for our concept of free will and moral/criminal responsibility. In this chapter, we briefly review philosophical theories concerning the relationship between free will and moral responsibility. On one hand, hard determinists and hard incompatibilists argue that free will is incompatible with a scientific worldview (i.e., knowledge provided by our best scientific theories) and therefore argue that free will is an illusion. If free will is an illusion, then no individual, including a psychopath, can be held responsible for his or her behavior because moral responsibility presupposes free will. Moreover, according to hard determinists and hard incompatibilists, knowledge about the genetic or neurobiological factors that contribute to deviant behavior is irrelevant to the debate on responsibility since no individual, regardless of genetic or neurobiological makeup, can be held responsible. For example, a hard determinist may argue that both the psychopath's and the non-psychopath's behavior is "100% determined by brain function, which is in turn determined by the interplay of genes and experience" (Farah, 2005: 38). On these views, the answer to criminal offenders with psychopathy and the potential threat to public safety may lie in non-punitive measures that aim to protect society and its members from harm. For example, some defend a consequentialist, deterrence-based view of incarceration aimed not at punishing psychopaths but preventing them from causing further harm to others, while others argue for the development of innovative and benign biosocial programs for crime prevention (Glenn & Raine, 2014). Compatibilists, on the other hand, argue that free will, and thus moral responsibility, is compatible with a scientific worldview. Compatibilist theories on the relationship between free will and moral responsibility specify the requirements that are necessary for holding an individual morally responsible. Compatibilists may argue that the ability for reasons-responsive behavior enables free behavior and thus moral responsibility. If psychopaths can be said to have the ability for *reasons-responsive behavior*, then these individuals are morally responsible and may be held criminally responsible and punished. If they are not responsible because they are impaired in or lack the capacity for reasons-responsive behavior, then it is this impairment, not causal determinism, that explains why they are not responsible.

In this chapter, we discuss one of the most influential compatibilist accounts on free will, Fischer and Ravizza's (1998) reasons-responsiveness theory, and review the empirical literature on psychopathy that addresses the requirements for moral responsibility that are put forward in their account. Based upon the literature, we will discuss whether psychopaths can be considered reasons-responsive individuals. Reasons-responsive compatibilist views seem to argue for the absence of moral responsibility or at least for diminished responsibility when considering psychopathy, due to the absence of the relevant kind of reasons-responsiveness that is necessary for moral responsibility (i.e., responsiveness to prudential *and* moral reasons). If moral reasons as genuine reasons that may motivate behavior are somehow *alien* to individuals with psychopathy, can we argue that these individuals are (fully) responsible for their immoral behavior? Based on empirical findings, we argue that psychopaths have core affective deficits, as well as cognitive deficits that may (partially or fully) impair moral rationality. We conclude that the hard determinist, hard incompatibilis, and reasons-responsive compatibilist view suggest that offenders with severe psychopathy should not be held criminally responsible, and that mild psychopathy should function as a mitigating factor allowing for partial criminal responsibility (as in the Netherlands).

Incompatibilist and compatibilist accounts of free will

Free will can be defined as "the unique ability of persons to exercise control over their conduct in the fullest manner necessary for moral responsibility" (McKenna, 2009), or alternatively, and somewhat less circular, as "the ability of persons to exercise full control over their conduct." The philosophical debate on free will is concerned with the notion of moral responsibility and the knowledge or presupposition that we need a concept of voluntary control/behavior (i.e., free will) in order to justify its use: "it is a presupposition that some sort of control is a necessary condition of morally responsible agency" (Fischer & Ravizza, 1998: 20). The crucial question, then, seems to be which kind of control is required for us to hold others morally responsible. Does it imply that I, as an agent, could have acted differently or that I have ultimate control over my behavior? And how does causal determinism come into play?

Causal determinism can be defined as "the metaphysical thesis that *facts of the past, in conjunction with the laws of nature, entail every truth about the future*" (McKenna, 2009). According to incompatibilists (i.e., libertarians, hard determinists, and hard incompatibilists), free will is not compatible with causal determinism (e.g., Clarke, 2000; Greene & Cohen, 2004; Kane, 1999; Wegner, 2002). Libertarians argue that because at least certain individuals behave freely and are responsible for at least some of their behavior, causal determinism must be false. They argue that the alternatives to causal determinism enable free will (e.g., the possibility of ontological indeterminacy in classical mechanics and/or the claim of ontological indeterminacy in quantum mechanics extending from the micro-level of atoms to the macro-level of human decision-making). The concepts of *acausality* (events that happen without a distinct cause), and/or *autocausation* (events that happen without an external cause) are invoked to allow for free will. Hard determinists argue that free will is an illusion due to the causal deterministic processes that are at work. Hard incompatibilists argue that both causal determinism and indeterminism (e.g., quantum physics) pose a threat to free will. According to hard determinists and hard incompatibilists, to have full control over one's conduct implies that an individual has the ability to act differently at a given point in time (i.e., has alternative possibilities), and/or that an individual can be considered the ultimate source of his or her actions (i.e., meaning that one's actions originate in oneself). This means that if at any point in time *we could not have acted differently*, and/or *we cannot be considered the ultimate source of our own actions*, then we cannot be held responsible for our behavior. Causal determinism rules out freedom of alternatives and ultimate source control, because it implies that any action we perform at a particular time is the only action we could have performed at that time and because it implies that the mental states that issue in our actions are causally determined by antecedent events (Glannon, 2011).

If one holds the position that neither causal determinism nor indeterminism provides an individual with free will in the relevant sense, then our current knowledge about the neurobiology of psychopathy, or any other psychiatric conditions, is irrelevant to moral responsibility. The hard incompatibilist view, which argues that neither determinism nor indeterminism give us the right kind of free will, basically entails that no individual has the right kind of free will or freedom to be held morally responsible. Hence, what the brain science tells us about the brain of the psychopath and how normal or abnormal the psychopath's brain might be is basically irrelevant. In a world without alternative possibilities, or without ultimate source control, no individual can be held responsible (in a scientifically relevant sense at least). Whether one wishes to hold individuals responsible based on reasons other than purely scientific considerations (e.g., the pragmatic value of having a notion of moral responsibility) is a different matter. For example, Dennett (2003) argues that "the fact that free will *is* worth wanting can be used to anchor our conception of free will" (p. 297). The pragmatic value of having a notion of moral responsibility raises questions about the relevance of the deterministic view for normative judgments of individuals' behavior. If no one has free will and no one can be held morally responsible due to biological and environmental factors that are beyond our control, then there seems to be no way of differentiating between an individual who can control his or her behavior and an individual who cannot (e.g., violent offender). Compatibilists disagree with incompatibilists with regard to the kind of free will that is required for moral responsibility. According to many compatibilists, moral responsibility does not presuppose alternative possibilities, nor does it presuppose ultimate source control. Moreover, unlike libertarians, the kind of control that compatibilists typically put forward as the required condition for morally responsible agency does not presuppose acausality or autocausation. Hence, they will typically defend a type of control that is compatible with a causally closed deterministic universe. For example, many compatibilists argue that having control over one's behavior implies that an agent plays a *crucial* role in the production of his or her actions, or put differently, that one's actions issue from one's self in a *suitable manner* (McKenna, 2009). Fischer and Ravizza (1998) distinguish *regulative control* from *guidance control*. Regulative control implies that an agent has the ability to regulate between different alternatives (which brings us back to the "alternative possibilities" demand), whereas guidance control implies that an agent guides or brings about his or her conduct (in a suitable manner) even if he or she has no other alternatives to the course he or she takes. Regulative control implies a dual type of control in which the agent has the power both to act freely (i.e., guidance control) and to do something else instead (Fischer & Ravizza, 1998).

To convince non-compatibilists, philosophers defending *regulative control* must show what is wrong with the consequence argument. The consequence argument claims that since (a) no one has power over the facts of the past and the laws of nature, and (b) no one has power over the fact that the facts of the past and the laws of nature entail every fact of the future (i.e., causal determinism is true), we can conclude that (c) no one has power over the facts of the future (see McKenna, 2009). The consequence argument shows that an individual does not have alternative options available within a causally determined world. Interestingly, Frankfurt devised a thought experiment that questions the need for alternative possibilities when one attributes moral responsibility to others (see Frankfurt, 1969). McKenna (2000: 92) gives the following Frankfurt-type example:

> Sam plans to kill the major and carries out his plan without any interference from "outside forces." Unbeknownst to Sam, Jack, a mad neurologist, wants Sam to kill the mayor and would prefer that Sam did it on his own. But, worried that Sam will change his mind, Jack implants a device in Sam's brain which allows Jack to monitor Sam's brain activity from afar. Should Sam give any indication to Jack that he (Sam) will do other than kill the mayor, Jack will activate his otherwise dormant device, bringing it about that Sam kills the major. But, as things go, Sam kills the mayor on his own. Jack never intervenes.

According to Frankfurt and others (e.g., Fischer & Ravizza, 1998; McKenna, 2009), the natural reaction to this type of scenario is to claim that Jack, even though he could not have acted differently, is nevertheless morally responsible for his behavior. This seems to imply that moral responsibility does not rely on the "freedom to do otherwise" (i.e., alternative possibilities), but rather on the capacity 'to act freely' (i.e., having the right kind of control over one's actions). Following Frankfurt, most compatibilists focus on the issue of control rather than alternative possibilities, and many argue that what is necessary for moral responsibility (and the type of free will that is required to hold someone responsible) is *guidance control* rather than *regulative control*. Unlike regulative control, guidance control is compatible with determinism.

Reasons-responsive compatibilism

Compatibilists like Wolf (1990), and Fischer and Ravizza (1998) argue that to have control over one's conduct (i.e., guidance control) and thus have the capacity for moral responsibility implies that an individual has the ability for reasons-responsive behavior. Reasons-responsiveness generally entails that individuals who are unresponsive to a range of rational considerations do not act of their own free will (e.g., individuals with OCD or schizophrenia), whereas agents who are responsive to a range of rational considerations do act of their own free will. Reasons-responsiveness gives rise to moral responsibility by locating "the control required for morally responsible agency in the capacity to respond to reasons for action" (McKenna, 2000: 89). For example, Fischer and Ravizza (1998) claim that moral responsibility does not entail the freedom to do otherwise. According to them, another type of freedom is required for the attribution of moral responsibility. They defend a *semi-compatibilist* account, in which determinism is incompatible with the freedom to do otherwise, but compatible with moral responsibility. On their account, guidance control refers to "the power to perform an action freely," whereas regulative control refers to "the power to perform an action freely" as well as the "power to act otherwise" (McKenna, 2000: 91). This difference is important according to Fischer and Ravizza because although determinism rules out alternative possibilities, it doesn't rule out a different kind of freedom, namely the freedom that falls under guidance control. What appears to be relevant in the Frankfurt-type examples, according to Fischer and Ravizza (1998) is whether or not Sam's actions result from a "mechanism which *is* reasons-responsive" (McKenna, 2000: 95). Rather than focusing on whether or not the agent is reasons-responsive, we need to discover if the mechanism that actually issues in the action (i.e., the action-sequence mechanism) *is* reasons-responsive. In the Frankfurt-type case, although Sam *himself* cannot be considered reasons-responsive (due to the implanted device that would take control if he did not kill the mayor on his own), he can nevertheless be considered morally responsible because his actions result from a mechanism that *is* reasons-responsive. To ascribe moral responsibility, we need to detect whether or not, in the actual sequence of events, the agent exhibited the right kind of control (i.e., based upon the presence of a mechanism which *is* reasons-responsive). In their *moderately reasons-responsive mechanism* account, Fischer and Ravizza (1998) draw a difference between "receptivity to reasons" on the one hand, and "reactivity to reasons" on the other hand. Receptivity to reasons implies that the agent recognizes those reasons that are captured by "intuitively plausible conditions of rationality" (McKenna, 2000: 97):

> In judging a mechanism's receptivity, we are not only concerned to see that a person acting on that mechanism recognizes a sufficient reason in one instance; we also want to see that the person exhibits an appropriate *pattern* of reason-recognition. In other words, we want to know if he recognizes how reasons fit together, sees why one reason is stronger than another, and understands how the acceptance of one reason as sufficient implies that a stronger reason must also be sufficient. (Fischer & Ravizza, 1998: 70–71)

Reactivity to reasons involves the capacity to translate reasons into choices and subsequent behavior. However, whereas *regular* receptivity to reasons is required, only *weak* reactivity to reasons is required on their account (Fischer & Ravizza, 1998). This means that an individual has to have the capacity or "cognitive power" to recognize actual incentives to do otherwise on a regular basis, but only has to display *some* reactivity to reasons in order to show that he or she has the "executive power" to react to an actual incentive to do otherwise. For example, if an addict is not able to give up his or her addictive behavior based upon rational reasons related to health and wellbeing (i.e., health-related incentives), but is able to give up his or her addictive behavior if the price of the addictive substance goes up (i.e., market-related incentives), then this individual exhibits weak reactivity to reasons and thus can be held morally responsible for not acting upon health-related incentives to quit his or her addiction. Or, for example, if a heroine-addicted female cannot give up her addiction for her own health and wellbeing, but can abstain from taking heroine when she discovers that she's pregnant, then, according to Fischer and Ravizza, she can be held morally responsible for her behavior at other times (before or after her pregnancy). Fischer and Ravizza (1998) explain their position on weak reactivity as follows: "That is, we believe that if an agent's mechanism [= process that leads up to an action] reacts to *some* incentive to (say) do other than he actually does, this shows that the mechanism *can* react to *any* incentive to do otherwise" (p. 73). We do not discuss the scientific validity of their view, but there does remain a lively debate as to whether or not the human (addicted) brain indeed functions in such a way (Kennett, 2010). Finally, Fischer and Ravizza (1998) argue that the kind of reasons-responsiveness that is required for moral responsibility needs to be categorized as a responsiveness to a range of reasons, including (some, but not necessarily all) *moral* reasons. On Fischer and Ravizza's (1998) view, some psychopaths can be considered morally responsible agents whereas others cannot. They argue that a psychopath who is not capable of recognizing that he or she has reasons for action deriving from other individuals' rights or interests has an impaired *receptivity* to moral reasons and cannot be held morally responsible. A psychopath who has an appropriate receptivity to moral reasons can be held morally responsible. The inclusion of moral reasons is important because it has been argued that *severe* psychopaths are unresponsive to moral reasons (Morse, 2008), whereas offenders with lesser psychopathy may be partly impaired in terms of their responsiveness to moral reasons (Morse, 2011a). On this view, the ability or inability to respond to moral reasons is a matter of degree and should be understood on a continuum involving degrees of impaired responsiveness.

In sum, if one argues that having full control over one's conduct implies having the ability for reasons-responsive behavior, then individuals do have free will and can be held morally responsible for their behavior. Therefore, within the compatibilist universe sketched above, we need to ask ourselves whether psychopaths are *reasons-responsive* individuals. Can empirical studies on psychopathy help us in answering these questions? Psychopaths appear to have the capacity to choose in accord with their mental states since it is commonly argued that these individuals do possess cognitive rational capacities. At the same time, these individuals appear to lack moral rational capacities, as has been suggested by Stephen Morse (2008), and as can be argued when considering the neurobiological impairments in individuals with psychopathy. This means that although psychopaths may be able to respond to prudential rational reasons, they are likely unable to respond to *moral* rational reasons. Hence, it can be argued that these individuals, depending on the severity of their disorder, may not be fully responsible.

Empirical research on psychopaths

Psychopaths have an intellectual understanding that society has standards for which actions are acceptable and which actions are not. For example, a psychopath can acknowledge that it is illegal to steal. However, research examining how psychopaths respond to various types of stimuli suggests that they lack responsiveness to reasons that non-psychopathic individuals rely upon when making decisions in the moral domain. These deficits include the following:

The inability to take the perspective of another and feel concern for his or her suffering

Several studies have found that psychopaths have deficits in this domain at various levels. At the most basic level, both children and adults with psychopathic traits show deficits in recognizing facial expressions of fear in other individuals (Blair et al., 2001; Blair et al. 2004), thus limiting their ability to recognize when another individual is in distress. Similarly, they demonstrate an impairment in recognizing fearful vocal affect (Blair et al., 2005). The consequences of these deficits can be seen in a recent study of youth with psychopathic traits, which found that these children are less likely to expect that aggression will result in a victim suffering and are less likely to expect that they will experience feelings of remorse (Pardini & Byrd, 2012). Like adults with psychopathic traits (Glenn et al., 2009a), they report lower levels of empathetic concern and lower levels of sadness in response to others' distress.

The identification of deficits in the recognition of fearful facial expressions and vocalizations parallels findings from patients with damage to the amygdala (e.g., Adolphs et al., 1999), a region of the brain involved in emotional processing. Indeed, brain imaging studies indicate that psychopathic individuals have structural and functional differences in the amygdala. Yang et al. (2009) found an 18 percent reduction in the volume of the amygdala in a group of psychopaths compared to non-psychopaths. Reduced functioning of the amygdala has also been observed in psychopathic individuals, particularly when they are presented with stimuli that are thought to invoke social emotions, such as during an affect recognition task (Gordon et al., 2004), during a socially interactive game (Rilling et al., 2007), and during the processing of emotional stimuli (Kiehl et al., 2001). In one study, brain functioning during the process of moral decision-making was examined. Individuals scoring higher in psychopathy demonstrated less functioning in the amygdala, particularly when contemplating hypothetical moral dilemmas involving direct harm to another individual (Glenn et al., 2009b). Research suggests that deficits in the amygdala may exist early in life and therefore may affect the process of moral socialization. Brain imaging studies in youth with callous-unemotional traits, which are thought to be analogous to psychopathic traits in adults, have found reduced functioning in the amygdala when viewing fearful facial expressions (Jones et al., 2009; Marsh et al., 2008).

The inability to take the emotional perspective of others may also result from deficits in the orbitofrontal/ventromedial region of the prefrontal cortex. The orbitofrontal cortex is important in understanding the emotional states of others (Shamay-Tsoory et al., 2005) and has been found to be active in several brain imaging studies presenting morally relevant stimuli (e.g., Borg et al., 2006; Harenski & Hamann, 2006; Moll et al., 2002; Robertson et al., 2007). Furthermore, patients with damage to the orbitofrontal region demonstrate altered patterns of moral decision-making (Koenigs et al., 2007; Ciaramelli et al., 2007). Two studies have found reduced gray matter in the orbitofrontal cortex in psychopathic individuals (de Oliveira-Souza et al., 2008; Yang et al., 2009). Reduced functioning in this region has also been observed in individuals demonstrating higher levels of psychopathic traits during a social interactive game, and during emotion-related tasks (Gordon et al., 2004; Muller et al., 2003; Schneider et al., 2000). Reduced activity in the ventromedial prefrontal cortex has also been observed in criminal psychopaths when evaluating pictures of moral violations (Harenski et al., 2010).

Together, these findings suggest that in psychopaths, regions of the brain that are important in emotional processing are compromised, resulting in a diminished ability to empathize and recognize the suffering of others. This means that they are less responsive to one of the primary reasons that most individuals consider when making moral decisions.

A lack of fear of the negative consequences of immoral behaviors

In some situations, the emotions of a particular victim may not be salient, but individuals may still be deterred from committing immoral acts because of a fear of being caught and/or the negative consequences (e.g., paying a fine or being arrested) that may result from their actions. Psychopaths, however, demonstrate deficits that suggest that they are markedly less responsive to the types of cues that would generate this anxiety regarding being caught. For example, psychopathic murderers fail to show the normative increase in heart rate upon viewing emotion-provoking pictures. Psychopathic individuals also demonstrate reduced physiological responses to a number of stimuli, including imagined threat scenes (Patrick et al., 1994) and anticipated threat (Hare 1965, 1982; Hare et al., 1978; Ogloff & Wong, 1990). They also demonstrate poor fear conditioning (Flor et al., 2002; Hare & Quinn, 1971), meaning that they have difficulty learning to associate a particular cue with a negative event (e.g., punishment). Finally, one of the most robust findings in the psychopathy literature is that psychopaths fail to show the augmented startle response that most individuals show after exposure to threatening or anxiety-provoking stimuli. These studies suggest that psychopaths may not have the same internal signals that deter most individuals from engaging in acts that violate the law.

Deficits in fearfulness of negative stimuli have also been linked to deficits in the amygdala. Birbaumer et al. (2005) found that psychopathic individuals had reduced functioning in the amygdala during a fear-conditioning task in which participants learn to associate a particular cue with an aversive stimulus. Deficits in fear conditioning may be present at a very early age. In a longitudinal study, Gao et al. (2010) found that poor fear conditioning at age 3 was associated with criminal offending at age 23. Similarly, in a 25-year longitudinal study, Glenn et al. (2007) found that adults who demonstrated more psychopathic traits at age 28 had less of a fearful temperament at age 3.

The ability to shift behavior away from reward-seeking and attend to peripheral cues (e.g., the suffering of others or the threat of being caught) that signal that the behavior should be discontinued

In addition to affective deficits in fear and empathy, psychopaths have also been found to have cognitive deficits in attention that may impair their ability to process the relevant cues. For example, in neuropsychological tasks psychopathic individuals are able to avoid monetary punishment if that is their only goal. However, if the task also involves a goal of earning monetary rewards, it seems that reward becomes their primary goal and they are unable to perceive and recognize peripheral signals indicating that they should change their behavior (Newman & Kosson, 1986). This type of cognitive deficit may lead to the reduced processing of information such as distress cues that promote empathy, or cues of threat or punishment that serve as important guides for behavior. The inability to pick up warning cues may significantly impair their ability to alter their course of action.

In addition to contributing to the affective deficits described in the previous sections, poor functioning in the prefrontal cortex may also contribute to the cognitive inability to attend to relevant stimuli. The orbitofrontal cortex is involved in processing reward and punishment information (Rolls, 2000) and inhibiting responses (Vollm et al., 2006). Patients with damage to the orbitofrontal cortex demonstrate impulsivity, poor planning, and disinhibited behavior (Damasio et al, 1990). As mentioned above, psychopaths have been found to demonstrate both structural and functional deficits in this region.

The inability to alter behavior may also stem from an increased sensitivity to reward in psychopathic individuals. Psychopathic traits have been associated with higher scores on behavioral approach and reward sensitivity (Wallace et al., 2009). On neuropsychological tests such as the Iowa Gambling Task, psychopathic individuals tend to make choices yielding large rewards but with more severe penalties (Blair et al., 2001; Mitchell et al., 2002). Brain imaging studies have also revealed increased functioning and volume of the striatum, a region of the brain involved in reward processing. Buckholtz et al. (2010) found that the impulsive-antisocial traits of psychopathy were associated with greater release of the reward-related neurotransmitter dopamine in the striatum in response to the administration of amphetamine. These traits were also associated with increased activity in the striatum during the anticipation of monetary reward. Two studies have observed increased volume in the striatum in individuals with psychopathic traits (Glenn et al., 2010; Schiffer et al., 2011).

Overall, the research presented above suggests that because of underlying neurobiological differences from normal individuals, psychopaths appear to lack responsiveness to many of the reasons that motivate individuals to behave morally. Much of this lies in core deficits in emotional processing – deficits which are not only observed in self-reports and observation of behavior, but which can be detected using physiological measures and brain imaging. Cognitive deficits in the processing of information may also contribute to impaired moral decision-making by increasing attention toward salient rewards and reducing attention to cues of punishment or cues that another is in distress. As we see in patients with damage to the orbitofrontal cortex who demonstrate both cognitive (poor planning, impulsivity) and affective (lack of empathy, emotional blunting) deficits, the same brain regions may influence both of these processes. A likely possibility is that cognitive and affective systems are highly dependent on one another, and are both necessary for proper moral development (Kennett, 2006). Indeed, a recent review on the neurobiology of morality concludes that it is most plausible to depict moral processes as requiring the engagement of both emotional and cognitive neural networks (Pascual et al., 2013). Longitudinal research suggests that neurobiological differences likely exist very early in life in individuals with psychopathic traits as adults, suggesting that the ability to respond to reasons that motivate individuals to behave morally may be compromised at an early age.

Discussion and future directions

Reasons-responsive compatibilist views seem to argue for the absence of moral responsibility or at least diminished responsibility in psychopaths, due to the absence of the relevant kind of guidance control. According to Fischer and Ravizza (1998), an individual is not morally responsible for a particular behavior if we can show that the behavior in question "is attributable to a significant brain lesion or a neurological disorder" (p. 35) that deprives these individuals of the right kind of reasons-responsiveness. In those cases, one cannot argue that the individual possesses guidance control over his or her behavior because responsibility-undermining factors are at work. Whereas normal individuals with normal brains can be said to have the right kind of reasons-responsiveness to be held morally responsible (Fischer & Ravizza, 1998; Glannon, 2011), individuals with brain impairments do not have the capacity to choose and act freely if their brain impairments deprive them of the right kind of reasons-responsiveness (i.e., the capacity for regular reasons receptivity and weak reasons reactivity).

According to Fischer and Ravizza, although smart animals, children, and (some) psychopaths can be said to exhibit a certain pattern of responsiveness to reasons, they are nevertheless not ordinarily judged as morally responsible. Although they may have the cognitive ability to respond appropriately to instrumental or prudential reasons, they do not seem to possess the cognitive ability to be guided by moral demands.

An *appropriate pattern* of responsiveness to moral reasons involves an ability to recognize that "other persons' claims give rise to moral reasons that *apply to him*" (Fischer & Ravizza, 1998: 77). This entails that it is not sufficient to *know* that certain acts involve a moral transgression (e.g., that according to "society" it is morally wrong to do such and such action). One additionally needs to be able to identify moral reasons for or against a certain action as *reasons that apply to oneself*. If an individual lacks such a minimal receptivity to reasons, he or she fails to be a moral agent at all. On their view, smart animals, children and (some) psychopaths cannot be considered moral agents and should therefore not be held morally responsible.

Based upon the above-mentioned empirical findings, it appears that psychopaths, at the very least, suffer from an impaired responsiveness to moral reasons in such a way that these individuals may *know* that certain acts are wrong, but may nevertheless be unable to fully grasp, both affectively and cognitively, why these acts are wrong and therefore unable to translate this knowledge into morally appropriate action. In line with Kennett (2006), the empirical literature suggests that the moral impairments in psychopathy are due to a combination of both affective and cognitive deficits. Individuals with psychopathy suffer to a greater or lesser degree from impairments in emotional responsiveness (affective deficits in empathy and fear) and impairments in cognitive functioning (attention deficits and reward-processing deficits), which in combination may lead to greater or lesser abnormalities in moral rationality/decision-making. Although Fischer and Ravizza (1998) limit their account of reasons-receptivity to *cognitive* capacities, it seems most plausible to assume that *affective* capacities are involved as well (Pascual et al., 2013). Both affective and cognitive capacities are essential for proper moral development and are very likely neurobiologically and experientially interdependent (Greene et al., 2001; Greene & Haidt, 2002; Kennett, 2006). On our view, an individual's *receptivity* and *reactivity* to moral reasons may be similarly interdependent. Although psychopaths may lack the necessary cognitive ability to be moved by moral demands, the empirical data suggest that psychopaths' affective deficits are central to their diminished (or absent) responsiveness to moral reasons. It appears that criminal psychopaths cannot "feel" the wrongness of their actions (or are impaired in this sense), which likely makes it impossible to adequately recognize moral reasons against such actions as reasons applying to themselves (i.e., as generating sufficient reasons for action), and to adequately react to moral reasons. In fact, it may be argued that in normal individuals, one's emotional responsiveness plays a major role both in the ability to identify with moral reasons as *reasons applying to oneself* and in the ability to react to moral reasons (Greene et al., 2001; Greene & Haidt, 2002). Abnormalities in emotional responsiveness, in combination with and potentially aggravated by cognitive impairments, may result both in impaired *receptivity* and in impaired *reactivity* to moral reasons. Together, the empirical findings are in line with an impaired *responsiveness* to moral reasons in psychopaths driven by abnormalities in emotional responsiveness and cognitive decision-making. Hence, on Fischer and Ravizza's account and in line with the empirical findings outlined above, criminal psychopaths may be partially or fully excused based upon diminished or absent responsiveness to moral reasons.

Although we have restricted our analysis to reasons-responsiveness compatibilist views, we briefly want to touch upon Frankfurt's hierarchical "mesh theory" account of free will and moral responsibility (Frankfurt, 1971). According to Frankfurt, moral responsibility requires that an individual's behavior is motivated by or originates from his or her second-order identification with his or her first-order desire to act in a certain way. Surely, psychopaths can be regarded as having the capacity to identify with their desires. Are they morally responsible after all? Frankfurt's view can be described as a hierarchical "mesh theory," in which moral responsibility depends on an appropriate "mesh" between one's behavior and one's true self. If an individual's behavior and the desires that function as motives for his or her behavior reflect how he or she wishes to be, then he or she can be considered morally responsible. The problem with this kind of mesh theory is the dependence of moral responsibility on one's psychological functioning *at a particular moment in time*. It does not seem to matter how an individual's psychological functioning came about or why it is the way it is. Fischer and Ravizza (1998) rightly criticize Frankfurt's mesh theory as incomplete because it does not account for the possibility of (prior) responsibility-undermining factors that may impact the psychological mechanisms (i.e., the processes that underlie human decision-making and behavior) by which an individual's current psychological functioning comes about. Fischer and Ravizza (1998) argue that such responsibility-undermining factors may potentially be identified in the case of psychopaths. It is likely that the normative power of reasons draws upon the normal functioning of both affective and cognitive processes involved in moral decision-making. The empirical data presented above suggests that individuals with psychopathy are to a greater or lesser extent impaired in each of these domains of normal psychological functioning. Moreover, if we consider psychopathy to be a neurodevelopmental psychiatric disorder (Gao et al., 2009; Rutter, 2012), the identification of the precursors to these traits early in life may lead to effective intervention that might prevent a person from developing psychopathy in adulthood. This may be key to successful crime prevention in adult life (Glenn & Raine, 2014).

Under current US criminal law there are two generic excusing conditions: lack of rational capacity and compulsion. Compulsion can be either externally (e.g., threats) or internally (i.e., strong internal desires) manifested (Morse, 2011b). Drawing upon a human rights-based framework, offenders who do not satisfy the required rationality criteria for legal culpability and who are not deemed legally responsible should not be sentenced and should instead receive adequate mental health treatment that may or may not involve involuntary civil commitment. Of course, with respect to psychopathy, a major challenge will be determining which individuals should be held responsible and which individuals should be excused. Psychopathic traits exist on a continuum in the population, as do many of the neurobiological deficits that we observe. The unfortunate truth is that attempting to draw a firm line between responsibility and non-responsibility will be futile (Eagleman, 2011). What we should take away from the neurobiological research on psychopathy is that not all individuals have the same capacity for making moral decisions. Rather than focusing on punishment of the individual who may have had limited capacity to behave morally, we should greatly increase our emphasis on rehabilitation efforts, while at the same time ensuring that society is protected, and that the feelings and the rights of victims are acknowledged. As outlined above, such an approach is in line with hard determinist, hard incompatibilist, and compatibilist views (e.g., Fischer & Ravizza, 1998; Greene & Cohen, 2004; Wolf, 1990) on free will and moral/criminal responsibility.

For example, the Netherlands allows for post-prison mandated mental health treatment, either residential or non-residential, of mentally ill offenders provided that such treatment has been deemed necessary at the time of sentencing. For non-violent crimes the maximum duration entails four years after the offender has completed his or her prison sentence. For violent crimes, the duration may be extended if certain conditions are met. Such post-prison treatment, possibly involving non-residential treatment, might provide a better "solution" for individuals with mild to moderate psychopathy compared to a prison sentence without any type of treatment at all (e.g., neurofeedback, cognitive behavioral therapy with or without psychopharmacological treatment, neurocognitive training, nutritional interventions). In comparison, for certain severe and violent psychopathic offenders it will not be warranted from a public safety perspective to release these individuals back into society and may thus result in very long or even lifelong civil commitment. Hence, for certain severe and violent psychopathic offenders, getting a prison sentence will likely lead to an earlier release compared to civil commitment. At the same time, giving these individuals a long prison sentence without any kind of treatment is problematic from the standpoint of public safety (these individuals will re-enter society at some point), as well as from the standpoint of offenders' human rights. Individuals with mental health disorders, including individuals with psychopathy, have a basic human right to receive adequate mental health treatment whether these individuals are offenders or law-abiding citizens.

Interestingly, affective and cognitive deficits and their underlying neurobiological abnormalities may potentially be addressed by modulating abnormal brain activation using fMRI neurofeedback (i.e., conditioning the brain areas involved to function differently). fMRI neurofeedback research in criminal psychopaths is currently focusing on the impaired fear system in psychopathy that comprises the orbitofrontal cortex, the amygdala, the anterior cingulate cortex (ACC), and the insula. The aim of the feedback is to increase the activity in those areas of the brain that form the fear-system in normal individuals, and to induce brain growth since these areas are typically reduced in volume in individuals with psychopathy compared to normal controls. In an ongoing study, Sitaram and colleagues have shown that offenders with psychopathy can learn to regulate their left anterior insula based upon a combination of emotional episodic memories and contingent feedback, which was found to increase the causal density (number of connections) in their emotional brain network and increase the causal flow (difference between ingoing and outgoing connections) of their left insula (Sitaram, 2007; Sitaram et al., 2009). Although highly experimental at present, this kind of research might provide us with effective treatment options for psychopathy in the future – hence, the need to discuss the ethical desirability of offering such neurotechnological or other sufficiently benign biosocial treatments to offenders either as an alternative to incarceration or requirement for probation and/or parole (Bublitz & Merkel, 2014; Focquaert, 2014).

REFERENCES

Adolphs, R., Tranel, D., Hamann, S., Young, A. W., Calder, A. J., et al. (1999). "Recognition of facial emotion in nine individuals with bilateral amygdala damage." *Neuropsychologia* **37**: 1111–1117.

Birbaumer, N., Veit, R., Lotze, M., Erb, M., Hermann, C., et al. (2005). "Deficient fear conditioning in psychopathy: a functional magnetic resonance imaging study." *Archives of General Psychiatry* **62**: 799–805.

Blair, R. J., Colledge, E., Murray, L., and Mitchell, D. G. (2001). "A selective impairment in the processing of sad and fearful facial expressions in children with psychopathic tendencies." *Journal of Abnormal Child Psychology* **29**: 491–498.

Blair, R. J., Colledge, E., and Mitchell, D. G. V. (2001). "Somatic markers and response reversal: is there orbitofrontal cortex dysfunction in boys with psychopathic tendencies." *Journal of Abnormal Child Psychology* **29**: 499–511.

Blair, R. J. R., Mitchell, D. G. V., Peschardt, K. S., Colledge, E., Leonard, R. A., et al. (2004). "Reduced sensitivity to others' fearful expressions in psychopathic individuals." *Personality and Individual Differences* **37**(6): 1111–1122.

Blair, R. J. R., Budhani, S., Colledge, E., and Scott, S. (2005). "Deafness to fear in boys with psychopathic tendencies." *Journal of Child Psychology and Psychiatry* **46**(3): 327–336.

Borg, J. S., Hynes, C., Horn, J. V., Grafton, S., and Sinnott-Armstrong, W. (2006). "Consequences, action, and intention as factors in moral judgments: an fMRI investigation." *Journal of Cognitive Neuroscience* **18**: 803–817.

Bublitz, J. C., and Merkel, R. (2014). "Crimes against minds: on mental manipulations, harms, and a human right to mental self-determination." *Criminal Law and Philosophy* **8**: 51–77.

Buckholtz, J. W., Treadway, M. T., Cowan, R. L., Woodward, N. D., Benning, S. D., Li, R., et al. (2010). "Mesolimbic dopamine reward system hypersensitivity in individuals with psychopathic traits." *Nature Neuroscience* **13**: 419–421.

Ciaramelli, E., Muccioli, M., Làdavas, E., and di Pellegrino, G. (2007). "Selective deficit in personal moral judgment following damage to ventromedial prefrontal cortex." *Social, Cognitive and Affective Neuroscience* **2**: 84–92.

Clarke, R. (2000) "Modest libertarianism." *Philosophical Perspectives* **14**: 21–45.

Damasio, A. R., Tranel, D., and Damasio, H. (1990). "Individuals with sociopathic behavior caused by frontal damage fail to respond autonomically to social-stimuli." *Behavioural Brain Research* **41**(2): 81–94.

de Oliveira-Souza, R., Hare, R. D., Bramati, I. E., Garrido, G. J., Azevedo, Ignácio F., et al. (2008). "Psychopathy as a disorder of the moral brain: fronto-temporo-limbic grey matter reductions demonstrated by voxel-based morphometry." *NeuroImage* **40**: 1202–1213.

Dennett, D. (2003). *Freedom Evolves*. Penguin Books.

Eagleman, D. (2011). "The brain on trial." *Atlantic Monthly* **308**: 112–123.

Farah, M. (2005). "Neuroethics: the practical and the philosophical." *Trends in Cognitive Sciences* **9**: 34–40.

Fischer, J. M., and Ravizza, M. (1998). *Responsibility and Control: A Theory of Moral Responsibility*. Cambridge University Press.

Flor, H., Birbaumer, N., Hermann, C., Ziegler, S., and Patrick, Christopher J. (2002). "Aversive Pavlovian conditioning in psychopaths: peripheral and central correlates." *Psychophysiology* **39**: 505–518.

Focquaert, F. (2014). "Mandatory neurotechnological treatment: ethical issues." *Theoretical Medicine and Bioethics* **35**: 59–72. DOI 10.1007/s11017-014-9276-6.

Frankfurt, H. (1969). "Alternate possibilities and moral responsibility." *The Journal of Philosophy* **66**: 829–839.

(1971). "Freedom of the will and the concept of a person." *The Journal of Philosophy* **1**: 5–20.

Gao, Y., Raine, A., Venables, P. H., and Dawson, M. E. (2010). "Association of poor childhood fear conditioning and adult crime." *American Journal of Psychiatry* **167**: 56–60.

Gao, Y., Glenn, A. L., Schug, R. A., Yang, Y., and Raine, A. (2009). "The neurobiology of psychopathy: a neurodevelopmental perspective." *Canadian Journal of Psychiatry* **54** (12): 813–823.

Glannon, W. (2011). *Brain, Body, and Mind: Neuroethics with a Human Face.* Oxford University Press.

Glenn, A. L., Raine, A., Venables, P. H., and Mednick, S. (2007). "Early temperamental and psychophysiological precursors of adult psychopathic personality." *Journal of Abnormal Psychology* **116**(3): 508–518.

Glenn, A. L., Iyer, R., Graham, J., Koleva, S., and Haidt, J. (2009a). "Are all types of morality compromised in psychopathy?" *Journal of Personality Disorders* **23**: 384–398.

Glenn, A. L., Raine, A., and Schug, R. A. (2009b). "The neural correlates of moral decision-making in psychopathy." *Molecular Psychiatry* **14**: 5–6.

Glenn, A. L., Raine, A., Yaralian, P. S., and Yang, Y. (2010). "Increased volume of the striatum in psychopathic individuals." *Biological Psychiatry* **67**: 52–58.

Glenn, A.L., and Raine, A. (2014). "Neurocriminology: implications for the punishment, prediction and prevention of criminal behaviour." *Nature Reviews Neuroscience* **15**: 54–63.

Gordon, H. L., Baird, A. A., and End, A. (2004). "Functional differences among those high and low on a trait measure of psychopathy." *Biological Psychiatry* **56**: 516–521.

Greene, J. D. and Cohen, J. D. (2004). "For the law, neuroscience changes nothing and everything." *Philosophical Transactions of the Royal Society B-Biological Sciences* **359**: 1775–1785.

Greene, J. D. and Haidt, J. (2002). "How (and where) does moral judgment work." *TRENDS in Cognitive Sciences* **6**: 517–523.

Greene, J. D., Sommerville, R. B., Nystrom, L. E., Darley, J. M., and Cohen, J. D. (2001). "An fMRI investigation of emotional engagement in moral judgement." *Science* **293**: 2105–2108.

Hare, R. D. (1965). "Psychopathy, fear arousal and anticipated pain." *Psychological Reports* **16**: 499–502.

(1982). "Psychopathy and physiological activity during anticipation of an aversive stimulus in a distraction paradigm." *Psychophysiology* **19**: 266–271.

Hare, R. D., Frazelle, J., and Cox, D. N. (1978). "Psychopathy and physiological responses to threat of an aversive stimulus." *Psychophysiology* **15**: 165–172.

Hare, R. D., and Quinn, M. J. (1971). "Psychopathy and autonomic conditioning." *Journal of Abnormal Psychology* **77**: 223–235.

Harenski, C. L., and Hamann, S. (2006). "Neural correlates of regulating negative emotions related to moral violations." *NeuroImage* **30**: 313–324.

Harenski, C. L., Harenski, K., Shane, M., and Kiehl, K. (2010). "Aberrant neural processing of moral violations in criminal psychopaths." *J Abnorm Psychol* **119**: 863–874.

Jones, A. P., Laurens, K. R., Herba, C. M., Barker, G. J., and Viding, E. (2009). "Amygdala hypoactivity to fearful faces in boys with conduct problems and callous-unemotional traits." *American Journal of Psychiatry* **166**: 95–102.

Kane, R. (1999) "Responsibility, luck and chance: reflections on free will and indeterminism." *Journal of Philosophy* **96**: 217–40.

Kennett, J. (2006). "Do psychopaths really threaten moral rationalism?" *Philosophical Explorations* **9**: 69–82.

(2010). "Drugs and disordered choices." *Australian Review of Public Affairs*. Available at www.australianreview.net/.

Kiehl, K. A., Smith, A. M., Hare, R. D., Mendrek, A., Forster, B. B., et al. (2001). "Limbic abnormalities in affective processing by criminal psychopaths as revealed by functional magnetic resonance imaging." *Biological Psychiatry* **50**: 677–684.

Koenigs, M., Young, L., Adolphs, R., Tranel, D., Cushman, F., et al. (2007). "Damage to the prefrontal cortex increases utilitarian moral judgements." *Nature* **446**: 908–911.

Marsh, A. A., Finger, E. C., Mitchell, D. G., Reid, M. E., Sims, C., et al. (2008). "Reduced amygdala response to fearful expressions in children and adolescents with callous-unemotional traits and disruptive behavior disorders." *American Journal of Psychiatry* **165**: 712–720.

McKenna, M. S. (2000). "Assessing reasons-responsive compatibilism." *International Journal of Philosophical Studies* **8**: 89–124.

McKenna, M. S. (2009) "Compatibilism." *The Stanford Encyclopedia of Philosophy*, Edward N. Zalta (ed.). Available at http://plato.stanford.edu/archives/win2009/entries/compatibilism/.

Mitchell, D. G. V., Colledge, E., Leonard, A., and Blair, R. J. R. (2002). "Risky decisions and response reversal: is there evidence of orbitofrontal cortex dysfunction in psychopathic individuals?" *Neuropsychologica* **40**(12): 2013–2022.

Moll, J., de Oliveira-Souza, R., Eslinger, P. J., Bramati, I. E., Mourão-Miranda, J., et al. (2002). "The neural correlates of moral sensitivity: a functional magnetic resonance imaging investigation of basic and moral emotions." *The Journal of Neuroscience* **22**(7): 2730–2736.

Morse, S. J. (2008). "Psychopathy and criminal responsibility." *Neuroethics* **1**: 205–212.

(2011a). "Mental disorder and criminal law." *The Journal of Criminal Law & Criminology* **101**: 885–968.

(2011b). "Genetics and criminal responsibility." *TRENDS in Cognitive Sciences* 15: 378–380.

Müller, J. L., Sommer, M., Wagner, V., Lange, K., Taschler, H., et al. (2003). "Abnormalities in emotion processing within cortical and subcortical regions in criminal psychopaths: evidence from a functional magnetic resonance imaging study using pictures with emotional content." *Biological Psychiatry* **54**: 152–162.

Newman, Joseph P., and Kosson, D. S. (1986). "Passive avoidance learning in psychopathic and nonpsychopathic offenders." *Journal of Abnormal Psychology* **95**: 252–256.

Ogloff, J. R., and Wong, S. (1990). "Electrodermal and cardiovascular evidence of a coping response in psychopaths." *Criminal Justice and Behavior* **17**: 231–245.

Pardini, D. A. and Byrd, A. L. (2012). "Perceptions of aggressive conflicts and others' distress in children with callous-unemotional traits: 'I'll show you who's boss, even if you suffer and I get in trouble'." *Journal of Child Psychology and Psychiatry* **53**(3): 283–291.

Pascual, L., Rodrigues, P., and Gallardo-Pujol, D. (2013). "How does morality work in the brain? A functional and structural perspective of moral behaviour." *Frontiers in Integrative Neuroscience* **7**(65): 1–8.

Patrick, Christopher J., Cuthbert, B. N., and Lang, P. J. (1994). "Emotion in the criminal psychopath: fear image processing." *Journal of Abnormal Psychology* **103**: 523–534.

Patrick, Christopher J., Bradley, M. M., and Lang, P. J. (1993). "Emotion in the criminal psychopath: startle reflex modulation." *Journal of Abnormal Psychology* **102**: 82–92.

Rilling, J. K., Glenn, A. L., Jairam, M. R., Pagnoni, G., Goldsmith, D. R., et al. (2007). "Neural correlates of social cooperation and non-cooperation as a function of psychopathy." *Biological Psychiatry* **61**: 1260–1271.

Robertson, D., Snarey, J., Ousley, O., Harenski, K., Dubois Bowman, F., et al. (2007). "The neural processing of moral sensitivity to issues of justice and care." *Neuropsychologia* **45**(8): 755–766.

Rolls, E. T. (2000). "The orbitofrontal cortex and reward." *Cerebral Cortex* **10**: 284–294.

Rutter, M. (2012). "Psychopathy in childhood: is it a meaningful diagnosis?" *The British Journal of Psychiatry* **200**: 175–176.

Schiffer, B., Muller, B. W., Scherbaum, N., Hodgins, S., Forsting, M., et al. (2011). "Disentangling structural brain alterations associated with violent behavior from those associated with substance use disorders." *Archives of General Psychiatry* **68**: 1039–1049.

Schneider, F., Habel, U., Kessler, C., Posse, S., Grodd, W., et al. (2000). "Functional imaging of conditioned aversive emotional responses in antisocial personality disorder." *Neuropsychobiology* **42**(4): 192–201.

Shamay-Tsoory, S. G., Tomer, R., Berger, B. D., Goldsher, D., and Aharon-Peretz, J. (2005). "Impaired 'affective theory of mind' is associated with right ventromedial prefrontal damage." *Cognitive Behavioral Neurology* **18**(1): 55–67.

Sitaram, Ranganatha (2007). "*fMRI brain–computer interfaces.*" 15th Annual Conference of the International Society for Neurofeedback & Research, Current Perspectives in Neuroscience: Neuroplasticity & Neurofeedback, San Diego, California.

Sitaram, Ranganatha, Caria, Andrea, and Birbaumer, Niels (2009). "Hemodynamic brain–computer interfaces for communication and rehabilitation." *Neural Networks* **22**: 1320–1328.

Vollm, B. A., Taylor, A. N., Richardson, P. Corcoran, R., Stirling, J., et al. (2006). "Neuronal correlates of theory of mind and empathy: a functional magnetic resonance imaging study in a nonverbal task." *NeuroImage* **29**(1): 90–98.

Wallace, J. F., Malterer, M. B., and Newman, J. P. (2009). "Mapping Gray's BIS and BAS constructs onto Factor 1 and Factor 2 of Hare's Psychopathy Checklist-Revised." *Personality and Individual Differences* **47**: 812–816.

Wegner, D. M. (2002). *The Illusion of Conscious Will.* Cambridge, MA: MIT Press.

Wolf, S. (1990). *Freedom within Reason.* New York: Oxford University Press.

Yang, Y., Raine, A., Narr, K. L., Colletti, P., and Toga, A. W. (2009). "Localization of deformations within the amygdala in individuals with psychopathy." *Archives of General Psychiatry* **66**: 986–994.

7 How mental disorders can compromise the will

Gerben Meynen

ABSTRACT

Mental disorders have a special characteristic: they may directly affect a person's will. For instance, some hallucinations take the form of commanding voices that the person cannot but obey. Depending on their content, these hallucinations may not only affect a person's decision-making but result in harmful actions as well. In criminal cases, the impact of mental disorders on a defendant's will may even lead to exculpation due to insanity. This chapter aims to clarify how mental disorders may compromise (freedom of) the will. I conclude that there are various ways in which psychiatric disorders may influence the will. Such impact may substantially interfere with a person's life and, in particular, with a person's ability to seek help or to follow treatment advice. Therefore, mental health care professionals should be able to recognize the challenges patients may face in this respect and to motivate them to start or continue treatment.

Introduction

Mental disorders have a special characteristic: they may directly affect a patient's will. For instance, a severely depressed patient may no longer have the will to play tennis, something she used to do twice a week. Surely, physical disorders may influence a patient's will as well. If a person suffers from back pain (sciatica), he may lose the will to play tennis, just like the depressed patient. Still, the impact on the will in mental disorders appears to be of a different nature. The back pain patient will probably explain his lack of will as follows: "Lately, I am suffering from a terrible back pain, and, *therefore*, I have decided, in accordance with my doctor's advice, not to play tennis – regrettably." This patient still has the wish to play tennis, but reason tells him that he should not play tennis and therefore he deliberately sets his mind on other activities. Apparently, there is a specific hindrance to playing tennis and the will is knowingly adapted accordingly. The depressed patient, however, is often less aware of why she lost the will to play tennis. It may be much harder for her to provide a clear reason, and it is unlikely that she will say: "*Because* I am suffering from a depression, I think it is better for this moment not to play tennis – regrettably." In the back pain case, the disease is a factor which is contemplated and taken into account, and then results in an explicit decision not to play tennis. Yet, in the severe depression case it looks like the will itself has been impaired, probably in a way that makes the patient lose the will to do many things, including playing tennis. The will is not encountering a specific hindrance, but it looks as if the will itself is somehow compromised. Indeed, phenomena like *apathy* or *avolition* may occur in depressed patients – avolition being a medical term meaning "lack of will."

Although this introductory and sketchy example about a physical and mental condition interfering with the will to play tennis is meant to suggest a difference between the impact on the will in both conditions, it is difficult – perhaps impossible – to clearly distinguish the impact of mental disorders from the impact of physical disorders on the will in all cases. (Some people assume that mental disorders are brain disorders, and in that sense they are physical as well; Andreasen 1984.) One of the reasons is that mental disorders take many forms, and, accordingly, the ways in which they affect the will are diverse. This chapter aims to identify some important ways in which mental disorders may compromise the will. I do not claim that all mental disorders affect the will in every case; this would require a separate argument (see Perring 2004 on involuntariness and mental disorder).

The influence of mental disorders on the will is of interest for at least three reasons. First, the will determines our actions, and therefore if the will is affected by a mental disorder, this may profoundly affect our actions. Since our actions shape our lives, mental disorders may profoundly affect people's lives by influencing their wills. Second, treatment of a mental disorder requires some action on the part of a patient, for instance, visiting a doctor, taking medication or participating in therapy sessions. If mental disorders affect a patient's will, they may affect the patient's ability to seek help and find treatment. Thirdly, we may be interested in the impact of a mental disorder on a person's will because this impact can allegedly be of such a nature that a person's free will is affected.

Not all willed action is "freely willed" action. For instance, our will may apparently be formed because we are somehow forced by external factors (e.g., threats by other people) or internal factors (e.g., obsessions) beyond our control. The question that has troubled many philosophers over the last two thousand years is whether our wills are ever *truly* free, or whether our wills are always forced or determined by factors beyond our control (Kane 1998, 2002). So, although the existence of a will is usually taken for granted, the existence of a *free* will is the topic of a vivid debate in philosophy. In the third section (Free will), based on an account suggested by Henrik Walter, I will identify three aspects, or elements, of free will: having alternative possibilities, acting for reasons, and being the source of the action. Usually, we become interested in a person's free will when questions arise about that person's responsibility for a particular action. In practice, the issue often comes up when making a distinction between *mad or bad*, for instance in the court of law, although it is a matter of debate whether free will is required for criminal responsibility (Morse 2007; Felthous 2008). Within the context of this chapter, I will consider the cases in which free will is affected by a mental disorder a subset of the cases in which the will is affected by a mental disorder.

What is the will? Within the context of forensic psychiatry, Alan Felthous conceives of the will as follows: "The will is simply the intentional faculty: Through motivation and decision the will settles upon and then implements an action" (2008, p. 23). This loose definition of will appears to be a helpful starting point. Felthous adds that we should not confuse *will* with *desire*: "More problematic is the common error of mistaking the will for desire" (2008, p. 23). Let us further explore and describe the concept of the will by distinguishing it from desire or wish. First, the will concerns the realm of our own actions. Desires and wishes may concern our own actions, but they may concern many other things as well. We may desire beautiful weather, but we cannot "will" beautiful weather because it is beyond our agential control. Second, the will is involved only if we have "settled upon" an action. For instance, we may wish to go fishing next year. Although this falls within the realm of our own actions, it becomes our will only if we form the intention or make the decision to go fishing next year. So, unlike mere desires and wishes, the will is closely tied to the choice of a particular course of action. Third, wish and desire appear to be related with things we like. Our wills may settle upon actions we do not particularly desire, yet we want to do them for one reason or another. I do not desire or wish to do the laundry, but I feel I have to (for certain reasons), and therefore my will settles upon doing the laundry.

On this account of will, three concepts are of immediate interest: intention, motivation, and, especially, decision-making. Within the context of this chapter, I will consider the term *decision-making* synonymous with *will-formation*. Decision-making will be understood in accordance with a model suggested by Kalis et al. (2008) in a paper on mental disorders, decision-making and weakness of will. They distinguish between three phases or stages of decision-making: the generation of options, the selection of one of the options, and, finally, transferring the selected option into action. Since in this chapter I will treat the terms will-formation and decision-making as synonymous, these stages will be considered relevant to will-formation as well (see also Kalis and Meynen 2014).

In the next section I will show the diversity of ways in which mental disorders may influence a patient's will. I then consider what the impact of these disorders on the will means for a patient's free will. In the final section, I identify the implications of this impact for treatment and discuss the relevance of future neurobiological research.

Various mental disorders and the will

The ways in which psychiatric disorders may affect the will are numerous. In this section, the following psychopathological phenomena will be considered: dementia, delirium, psychosis, mood disorders, anxiety disorders, drug-related conditions, Tourette's syndrome, impulse-control disorders, and, finally, personality disorders. There are many more disorders and symptoms, but these conditions have been selected for their clinical relevance or prevalence, or because they are of particular interest from the perspective of the will. Together, these mental disorders cover most of the conditions encountered in everyday psychiatric practice. Some of the disorders are discussed in more detail in other chapters in this volume: compulsive behavior, generalized anxiety disorder, addiction, and psychopathy. The discussion of the impact of the various disorders is, first of all, meant to provide an overview of the diversity of these symptoms and the diversity of their potential impact on decision-making. Notably, even if two patients have the same diagnosis, for example depression, their symptoms may vary considerably. Consequently, the impact of the disorder on will-formation may be very different as well.

Dementia and delirium

Dementia and delirium are among the most serious mental conditions (Sadock and Sadock 2005). Depending on the brain areas affected, the impact of dementia on a person's will may be profound and multifaceted. For instance, in Alzheimer's disease, damage in the temporal cortex and hippocampus is related to amnesia. Such amnesia may interfere with decision-making because a patient may simply forget the options or forget the reasons for choosing them (Kalis and Meynen 2014). Consequently, the will cannot be formed effectively. The formation of intentions may also be hampered because people lack planning capacities, or overview. Damage in the prefrontal cortex is related particularly to difficulty in planning one's actions. In addition, dementia patients may become apathetic, and consequently will-formation can be reduced. Although in dementia, various brain areas may be affected simultaneously, researchers have tried to link impaired decision-making in dementia to certain brain areas. Strenziok et al. (2011) found that altered stimulus-reinforcement learning (a component of accurate decision-making) in frontotemporal dementia was related to atrophy in the right lateral orbitofrontal cortex (OFC).

Delirium is often the result of a serious physical condition which at some point affects the mind (Sadock and Sadock 2005). For instance, delirium may occur in infectious diseases or after head trauma. Characteristics of a delirium are lowered levels of consciousness, loss of the ability to focus one's attention, and disorientation to time, place, and/or person. Lowered levels of consciousness substantially influence will-formation: in a drowsy state, decision-making is problematic. The inability to focus one's attention will also hamper the process of decision-making, because it is more difficult to integrate the relevant information. Fortunately, unlike dementia, which is a neurodegenerative condition, the features of a delirium often resolve completely. So, after a couple of days, especially when the underlying physical condition has been treated effectively, the integrity of the decision-making process may be completely restored.

Psychosis

Psychosis may take different forms (Sadock and Sadock 2005). Three important manifestations of psychosis are: delusions, hallucinations, and thought disorder. Psychotic symptoms may occur independently of another mental disorder, but they frequently accompany other disorders as well, such as delirium (e.g., visual hallucinations) and severe depression (e.g., delusions).

Delusions may deeply affect a person's will. A delusion is often considered to be a false belief (see, however, Fulford 1993). Beliefs (together with desires) have a strong impact on human decision-making. And if our beliefs are incorrect they may lead to inappropriate – and dramatic – action.

Case: John, a 28-year-old clerk, does not have much contact with other people. The only person he talks to, from time to time, is his neighbor Fred. Since several months, John is convinced that microscopic aliens are threatening him and trying to invade his body in order to take control over his mind. Fred, John believes, is coordinating their actions, and Fred himself is, in fact, an alien in disguise. John turns to the police, several times, but they are unable to help him. He also contacts some organizations in his city, but nobody seems to take his concerns seriously. After several fearful months it becomes evident to John that taking out Fred is the only way to stop the aliens. Two months later, John buys a gun and kills his neighbor Fred.

What makes a delusion so peculiar is its immunity to falsification by clear evidence of the contrary. In fact, nobody has been able to convince John that there were no such aliens, neither the police, nor Fred (the fact that Fred denied the very possibility of such an alien attack had made John even more suspicious about Fred's role in the matter). Such an immunity to falsification or correction is unusual for (most of) our beliefs. This characteristic of a delusion, however, makes it more likely that over time such an unshakable belief may affect a person's decision-making. And there are additional factors that further increase this likelihood. First, delusions often concern beliefs about the person himself, like *I* am persecuted, or *I* am the Chosen one, or *I* have a disease, or Lady Gaga loves *me*. Second, their content is often disturbing and may call for action (like protecting oneself, preaching, visiting a doctor, and writing letters to Lady Gaga). The fact that I am *persecuted* is not "nice to know" information, but requires immediate action on my part. Given these two characteristics of delusions, they may well influence a person's decision-making or will-formation. Notably, in criminal law, successful insanity defenses often concern cases in which the defendant was suffering from a (paranoid) delusion.

Hallucinations may occur in any sensory modality: visual, auditory, haptic, olfactory, and gustatory (Sadock and Sadock 2005). A common type of auditory hallucination is "hearing voices." These voices may have different content, but, especially in schizophrenia, they may be of a commanding nature. They may say things like "Go outside!" "Stop talking!" or "Kill that person!" Often, such commands can be disobeyed by the patient. Still, there are (rare) cases in which the patient must obey them. Suppose that the content of a voice would be "Kill that person!" In that case, the will unavoidably settles on that action. Notably, the impact on will-formation by these hallucinations is very different from the impact of dementia (e.g., there is no amnesia), of delirium (e.g., there is no lack of attention), and of delusions (there is no false belief guiding the action). Apparently, in this case there is a hallucination containing a command which is of such a nature that it "hijacks" the decision-making process. Apparently, the "voice" generates and simultaneously selects the behavioral option; and action is initiated (on the nature of auditory hallucinations, see, e.g., Meynen 2010b). It is as if an alien influence hijacks the patient's will. This is a profound and potentially dangerous way in which mental disorders may affect will-formation (see Kalis and Meynen 2014).

Thought disorder is another feature of psychosis. One manifestation is incoherent thinking. The various lines of thought are no longer successfully integrated; a patient's thinking becomes inconsistent. In some cases of such incoherence, the will may settle very easily on action, without the proper cognitive processing of the variety of options. In fact, the integrity of our thinking process, in the sense of accurate integration of various strands of thoughts, is essential to rational decision-making.

In sum, psychotic features take various forms and may strongly influence a patient's will in different ways. In fact, these features can impair the will to varying degrees in different individuals; in most cases, even though psychoses may severely impair the will, they do not completely hijack or undermine it.

Mood disorders

Mood disorders basically involve low mood (depression and dysthymia) and elevated mood (hypomanic or manic episodes in bipolar disorder), while mixed episodes may also occur, in which features of elevated mood and depression co-occur. As mentioned in the example in the Introduction about the will to play tennis, one of the ways in which a depression influences a patient's will is by affecting one's motivation. Motivational changes in depression were found to be related to neural responses in, among other areas, the amygdala and OFC, which are considered the "relevance detector" of the brain (Diekhof et al. 2008). But other features of depression may interact with will-formation as well. Patients may have problems reading and watching television just because they cannot muster the concentration required for these activities (Marazziti et al. 2010). In addition, depressed patients may adopt a negative view of opportunities offered to them. Options may appear far less promising to a depressed patient than to a person with normal mood (Kalis and Meynen 2014). A practical problem is that treatment options may appear less attractive to them as well. They may think: "If 70% of the patients respond to this treatment, I will certainly be among the other 30%," and refuse potentially beneficial treatment. Given such an impact on decision-making in depression, we may even question a patient's competence to decide about treatment options (Meynen 2011). In the end, it may be difficult for a patient to actually *do* what he or she has chosen to do. This means that when a choice has been made, the final phase of decision-making – translating the choice into action – is not completed. Some may call this weakness of will (Kalis et al. 2008; Mele 2012) on the part of the patient. Apart from weakness of will, lack of will (*avolition*) may also occur in depression (Nitschke and Mackiewicz 2005).

But the counterpart of depression, hypomania, may also affect a person's will. The term for conditions characterized by manic episodes and periods of hypomania (often interspersed with depression) is bipolar disorder.

Case: Susan is a young lawyer who has a lot of energy lately, working 12 hours a day, writing poems and a blog, and sending 40 tweets per day. She is actually thinking faster than usual, making interesting associations, which are much appreciated by the readers of her blog. In addition, her social life is booming (she talks a lot, is very witty), while the quality of her work and poems is very good. One editor has already expressed interest in her work. Moreover, she feels great. Everything seems perfect. Her parents are a bit worried, though. To them, Susan's behavior looks much like before her depression, almost three years ago.

In manic episodes in bipolar disorder, people may come up with many ideas (first phase: generation of options), sometimes very original, which may strike patients as very promising and they choose some (second phase: option selection). They may feel an enormous energy to translate all these ideas into willful action (third phase) (see also Kalis and Meynen 2014). This may have positive as well as negative (sometimes disastrous) consequences. As far as positive consequences are concerned, a link between bipolar disorder and creativity is generally assumed (Andreasen 2008). On the negative side, people may start buying expensive objects (like houses) they cannot afford, because they feel that this is a brilliant thing to do – and because of a high energy level due to hypomania, they do these things immediately. In hypomanic episodes there is less need for sleep, so will-formation may continue during night-time – as well as willful actions, like calling your boss in the middle of the night to share a 'brilliant' idea. Apart from bipolar disorder, other psychiatric disorders have been related with creativity as well (Hare 1987). So, there also appears to be a positive influence on will-formation by mental disorders.

Anxiety disorders and obsessive-compulsive disorder

There are different types of anxiety disorders: phobia, social anxiety disorder, generalized anxiety disorder (GAD), and panic disorder

(American Psychiatric Association 1994; Sadock and Sadock 2005). The impact of anxiety disorders and obsessive-compulsive disorder (OCD) on decision-making has also been studied neurobiologically. For instance, decision-making in OCD has been found to be specifically related to functioning of the ventromedial prefrontal cortex (Cavedini et al. 2006). In general, anxiety disorders share not only the element of fear but also the element of *avoidance* behavior, which is motivated by fear. The object of fear can be manifold, for instance mice (specific phobia), social situations (social anxiety), disasters that may allegedly occur (GAD), and heart attack or losing control (panic disorder). Avoidance behavior is, in principle, willful, deliberately chosen behavior to avoid harm and/or to diminish anxiety. Yet, although, in general, avoidance behavior is deliberate action, patients may feel that they are caught in such behavior, like the washing rituals in OCD, and that their will is no longer free in this respect: they have to will this behavior, because if they refrain from doing it, the fear only increases.

Still, one of the most widely used – and effective – therapies for anxiety disorders is cognitive behavioral therapy (CBT) (Otte 2011). A CBT therapist characteristically challenges patients to will *other* behavior, more precisely to resist the response to avoid fearful situations and stimuli, and even to willfully engage in these situations (so, to approach a mouse or to visit a party). This treatment is called "exposure *in vivo* with response prevention." It implies that the patient *exposes* him- or herself to the object of anxiety, but refrains from the usual response to escape the situation or to get away from the object of fear. In other words, patients are asked to explore different behavioral repertoires (the ones they deliberately avoided up till now). This indicates that, in principle, anxiety patients have the capacity to decide differently (see also Meynen 2013a).

Unlike delusions, anxiety disorders usually leave the possibility open that patients *reflect* on their compulsive behavior. Such reflective capacity is used in CBT to provide room for alternative behavioral responses. What appears to be important in these anxiety disorders is a (sometimes overwhelming) negative feeling – fear – to which a person responds willfully by avoidance behavior hoping that this emotion will become less intense. In the long run, however, the impact of an anxiety disorder usually gradually increases as a result of such avoidance behavior. Note that this is different from depression: the depressed patient is not *avoiding* the depressed feelings. In general, in anxiety disorders, crucial aspects of mental functioning which are affected in, e.g., delirium, psychosis, and severe mood disorders, remain completely intact. Given the intensity of anxiety, in CBT it is often needed to foster and strengthen the will as much as possible by explaining to the patient how anxiety works over time, and by motivating patients to really engage in these exposure programs. Still, not all CBT interventions are successful, and in a considerable percentage of patients there appears to be very little room for exploring alternative courses of action.

Drug-related disorders

With respect to drugs it is helpful to distinguish between three conditions: being under influence/being intoxicated, withdrawals states, and addiction. Notably, a person who is addicted may or may not be intoxicated and may or may not be in a withdrawal state. Each of these conditions can (strongly) affect the will. Many people are familiar from personal experience with the impact of substances such as alcohol on a person's will, although people may respond very differently. Some people feel tired when drinking too much, other people become euphoric. Both conditions affect the will to some extent. Intoxication and withdrawal may even lead to a delirium (see above). Currently, much neuroscientific work is done on impaired decision-making in addiction, in particular by Nora Volkow. Decision-making in addicted patients appears affected in different ways. Volkow et al. write:

> Based on brain imaging findings, we present a model according to which addiction emerges as an imbalance in the information processing and integration among various brain circuits and functions. The dysfunctions reflect (a) decreased sensitivity of reward circuits, (b) enhanced sensitivity of memory circuits to conditioned expectations to drugs and drug cues, stress reactivity, and (c) negative mood, and a weakened control circuit. Although initial experimentation with a drug of abuse is largely a voluntary behavior, continued drug use can eventually impair neuronal circuits in the brain that are involved in *free will*, turning drug use into an automatic compulsive behavior. (Abstract, Volkow et al. 2010, emphasis added)

Interestingly, this quote has it that after continued drug use people's brain circuits involved in free will (see next section) may be impaired. This suggests *profound* impairment of will-formation in these patients. At present, much neuroscientific work done on addiction seems to reveal substantial decision-making impairments (Hall and Carter 2013). Meanwhile, there have been challenges to this view by philosophers and psychologists, notably Gene Heyman and Herbert Fingarette who argue that addictions result from voluntary choices (see also other chapters in this volume)(Fingarette 1989; Heyman 2009). In fact, Fingarette emphasized in *Heavy Drinking: The Myth of Alcoholism as a Disease* (1989) the responsibility of people for their drinking behavior.

Tourette's syndrome

In this section, we consider another disorder which has, as it turned out, a peculiar phenomenology as far as the will is concerned: Tourette's syndrome. People assumed that the tics in the neuropsychiatric Tourette's syndrome were involuntary, just like epileptic seizures (see also Meynen 2010a). The tics, it was assumed, bypassed a person's decision-making. However, in 1991 Lang published a study reporting on patients' subjective perception of their tics. Surprisingly, although about 30 percent perceived the tics as involuntary, the majority of tic-disorder patients reported that their tics were voluntary rather than involuntary; the tics were intentional actions. Patients do not wish to have Tourette's or to produce tics, yet the coming about of a tic is not involuntary (Lang 1991; Verdellen 2007). This is an interesting finding, for different reasons. One reason is that it shows that we may err as far as the (in)voluntariness of certain psychopathological behavior is concerned. This also implies a caveat with respect to this section of the chapter; things may not be how they seem. Another reason is that this study demonstrates that asking patients questions about their own perception of psychopathological phenomena may reveal new aspects of the disorder. In fact, Lang's finding shows the need for research on patients' experiences concerning the impact of mental disorders on their wills (Meynen 2010a). Still, not all Tourette's patients experienced their tics as intentional; in some cases will-formation is apparently bypassed.

Now we know that some Tourette's patients experience their tics as intentional, we may ask why and how the intention is formed to move a part of the body or to make a certain sound in Tourette's? Apparently, these tics are the intentional response to so-called premonitory sensations (Verdellen et al. 2008). On this account, there is a particular type of sensation in a Tourette's patient's body which generates the *urge* to act and to which the patient willfully responds by performing the tic/act (Verdellen 2007). Based on this finding, people inferred that if tics are the result of actual will-formation, this decision-making process might be targeted via CBT (as in anxiety disorders). Such a treatment was developed, and it shows promising results (Verdellen et al. 2008; Meynen 2010a).

Impulse-control disorders

Brewer and Potenza point to the importance of the amygdala in decision-making and impulsivity, and interestingly, they also state that "[e]merging data on the neurobiology of impulsivity and impulse control disorders (ICDs) suggest parallels with drug addictions" (2008, p. 69). Kleptomania – just like pathological gambling and pyromania – is one of the impulse-control disorders. It is legally relevant, because it comes down to the urge to commit a *crime*, to *steal*. Typically, the stolen object is not even desired for itself. It is basically about the *act* of stealing, which is very different from normal stealing, where a thief desires the object and the act of stealing is simply a means to obtain the object. How to understand this disorder with respect to the will? We may feel that in kleptomania the will is entirely bypassed as in epileptic seizures: there is no control, no acting for reasons. However, there is an alternative view (see also Meynen 2013a) which assumes that the disorder produces a strong and unrelenting pathological *urge* to steal (see Grant et al. 2009). This urge can in principle be resisted, but it is very hard to resist. And it might be that a patient suffering from kleptomania resisted the urge most of the time, although it was very hard, but just this time he or she gives in. Mental disorders may produce strange and extreme urges that may be very hard to resist. Perhaps such an urge may also exist in addiction, and we could speculate that the quote by Brewer and Potenza (above) supports such a similarity. Notably, the claim that it is very hard to resist an urge leaves open the possibility that it is not impossible to resist it. This suggests degrees of control of behavior and, perhaps, degrees of legal responsibility for that behavior. In criminal law cases, it could mean the difference between mitigation and excuse.

Personality disorders

The *Diagnostic and Statistical Manual of Mental Disorders* (DSM-IV) identifies ten different personality disorders (American Psychiatric Association 1994). Their features, although in part overlapping, are very different as well. Even people diagnosed with the same personality disorder may exhibit quite different features. Characteristically, in personality disorders there is an *enduring pattern* of certain maladaptive behaviors and coping mechanisms. Many features of such disorders affect the will, like paranoid thoughts in schizotypical personality disorder and lack of impulse control in borderline personality disorder and antisocial personality disorder. In part, features of the disorders discussed above can also be part of personality disorders. The personality disorder which has probably generated most research and discussion, as far as forensic psychiatry and criminal responsibility are concerned, is antisocial personality disorder, in particular the psychopathic traits. It seems hard to relate psychopathy directly to any of the influences on the will described above. As psychopathy and its impact on the will is the topic of Chapter 10, I will not discuss it here.

Types of influence

Mental disorders, as we have seen, may affect the will in many and very different ways. If we would try to identify *types* of influence on will-formation, tentatively, we can distinguish at least the following groups.

Epistemic problems (delusions).
Hijacking of the will (certain commanding voices).
Bypassing the will in some tics in Tourette's.
"Subtle" changes in the decision-making process, such as motivation, energy level, positive or negative coloring of options (mood disorders: depression, hypomania)
Inducing an either repulsive (e.g., fear of mice) *or somehow attractive factor* (e.g., urge to steal in kleptomania) that pushes and pulls the formation of the will.

These types of influences are likely to affect and impair will-formation to different degrees. While, for instance, hijacking of the will is a profound way in which the will may be affected by mental disorders (see also next section on free will), the mere introduction of an either repulsive or attractive factor appears to leave will-formation largely intact. Still, especially over a longer period of time, the presence of such a repulsive or attractive factor could have a major impact on a person's life.

Free will

In this section, we aim to explore the connection between the impact of a disorder on the will and the impact on free will. Free will is a much-debated topic, and it has been a much-debated topic in metaphysics for centuries (Kane 2002). In this chapter, I do not take an explicit stance on the question of whether free will exists, or on its compatibility with determinism. I will stay away from metaphysical issues as much as possible (see Meynen 2013a). Currently, the relationship between free will and neuroscience is frequently discussed; various neuroscientific experiments allegedly show that free will is illusory, such as Libet's experiments on the *readiness potential* and conscious will to act (Libet 1999). With respect to the interpretation of these experiments, however, opinion is still divided (Radder and Meynen 2012). Although I discuss neuroscientific findings, I will not discuss the relationship between neuroscience and free will.

The concept of free will appears to be closely related to moral responsibility. As Tim O'Connor writes, "most philosophers suppose that the concept of free will is very closely connected to the concept of moral responsibility. Acting with free will, on such views, is just to satisfy the metaphysical requirement on being responsible for one's action" (2010). Free will is not the only factor relevant to responsibility. As O'Connor points out: "Clearly, there will also be epistemic conditions on responsibility as well, such as being aware – or failing that, being culpably unaware – of relevant alternatives to one's action and of the alternatives' moral significance." So, if a person was incapable of knowing that his or her action could be harmful, we may exculpate that person. On this account what is required for moral responsibility is free will *and* epistemic conditions (see also Meynen 2013a). Notably, although epistemic factors are to be distinguished from the metaphysical factors of free will, we should realize that a person's will can be profoundly influenced by such epistemic factors, as we have seen in the previous section with respect to delusions.

Mental disorders may not just affect the will, but also, it is often assumed, free will (Meynen 2010a; Glannon 2011). Indeed, many conditions, pathological and non-pathological, may affect our wills. For instance, if I get sleepy late at night, then my will to work on a paper is likely to be affected. But probably we would not consider my free will to be affected at this point. Still, it may be hard to clearly draw the line between cases in which just the will is affected (because a person is sleepy) and cases in which "free will" is affected (for instance in a severe depression). There are at least two ways to look at this. First, it may be that there is some *threshold*. For instance, if a person is just a little sleepy, the will is likely to be affected to some extent, but free will remains intact. Yet, if a person is *very* sleepy, almost falling asleep, then the threshold has been reached and free will is undermined. Second, on an alternative account, we may assume that there is no such threshold but a *scale*. This could imply that even if the will is slightly affected, to some extent free will is affected as well (although largely left intact). This would mean that there is a grey area in which free will is partly undermined and partly intact. I leave it to the reader to adopt a stance on this matter. My approach in this chapter is compatible with both views (threshold and scale).

It is hard to clearly define free will. Based on an account suggested by Henrik Walter (Walter 2001; Muller and Walter 2010), three central aspects or elements of free will can be distinguished (Meynen 2010a, 2013a). The first element is to be able *to act otherwise* (if there are no alternatives, an action is not a free action); the second element is acting *for a reason* (unintentional action is not considered free action); the third element is that the person is the *originator* of the action (a person should not be manipulated or forced to act). Many features discussed in the previous section can be linked to one of these elements of free will. In what follows, I will provide examples derived from psychopathology for each of these three elements (see also Meynen 2013a).

Being able to act otherwise. Above, we used the term hijacking of will-formation with respect to commanding voices. A patient who experiences such a commanding voice, as it appears, no longer has the possibility to do otherwise; he or she *cannot but* obey the voice. This may be the clearest example from clinical psychiatry of a condition that does not leave other behavioral options open to a patient (see also Meynen 2013a). Notably, many other disorders appear to leave alternative options open. For instance, CBT for anxiety disorders makes use of the fact that, at least to some extent, many patients can refrain from avoiding-behavior, in other words, that, apparently, they can act otherwise.

Acting for reasons. Most of the times, psychiatric disorders affect a person's behavior in a way that leaves the element of 'acting for reasons' intact. A person suffering from panic disorder can clearly explain why she fled from the cinema: she was panicking and afraid to lose control. In some disorders, meanwhile, behavior may arise that is not the result of reasoning and cannot be properly explained and understood in terms of reasons. This may happen during a delirium with lowered states of consciousness or in conditions of dementia, and incoherence. Tics in Tourette's, at least as long as they are not performed in response to premonitory sensations (see above), may also be considered not to be performed for a reason; they just happen.

Being the originator. This element refers to authorship and, in a way, authenticity of an action. Although a patient has alternative possibilities, and although his or her actions are motivated by reasons, we may feel that, due to a mental disorder, the patient is not "him- or herself." Consider a mother whose depression causes her to neglect her children – we may not blame her, saying: "she is not herself lately." She does what she does, but it is not *her.* This could also be the case in hypomanic states: cognitive functioning is technically intact, but the person is different from who he or she used to be. If this is the case, we may feel that the disorder is bringing about the behavior. Consequently, the patient is not acting freely, and may not therefore be blamed for violating a moral or legal obligation. Alternatively, we could interpret a hypomanic state as a condition in which rational control over the alternative options is diminished (so, in terms of *being able to act otherwise*), and that, therefore, the patient is less free.

Since mental disorders may have different features simultaneously, they may affect more than one aspect of free will at one point in time. In addition, even one symptom can be categorized under more than one element: some tics in Tourette's syndrome could be classified under "no reason" and probably also under "no alternative."

Finally, there is one important feature of various mental disorders that we have not mentioned with respect to one of the three elements of free will: delusion. As discussed above, in my view, delusions are primarily relevant to responsibility as an *epistemic* factor. Interestingly, the most famous legal standard for the insanity defense, the M'Naghten Rule, focuses on knowledge issues, rather than on the three elements of free will discussed above:

> At the time of committing the act, the party accused was laboring under such a defect of reason, from disease of the mind, as not to *know* the nature and quality of the act he was doing; or if he did know it, that he did not *know* what he was doing was wrong. (M'Naghten's Case, 10 Cl. & Fin. 200, 8 Eng. Rep. 718 [H.L. 1843], emphasis added)

This suggests that the epistemic factor (knowledge) is crucial as far as the impact of a mental disorder on criminal responsibility is concerned. Another conclusion could be: this legal rule is overlooking many of the effects mental disorders may have on a person's will (Elliott 1996). For instance, we may feel that this rule unjustly overlooks a condition like kleptomania: these patients clearly know very well what they are doing. Still, their will to steal appears to be substantially influenced by the disorder. If they had not have suffered from kleptomania, they would never have felt this enormous urge to steal, for instance, this worthless toothbrush.

Although there are exceptions, the interesting thing about mental disorders is that they influence behavior *via* the will. Neurological disorders such as epilepsy also influence behavior, but they usually *bypass* the will. However, some voluntary control is apparently also possible over some epileptic seizures (Glannon 2011).

Implications

Life, law, treatment

The many ways in which mental disorders may affect a patient's (free) will have profound consequences.

First, they may affect a person's *daily life*. Some disorders almost continuously affect the will, for instance a severe depression. Other disorders may influence the will only in specific situations, like fear of mice (phobia). Some disorders may even influence a person's behavior in such a way that he or she commits a crime. Briefly, by influencing a patient's will, a mental disorder may profoundly affect a patient's life.

Second, a mental disorder may undermine a person's will to seek help or to follow *treatment*. Of course, treatment is part of a person's life, but I highlight this aspect because it is especially relevant from a healthcare professional's point of view. A person with an addiction may start to realize that he or she has a problem but may not yet have the will to seek treatment. So, healthcare professionals have to be aware that patients may not be ready for therapy. In such a case, the wise thing to do is not to propose therapy straightaway but, first, to motivate the patient. In addition, due to avolition, depressed patients may be incapable of forming the will to seek help for their problems. In general, treatment requires appropriate will-setting on the part of the patient. If a mental disorder affects the will, then it may thus affect the will-formation needed to seek help and to work on cure and recovery. In fact, this means that by affecting the will, a mental disorder may deprive a patient of the means to get rid of the disorder. Therefore, in psychiatry, healthcare professionals should be able to recognize such impact on the will. In addition, they should possess specific skills to motivate patients to start or continue treatment. An ultimate consequence of the fact that mental disorders may undermine the will to seek help can be *compulsory* measures/treatment. In psychiatric practice, compulsory measures, regulated by health law, often have to do with a dangerous situation brought about by the way in which a mental disorder interferes with a person's decision-making. For instance, a severe depression may affect will-formation in such a way that a patient decides to commit suicide. In such a case, compulsory interventions may be justified in order to prevent the patient from harming himself.

Finally, although it is important to recognize the impact psychiatric disorders may have on a patient's will, we should be aware that a psychiatric patient – as any other patient – is, in principle, capable of making autonomous choices and that their autonomy has to be respected. Respect for the patient, meanwhile, also implies that the healthcare professional should recognize the above-mentioned challenges a patient may face due to the effects of the disorder on his or her will.

Research

Given the importance of our wills, and given the many ways in which mental disorders may influence the will, neuroscientific research on the impact of mental disorders on patients' decision-making is of utmost importance (see Meynen 2013b). Notably, in practice, the impairment of the will can be considered *part* of the disorder, as in severe depression. Therefore, by elucidating will-formation in depressed patients, the disorder itself can be further understood and perhaps more effectively treated.

In addition, the negative consequences of a mental disorder are for a substantial part mediated via the impact on the patient's will. A considerable problem in depression concerns the fact that the depression may affect a patient's will: the patient develops fewer activities and may lose his job. In general, the disorder and the impact on decision-making are closely related, and several aspects of the disorder together may impair aspects of decision-making.

Fortunately, neuroscientists have become interested in the impairments in decision-making in mental disorders (see findings in the previous section). Nora Volkow is a good example of a researcher who tries to elucidate the impact of a group of mental disorders (addiction and impulse control disorders) on decision-making. Moreover, Volkow's work appears to bring about a shift in the perception of addictive behavior: addiction as a brain disease significantly impairing a patient's will-formation – as opposed to authors like Fingarette and Heyman (see previous section on mental disorders and the will).

Still, as mentioned above, at present little with respect to the brain and the will is known for certain. The psychopathological phenomena described in the previous section still constitute a puzzle as far as their neurobiological correlates are concerned. Meanwhile, the expanding field of neuroscience with the continuous development of new (imaging) techniques appears to be in the best position to further our understanding of the impact mental disorders may have on the will. Notably, neuroscience can also try to clarify how original and creative decision-making, as it may occur in hypomanic states, comes about.

Conclusion

Mental disorders may have a substantial behavioral impact because of their ability to influence a person's will. Such influence takes many forms, and it may interfere with a patient's life and, in particular, with a patient's ability to seek help or to follow treatment advice. In some cases, the impact on the will results in dangerous situations for the patient him- or herself or for other people – and coercive measures may be the only option left. Nevertheless, in principle, psychiatric patients are, just like other patients, autonomous agents, and their autonomy ought to be respected. At the same time healthcare professionals should be aware of the specific challenges these patients may face because of the influence of the mental disorder on their wills. Further brain research on the impact of mental disorders on will-formation is needed.

REFERENCES

American Psychiatric Association (1994) Diagnostic and Statistical Manual of Mental Disorders-IV *(DCM-IV)*. Washington, DC: American Psychiatric Association.

Andreasen, N. C. (1984) *The Broken Brain: The Biological Revolution in Psychiatry*. New York: Harper & Row.

(2008) The relationship between creativity and mood disorders. *Dialogues in Clinical Neuroscience* 10(2): 251–255.

Brewer, J. A. and Potenza, M. N. (2008) The neurobiology and genetics of impulse control disorders: relationships to drug addictions. *Biochemical Pharmacology* 75(1): 63–75.

Cavedini, P., Gorini, A., and Bellodi, L. (2006) Understanding obsessive-compulsive disorder: focus on decision making. *Neuropsychology Review* 16(1): 3–15.

Diekhof, E. K., Falkai, P., and Gruber, O. (2008) Functional neuroimaging of reward processing and decision-making: a review of aberrant motivational and affective processing in addiction and mood disorders. *Brain Research Reviews* 59(1): 164–184.

Elliott, C. (1996) *The Rules of Insanity: Moral Responsibility and the Mentally Ill Offender*. Albany: State University of New York.

Felthous, A. R. (2008) The will: from metaphysical freedom to normative functionalism. *Journal of the American Academy of Psychiatry and the Law* 36(1): 16–24.

Fingarette, H. (1989) *Heavy Drinking: The Myth of Alcoholism as a Disease*. Berkeley: University of California Press.

Fulford, K. W. M. (1993) Mental illness and the mind-brain problem: delusion, belief and Searle's theory of intentionality. *Theoretical Medicine* 14: 181–194.

Glannon, W. (2011) Diminishing and enhancing free will. *AJOB Neuroscience* 2(3): 15–26.

Grant, J. E., Kim, S. W., and Odlaug, B. L. (2009) A double-blind, placebo-controlled study of the opiate antagonist, naltrexone, in the treatment of kleptomania. *Biological Psychiatry* 65(7): 600–606.

Hall, W. and Carter, A. (2013) How may neuroscience affect the way that the criminal courts deal with addicted offenders? In N. A. Vincent (ed.) *Neuroscience and Legal Responsibility*. New York: Oxford University Press.

Hare, E. (1987) Creativity and mental illness. *British Medical Journal (Clinical Research Ed.)* 295(6613): 1587–1589.

Heyman, G. M. (2009) *Addiction: A Disorder of Choice*. Cambridge, MA: Harvard University Press.

Kalis, A. and Meynen, G. (2014) Mental disorder and legal responsibility: the relevance of stages of decision making. *International Journal of Law and Psychiatry*. Doi: 10.1016/j.ijlp.2014.02.034.

Kalis, A., Mojzisch, A., Schweizer, T. S., and Kaiser, S. (2008) Weakness of will, akrasia, and the neuropsychiatry of decision making: an interdisciplinary perspective. *Cognitive, Affective & Behavioral Neuroscience* 8(4): 402–417.

Kane, R. (1998) *The Significance of Free Will*. New York: Oxford University Press.

(2002) *The Oxford Handbook of Free Will*. Oxford University Press.

Lang, A. (1991) Patient perception of tics and other movement disorders. *Neurology* 41 (2, Pt 1): 223–228.

Libet, B. (1999) Do we have free will? *Journal of Consciousness Studies* 6(8–9): 47–57.

Marazziti, D., Consoli, G., Picchetti, M., Carlini, M., and Faravelli, L. (2010) Cognitive impairment in major depression. *European Journal of Pharmacology* 626(1): 83–86.

Mele, A. R. (2012) *Backsliding: Understanding Weakness of Will*. New York: Oxford University Press.

Meynen, G. (2010a) Free will and mental disorder: exploring the relationship. *Theoretical Medicine and Bioethics* 31(6): 429–443.

(2010b) Wegner on hallucinations, inconsistency, and the illusion of free will: some critical remarks. *Phenomenology and the Cognitive Sciences* 9: 359–372.

(2011) Depression, possibilities, and competence: a phenomenological perspective. *Theoretical Medicine and Bioethics* 32(3): 181–193.

(2013a) Why mental disorders can diminish responsibility: proposing a theoretical framework. In A. W. Musschenga and A. Van Harskamp (eds.), *What Makes Us Moral: On the Capacities and Conditions for Being Moral*. Berlin: Springer.

(2013b) A neurolaw perspective on psychiatric assessments of criminal responsibility: decision-making, mental disorder, and the brain *International Journal of Law and Psychiatry* 36(2): 93–99.

Morse, S. J. (2007) The non-problem of free will in forensic psychiatry and psychology. *Behavioral Sciences and the Law* 25(2): 203–220.

Muller, S. and Walter, H. (2010) Reviewing autonomy: implications of the neurosciences and the free will debate for the principle of respect for the patient's autonomy. *Cambridge Quarterly of Healthcare Ethics* 19(2): 205–217.

Nitschke, J. B. and Mackiewicz, K. L. (2005) Prefrontal and anterior cingulate contributions to volition in depression. *International Review of Neurobiology* 67: 73–94.

O'Connor, T. (2010). Free will. Retrieved February 2, 2011, from http://plato.stanford.edu/entries/freewill/.

Otte, C. (2011) Cognitive behavioral therapy in anxiety disorders: current state of the evidence. *Dialogues in Clinical Neuroscience* 13(4): 413–421.

Perring, C. (2004) Conceptual issues in assessing responsibility for actions symptomatic of mental illness. *International Journal of Law and Psychiatry* 27(5): 489–503.

Radder, H. and Meynen, G. (2012) Does the brain "initiate" freely willed processes? A philosophy of science critique of Libet-type experiments and their interpretation. *Theory & Psychology* 23(1): 3–21.

Sadock, B. J. and Sadock, V. A. (2005) *Kaplan & Sadock's Comprehensive Textbook of Psychiatry*, 8th edn. Philadelphia: Lippincott Williams & Wilkins.

Strenziok, M., Pulaski, S., Krueger, F., Zamboni, G., Clawson, D., and Grafman, J. (2011) Regional brain atrophy and impaired decision making on the balloon analog risk task in behavioral variant frontotemporal dementia. *Cognitive and Behavioral Neurology* 24(2): 59–67.

Verdellen, C. W. (2007) *Exposure and Response Prevention in the Treatment of Tics in Tourette's Syndrome*. Amsterdam: Boom.

Verdellen, C. W., Hoogduin, C. A., Kato, B. S., Keijsers, G. P., Cath, D. C., and Hoijtink, H. B. (2008) Habituation of premonitory sensations during exposure and response prevention treatment in Tourette's syndrome. *Behavior Modification* 32(2): 215–227.

Volkow, N. D., Wang, G. J., Fowler, J. S., Tomasi, D., Telang, F., and Baler, R. (2010) Addiction: decreased reward sensitivity and increased expectation sensitivity conspire to overwhelm the brain's control circuit. *Bioessays* 32(9): 748–755.

Walter, H. (2001) *Neurophilosophy of Free Will: From Libertarian Illusions to a Concept of Natural Autonomy*. Cambridge, MA: MIT Press.

8 Are addicted individuals responsible for their behaviour?

Wayne Hall and Adrian Carter

ABSTRACT

For two centuries, clinicians have argued that chronically addicted individuals suffer from a disease that is produced by the effects that chronic alcohol or drug use has on their brains. Neuroscience research has provided support for this view by describing the brain mechanisms that are believed to underlie chronic addiction. Research on animals has revealed the neurochemical circuitry on which psychoactive drugs of dependence act and produced animal models of human addiction that reproduce features of human addiction, such as drug tolerance and withdrawal symptoms, and rapid reinstatement of drug use after periods of abstinence. Human neuroimaging studies suggest that similar neurobiological processes operate in the brains of addicted humans. Leading proponents of neurobiological research on addiction have argued that it shows that addiction is a chronic brain disease. In this paper we critically examine the research used to support this claim and discuss its implications for ascribing responsibility to addicted persons for criminal acts that they commit to enable their drug use. We also assess whether the evidence for a brain disease model of addiction justifies the compulsory treatment of severely addicted persons for paternalistic reasons, that is, for their own good.

Neuroscience research on addiction promises to illuminate a long-standing debate in philosophy and the law about whether addicted persons are morally and legally responsible for their drug use and for any criminal offences that they may commit in order to obtain and use addictive drugs. We describe two conflicting views that have dominated discussions of this issue: the moral view that drug use is always a free choice for which individuals are, and should be, held fully morally and legally responsible; and the brain disease model in which chronic drug use is hypothesized to produce changes in brain function that impair the capacity of addicted persons to control their drug use, and so reduce their responsibility for their behaviour. We explore the evidence and arguments marshalled for each view and the competing interpretations of neuroscience and epidemiological research that the proponents of each view deploy. We also consider attempts that have been made to develop an account that does justice to the research evidence without accepting a strong form of the brain disease model that eliminates responsibility. We discuss how these views fit with legal and social practices towards addiction in two areas: the ways in which criminal courts deal with addicted offenders; and civil legislation which in some jurisdictions allows severely addicted persons to be compulsorily treated for their own good.

What is addiction?

The concept of addiction is invoked to explain the otherwise puzzling behaviour of some drug users who persist in using drugs despite the serious personal problems that their drug use causes to themselves and people close to them. They often profess an apparently sincere wish to stop and may have a history of multiple failed attempts to cease using drugs (Ross et al., 2008). These features are reflected in official classifications such as DSM-IV (American Psychiatric Association, 1994) which defines *substance dependence* as 'a cluster of cognitive, behavioral and physiologic symptoms indicating that the individual continues use of the substance despite significant substance-related problems' (p. 176). A diagnosis of substance dependence requires that *three* or more of the following seven criteria occur within the same twelve-month period: increased tolerance (e.g. use of markedly increased amounts of the drug to achieve the desired effect); withdrawal symptoms on abstinence; taking the drug in larger amounts or over a longer period than intended; a persistent desire and/or unsuccessful efforts to cut down or control the drug use; a great deal of time spent obtaining, using and recovering from using the drug; giving up important social, occupational or recreational activities; continued drug use despite knowledge of persistent or recurrent physical or psychological problems likely to have been caused or exacerbated by the substance(American Psychiatric Association, 1994).

Two explanations of this behaviour have often been debated: the moral and medical models. The moral model is the dominant common-sense view that addicted drug users simply choose to use drugs and so should be held fully morally and legally responsible for their behaviour in the same way as any other person who engages in acts that harm themselves or others (Satel, 2001; Szasz, 1975). The second view is a brain-centred disease model in which addictive drug use is a pattern of behaviour that is seen to be caused by enduring changes in brain function that are produced by the effects of chronic drug use (Courtwright, 2010; Leshner, 1997; Volkow and Li, 2004).

The moral model of problem drug use has dominated popular discourse on drug use and public policies towards it. It explains addictive patterns of drug use in much the same way as it explains other socially disapproved behaviour, that is, as a voluntary behaviour in which the drug user chooses to engage. On this view, addiction is dismissed as a self-interested excuse that drug users invoke to evade moral and legal responsibility for the consequences of their drug use. Acceptance of this view entails the implication that drug users who break the criminal law (e.g. to fund their drug use) should be prosecuted by the courts and imprisoned, if found guilty (Szasz, 1975).

A medical model of addiction acknowledges that all drug users initially choose to use drugs but argues that a minority who become chronic drug users develop a medical disorder. In these cases, addiction requires treatment if the sufferer is to become and remain abstinent (Leshner, 1997; Volkow and Li, 2004). The disease model of addiction was first proposed at the end of the eighteenth and beginning of the nineteenth centuries to explain uncontrolled and self-destructive alcohol use, well before there were any plausible biological hypotheses for such a disease model (Courtwright, 2010). In the last four decades, neuroscience research has provided renewed support for a disease model by providing detailed analyses of the changes in the brain processes of chronic drug users. Its advocates argue that these changes explain the difficulty that addicted persons experience in ceasing drug use and in remaining abstinent, if they do manage to stop using.

In this chapter we critically evaluate the evidence for the claim that *addiction is a brain disease* and discuss its implications for the debate about whether addicted persons are morally and legally responsible for their drug use and any criminal offences committed to fund it. We first briefly summarise and then critically examine the type of evidence offered in support of this view of addiction before examining more critical views on the model. We then consider how these competing views fit with current legal practice in dealing with addicted offenders. We conclude with a discussion of a renewed interest in a late nineteenth-century social practice in some developed countries, namely, legislating to allow involuntary treatment of addiction for paternalistic reasons, that is, compulsory addiction treatment in the best interests of the addicted person.

The case for a brain disease model of addiction (BDMA)

For over 200 years the primary reason for proposing a disease model of addiction has been the chronicity of alcohol or drug use in patients treated for addiction (Courtwright, 2010). Physicians who treated patients for 'inebriety' – chronic, heavy alcohol use – in the second half of the nineteenth century hypothesised that chronic alcohol use changed inebriates' brains in ways that made it difficult for them to desist from drinking (Lewis, 1992). At the end of the twentieth century, leading US addiction researchers similarly stressed the chronicity of addiction as a central argument for accepting a disease model of addiction (McLellan et al., 2000). Neuroscience researchers in the field of addiction (e.g. Leshner, 1997) have argued that the chronicity of treated addiction is explained by persistent changes in brain structure and function arising from chronic drug use.

Three types of evidence are invoked to support the brain disease model of addiction: (1) animal models of addiction that have enabled researchers to identify the neurocircuitry on which major drugs of addiction act and the major neurotransmitters and receptors that mediate their actions; (2) neuroimaging studies of the effects of drugs on the brains of normal human volunteers, actively addicted persons and abstinent addicted persons; and (3) behavioural genetic studies of addiction in humans and animals.

Animal models of addiction

Neuroscience theories of addiction rely heavily on animal models of addiction, especially studies in which rats are trained to self-administer psychoactive drugs (Koob and Le Moal, 2006). These models possess considerable face validity for human addiction in that rats will self-administer addictive drugs at high frequencies (e.g. by pressing a bar) and will continue to do so long after delivery of the drug ceases. These responses can be rapidly reinstated after long periods in which no drug has been delivered by giving a priming dose of the drug, or presenting painful stimuli or cues (e.g. a light) that was associated with drug delivery (Koob and Le Moal, 2006). The self-administration of addictive drugs is also reduced by direct electric stimulation of 'reward centres' in the animals' forebrains, suggesting that the animals find the effects of these drugs rewarding (Koob and Le Moal, 2006).

Animal models can reproduce several key features of human addiction, namely, the development of drug tolerance, dose escalation, withdrawal symptoms and rapid reinstatement after abstinence. Animals given free access to drugs, for example, will increase the frequency and amount of drug that they self-administer and work increasingly harder to obtain drugs (e.g. enduring painful stimuli), indicating tolerance to drug effects. These animal models also have predictive validity in that the drugs that are most readily self-administered by animals are those to which humans become readily addicted.

Animal models of addiction have allowed researchers to identify the brain circuitry on which the major drugs of addiction act, namely, the dopaminergic 'mesolimbic brain reward system' (Koob and Volkow, 2010). This system consists of the ventral striatum, nucleus accumbens, amygdala, frontal cortices and interconnected structures in the forebrain. All of these structures are mediated by the neurotransmitter dopamine and lesions in these structures, or use of drugs to block dopamine receptors in these circuits, abolishes drug self-administration (Koob and Le Moal, 2006).

Human neuroimaging studies

Over the past two decades human neuroimaging studies of the effects of psychoactive drugs on brain function have provided support for the relevance of animal models to human addiction (Koob and Le Moal, 2006; Koob and Volkow, 2010). Radioactively labelled tracers have identified the molecular sites in the human brain on which drugs of addiction act, and these have proven to be in brain systems that are analogous to those identified in animals. Functional magnetic resonance imaging (fMRI) studies have identified differences in the way that these specific brain regions respond to drugs in addicted and non-addicted persons (Volkow et al., 2010).

Neuroimaging studies have provided support for the hypothesis that drugs of addiction act on the dopaminergic mesolimbic reward system in both humans and animals. They have also identified dopamine-mediated changes in key cortical areas (especially in the orbital frontal cortex) that have been implicated in decision-making and impulse control. Many of these changes in brain function persist after addicted persons have been abstinent for sustained periods of time (Volkow et al., 2010). The latter finding has led researchers to hypothesise that these brain changes explain the high rates of relapse to drug use in persons who have been treated for addiction (Volkow et al., 2010).

Human genetics of addiction

Twin and adoption studies reveal that genetic factors make a substantial contribution to the risk of developing addiction (Agrawal et al., 2012;

Kendler et al., 2012). The percentage of variation in the risk of alcohol, nicotine and cannabis dependence that is explained by genetic factors is estimated to be between 40–60 per cent (Agrawal et al., 2012; Sutherland et al., 2012). Researchers have searched for alleles that explain the genetics of addiction susceptibility. The leading candidates have been genes that influence drug metabolism and brain levels of the neurotransmitters, receptors and transporters on which these drugs act. Genome-wide association studies (GWAS) have found modest correlations between genetic markers (single nucleotide polymorphisms) and indicators of drug use and addiction. Pharmacogenetic studies have suggested that addicted patients with different genotypes respond differently to different types of drug treatment. Some of these genes influence brain function in the mesolimbic reward system, a finding that fits well with the hypothesis that addiction is a result of changes in these regions of the brain produced by chronic drug use.

Drug-induced compulsive behaviour in patients with Parkinson's disease

Clinical studies of Parkinson's patients have recently provided a novel form of support for the claim that addictive forms of behaviour can be caused by the chronic use of drugs that act on the mesolimbic dopaminergic reward system. Patients with Parkinson's disease (PD) are treated with dopamine replacement therapy (DRT) that often involves administering dopamine agonists that act on the mesolimbic reward system. A substantial minority (as many as one in six) of these patients develop compulsive disorders, such as compulsive gambling, sexuality and overeating (Weintraub et al., 2010). There are good reasons for believing that use of DRT is a contributory cause of these compulsive disorders, namely, that they develop after DRT is initiated or doses of DRT are increased; they usually rapidly remit after the cessation of DRT or a reduction in DRT dose; and similar disorders have been reported in patients who do not have Parkinsons' disease who are treated with these drugs (Ambermoon et al., 2011).

These disorders are especially interesting because they occur in adults who do not have many of the usual risk factors for addiction, namely, being young, anti-social males who initiate drug use at an early age and primarily used drugs for their euphoric effects. In the case of the Parkinson's patients, these disorders arise from medical treatment rather than recreational drug use, and they occur in adults in their 60s and 70s, well past the usual age in which addictive disorders develop. One puzzle is explaining why most of these disorders are compulsive forms of addictive behaviours, such as problem gambling or compulsive sexuality, rather than compulsive forms of drug use.

Criticisms of the brain disease model of addiction

The claim that addiction is a disease has been strongly criticised (e.g. Heyman, 2009; Szasz, 1975). These critics contest the claim that addiction is a chronic relapsing disorder by citing evidence that addictive drug use is affected by its consequences in ways that do not fit well with the brain disease model of addiction (Heyman, 2009).

First, these critics argue that the high rates of remission of addictive disorders found in epidemiological surveys are inconsistent with the claim that addiction is a chronic and relapsing disorder (Heyman, 2009; Kincaid and Sullivan, 2010). As these critics point out, epidemiological surveys typically find that the majority of adults who have ever met criteria for alcohol or drug dependence (70–80%) were *not* dependent at the time of the interview (Heyman, 2009). And more importantly, most former addicts had stopped using their drug of dependence more than three years before, usually without any form of addiction treatment (Heyman, 2009).

Survey data can inflate estimated rates of recovery in addiction; self-report may be affected by selective recall and more severe cases of addiction are likely to be under-represented in such surveys (Degenhardt and Hall, 2012). Nonetheless, longitudinal studies of representative samples do suggest that recovery from addiction is a common outcome. Longitudinal studies that follow adolescent drug users into adulthood find that substantial proportions of young people who meet criteria for dependence on alcohol, cannabis and other drugs in late adolescence and early adulthood (Fergusson et al., 2008; Swift et al., 2008) cease problematic drug use in their mid- to late 20s. This often occurs in the absence of treatment, in response to life events such as entering the workforce, marrying and having children (Bachman et al., 1997). This suggests that one's perception of increased responsibility for or a felt obligation to family members and co-workers might influence this behaviour.

Second, these critics point out that rates of recovery are substantial even in persons with addiction to heroin, the 'hardest drug'. Robins and colleagues (1974, 1993), for example, interviewed heroin-using US servicemen who served in Vietnam three years after they had returned to the USA. Most of those who regularly used heroin in Vietnam and who reported symptoms of dependence ceased using heroin before they returned to the USA and most did not become re-addicted to heroin after their return.

Third, evidence shows that addictive drug use can be affected by small financial incentives in persons who are treated for their addiction (Heyman, 2009). For example, giving patients food vouchers or small amounts of money (e.g. $20) for providing clean urine samples substantially reduces drug use in persons being treated for addiction (Heyman, 2009; Higgins et al., 2010). The responsiveness of addictive drug use to these modest incentives is hard to reconcile with the view that addictive drug use is a compulsive form of behaviour driven by impaired brain reward and cognitive control systems over which addicted individuals have little or no control.

Reconciling these competing views of addiction

These conflicting views of addiction can be reconciled by recognising that addictive disorders vary in severity and that it is only the most severe cases of addiction that are most usefully thought of as brain disorders (Kincaid and Sullivan, 2010; Ross et al., 2008). This explanation makes sense of the following features of the epidemiology of addictive disorders: mild to moderate addictive disorders are much more common in the population than the more severe forms of addiction; the milder disorders are most common in young adults, most of whom will cease problem drug use under the influence of marriages, mortgages and children (Bachman et al., 1997); only a minority of young adults who develop an addictive pattern of drug use will continue to use drugs into their early 30s (Bachman et al., 1997); and persons with these more persistent and severe disorders are more likely to seek or be coerced into seeking treatment (McLellan, et al., 2000). It is these more severe cases of addiction that are most likely to display the chronic, relapsing disorders that are associated with alterations in brain function of the type described in the brain disease model of addiction (Kincaid and Sullivan, 2010; Ross et al., 2008).

A modified brain disease model of addiction of this second type fits better with the epidemiology of addictive disorders, but it differs in important ways from the strongest form of the model encapsulated in the claim that 'addiction is a chronic relapsing brain disease' (Koob and Le Moal, 2006; Koob and Volkow, 2010). The modified model applies to the minority of addicted persons with severe, chronic relapsing disorders. This means that survey estimates of the prevalence of drug dependence in the population substantially over-estimate the prevalence of chronic forms of addiction. That is, the lifetime prevalence of *any form* of addictive disorder is far higher than the prevalence of addiction that is severe enough to warrant being described as a chronic, relapsing disorder.

Are addicted persons responsible for their behaviour?

These competing models of addiction have implications for views about the responsibility of addicted individuals for their drug use, and crimes they commit to facilitate their drug use. Views on these issues inform public policy responses to addiction. Should addicted persons who commit criminal offences to support their drug use be held legally responsible for these criminal offences? Should addicted offenders be given more lenient sentences by the courts than offenders who commit the same offences but do not use addictive drugs? Should persons with severe addiction be compulsorily treated for their own good?

Three views have dominated discussions of whether addicted persons are responsible for their drug use and criminal behaviour engaged in to facilitate it. The first view is a strong form of the brain disease model in which addicted persons are not responsible for their drug use because it is compulsive. The second view is the common-sense moral model according to which addicted persons are fully responsible for their decision to use drugs. A third set of views attempts to find some compromise between these two views by arguing that addicted persons' control over their drug use is impaired but not sufficiently to excuse criminal acts committed to facilitate their drug use.

Addiction as involuntary behaviour

Alan Leshner's 1997 article in Science is often seen as the key source for the view that an addicted person's drug use is compulsive. Leshner acknowledged that drug use is initially voluntary, but he argued that control over drug use is eroded by sustained drug use. Once drug use becomes chronic, a metaphorical switch is flicked in the person's brain after which drug use is no longer under the individual's control. As indicated above, the major evidence that Leshner cited were animal models of addiction and brain scans of addicted persons.

Leshner did not explicitly discuss the criminal responsibility of addicted offenders. So it is not clear if he believes that the brain disease model exculpates addicted offenders. He may be prepared to argue only that addicted drug users are compelled to use drugs when presented with the opportunity to do so. Louis Charland (2002) has expressed this view in arguing that heroin-addicted persons are incapable of giving free and informed consent to participate in heroin prescription trials because they are incapable of saying no to the offer of free heroin. Even those who are very sceptical of the claims made for the brain disease model of addiction are prepared to allow that an addicted person who is experiencing withdrawal symptoms may find it difficult to avoid using a drug if offered it (Morse, 2004).

Some proponents of a brain disease model distinguish between excusing an addicted person for continuing to use drugs and excusing them for any criminal acts engaged in to enable such drug use. For example, Hyman (2007), who provides a more nuanced brain disease model of addiction, does not accept that it exculpates addicted persons. He argues that the model does not 'reduce addicted persons to zombies ... other goals are not extirpated'. He argues on prudential grounds that they should be held responsible for their acts: 'For many reasons, it may be wise for societies to err on the side of holding addicted individuals responsible for their behaviour and to act as if they are capable of exerting more control than perhaps they can ... with a view to rehabilitation ... and protection of society rather than moral opprobrium' (Hyman, 2007, p. 10).

Legal critics of the brain disease model argue that its acceptance does not establish that addictive drug use is involuntary in the same sense as a reflex or an epileptic fit (Morse, 2004). Morse and other critics (e.g. Foddy and Savulescu, 2006) argue that the drug-seeking and drug-taking by addicted persons involve conscious choices and elaborate planning. Also, their behaviour often changes in response to characteristics of the social contexts within which the person operates and the social consequences of their drug use.

Moral views of addiction

The framing of the debate about the responsibility of addicted persons as a choice between medical and moral views has had the unfortunate consequence that rejection of the strongest form of the brain disease model (that addicts cannot be held responsible for their behaviour) is seen as entailing acceptance of the moral view of addiction. We do not think we should accept this inference.

We find the most uncompromising form of the moral model – libertarianism – implausible (e.g. Foddy and Savulescu, 2006; Szasz, 1975). Libertarians claim that all drug use is freely chosen and engaged in for the person's pleasure. Addicted drug users, on their account, are simply persons who value their pleasure more highly than their health and well-being, or that of family and friends, and neighbours. Libertarians accordingly conclude that drug users who harm others should be held fully responsible for their actions, and punished in the same way as persons who harm others but do not use drugs.

We accept that the brain disease model poorly describes most of those who qualify for a diagnosis of addiction in epidemiological surveys. However, we do not think its weaknesses support a libertarian view. The brain disease model provides a better fit to the minority of persons who have severe chronic addictive disorders whose behaviour is not explained by asserting that they simply value pleasure more highly than their health. Persons with these severe disorders persist in using drugs despite causing serious harm to themselves and others about whom they profess to care. More importantly, they have often made multiple failed attempts to quit or cut down and they unhappily continue to use in the face of severe adverse social consequences. These include the loss of relationships, custody of children and employment, and imprisonment for drug-related offences. The occurrence of dopamine-induced compulsive disorders in patients with PD also challenges the libertarian view that addiction is always a self-interested excuse for pleasure-seeking behaviour.

Addiction as impaired control

A number of philosophers and ethicists have attempted to develop an alternative to what they see as the weaknesses of the moral and medical views of addiction (e.g. Bonnie, 2002; Carter and Hall, 2012; Levy, 2012; Morse, 2004; Yaffe, 2001). These authors generally agree that addicted persons have impaired control over their drug use and that this makes it more difficult, but not impossible, for them to control their drug use. On this view addicted persons, face a harder choice than non-addicted persons, namely, the choice between desisting from using drugs and experiencing craving and aversive withdrawal symptoms. But these authors argue that these craving and withdrawal symptoms are not sufficiently coercive to excuse the commission of criminal acts (Bonnie, 2002; Morse, 2004). On this view, addiction is seen as reducing responsibility and justifying lesser penalties, thereby mitigating rather than exculpating addicted persons who perform criminal acts.

Authors who differ in their preparedness to accept a brain disease model of addiction seem to converge on this position. As noted above, Hyman (2007) is persuaded by the evidence for a brain disease model, but he argues nonetheless that we should err in the direction of holding addicted persons responsible for their behaviour in the addicted person's own interests and for the protection of society. Morse (2004) argues that the evidence offered for a brain disease model of addiction is not sufficient to show that the behaviour of addicted persons is involuntary. Nor does it show that craving constitutes sufficient duress to provide an excuse. Satel (1998) also rejects the brain disease model but concedes that addicted persons often have to struggle to become and remain abstinent. She argues that addicted offenders can be best assisted to cease using drugs by being coerced into treatment and forced to comply with its demands under the threat of legal or other sanctions (e.g. loss of a licence to practice in the case of addicted doctors). Vaillant (2001) argues for a similar position, citing long-term follow up studies of alcohol- and heroin-addicted persons that support the policy of coercing addicted persons into treatment, and providing immediate sanctions for drug use.

Criminal courts and the responsibility of addicted offenders

The criminal courts in developed countries routinely make judgments about addicted offenders' responsibility for criminal offences. This is because a substantial proportion of persons charged with criminal offences, such as drug dealing and property offences, are addicted to drugs (Hall and Lucke, 2010). It is therefore worth exploring how the criminal courts deal with such offenders.

Criminal courts in Australia and the USA often accept a compromise position: they do not accept that addiction is an excuse for committing criminal offences; however, they often treat addiction as a mitigating factor in sentencing in offering addicted offenders a choice of imprisonment or legally coerced addiction treatment, with imprisonment if they fail to comply with treatment (Hall and Lucke, 2010). We have argued elsewhere that this approach is best described as legally coerced addiction treatment. It differs from compulsory or mandatory treatment because offenders are offered a constrained choice of imprisonment or treatment rather than being sentenced to treatment and offered no choice (Hall and Lucke, 2010).

The justification for coerced addiction treatment fits best with a consequentialist theory of punishment in which the primary aim of punishment is reducing criminal offending. Addiction treatment, it is argued, is more effective in reducing recidivism in addicted offenders than imprisonment (Chandler et al., 2009). This argument has particular weight in the case of heroin-addicted offenders who, if untreated, are likely to return to heroin use and reoffend after release (Hall, 1996). Providing addiction treatment under coercion in the community is also a more cost-effective way of reducing recidivism than imprisonment (Moore et al., 2007). The advent of HIV/AIDS among injecting drug users adds a strong public health argument to the case for coerced treatment, namely, that it will reduce HIV and hepatitis transmission to other inmates via needle-sharing in prison (Dolan, 1991).

Legally coerced addiction treatment raises important ethical and philosophical issues that we do not have the space to discuss here (Carter and Hall, 2012). We endorse a 1986 World Health Organization (WHO) consensus view (Porter et al., 1986) that *legally coerced* drug treatment is legally and ethically justified if: (1) the rights of the individuals are protected by 'due process'; and (2) if effective and humane treatment is provided.

The effectiveness of coerced community-based addiction treatment was assessed in heroin- and cocaine-dependent offenders in the USA in the 1970s and 1980s (e.g. Hubbard, 1989; Simpson and Friend, 1988). In these studies drug-dependent offenders who entered Therapeutic Communities (TCs) and drug-free out-patient counselling on probation or parole did as well as those who entered these treatments without such legal pressure (Hubbard, 1989). Methadone maintenance treatment (MMT) reduced recidivism in heroin-addicted prisoners (Gordon et al., 2008) and among heroin-addicted persons coerced into entering MMT in California (Brecht et al., 1993).

Drug courts, the latest form of coerced addiction treatment, were introduced in the USA in the late 1980s (Belenko, 2002). They quickly spread throughout the USA and were established in Australia, the United Kingdom and Canada. In drug courts, judges supervise an offender's addiction treatment, monitor their progress via urinalyses and can impose short periods of imprisonment if drug use is detected or the offender fails to comply with treatment. Typically US drug courts order drug-free treatment for six to twelve months where success is defined as abstinence for some minimum period such as six months.

It has been difficult to evaluate the effectiveness of drug courts (Belenko, 2002). Much of the US research has used quasi-experimental designs with poorly constructed comparison groups and only measured treatment retention and drug use while in treatment (Belenko, 2002; Wild et al., 2012). On balance, observational studies suggest that drug courts reduce recidivism over one to three years (Belenko, 2002). However, their effects are modest, as one would expect given the type of recidivist offenders with which they typically deal. A meta-analysis of fifty-seven quasi-experimental studies of drug courts (primarily in the USA) found that they reduced the recidivism rate from 50 per cent to 42 per cent (Aos, Miller and Drake, 2006).

Involuntary or compulsory treatment of addiction

The criminal courts have largely rejected the strong form of the brain disease model in disposing of addicted offenders. But there is another area of medico-legal practice where this model has been implicitly accepted. For over a century the civil law in a number of jurisdictions has permitted persons with severe forms of addiction to be compulsorily treated for their own good. Involuntary treatment of inebriety, for example, was introduced in Australia in the late nineteenth century (Lewis, 1992) but largely fell into disuse in the twentieth century (Webb, 2003). Switzerland allows civil commitment of addicted persons, but these admissions constituted less than 2% of admissions in the late 1990s (Grichting et al., 2002). Sweden also had a compulsory treatment system for alcohol and drug dependence for over a century, but the use of these provisions has declined in the past decade (Palm and Stenius, 2002). Many US states also allow the civil commitment of addicted persons, but these provisions have rarely been used (Gostin, 1991).

Compulsory addiction treatment for paternalistic reasons is again being trialled in the Australian states of New South Wales (NSW) and Victoria (NSW Parliament Legislative Council Standing Committee on Social issues, 2004; Webb, 2003). The rationale for its revival echoes that used to justify involuntary treatment of adults with serious mental illnesses. We first briefly review the arguments for the latter practice before assessing how well the case for involuntary psychiatric treatment fits the circumstances in which involuntary addiction treatment is advocated.

The case for involuntary psychiatric treatment

Libertarians (such as Thomas Szasz) argue that mental illness does not exist and hence it cannot be used to justify involuntary psychiatric treatment. Libertarians apart, it is generally accepted that adults with serious mental illnesses such as schizophrenia, bipolar disorder and severe depression are not fully autonomous when they are acutely mentally ill (McMillan, 2007). Opinions nonetheless differ on the advisability of involuntarily treating these persons (Prinsen and Van Delden, 2009) and the conditions under which such treatment should be provided, if it is allowed (Janssens et al., 2004).

The consensus view expressed in the law of many developed countries has been that the state is justified in using legal powers (under appropriate safeguards) to compulsorily treat persons with these mental illnesses for their own good and/or to protect others (McMillan, 2007). Involuntary treatment is usually provided under legislation that requires a medical practitioner to certify that the person has a serious mental illness and that it requires treatment in order to protect the person or others. This recommendation usually has to be supported by a psychiatrist and is subject to a judicial or quasi-judicial review (usually within a short period of admission), often with legal or other representation of the patient. Involuntarily treated patients are expected to receive effective and humane treatment using the least restrictive alternative, such as supervised treatment in the community. Patients who are detained and treated in this way are regularly reviewed by an independent tribunal.

This consensus view has recently come under renewed criticism (see Sheehan, 2009 for a recent review). The main criticism is that there is no evidence to support the major warrant for compulsory treatment, namely, that the loss of liberty is justified because it improves the health and quality of life of patients who receive such treatment (Burns and Dawson, 2009). As these critics point out, there are few randomised controlled trials supporting compulsory treatment, and the observational evidence for its effectiveness is weak and largely from poorly controlled studies (Burns and Dawson, 2009; Sheehan, 2009).

The case for involuntary treatment of addiction

The ethical acceptability of involuntary treatment for addiction is even more contested than that for serious psychiatric disorders (Gostin, 1991; Janssens et al., 2004). The case for involuntary addiction treatment is prima facie most plausible in the cases of drug-dependent people who are severely intoxicated and incapable of protecting themselves. In these cases, short-term involuntary medical treatment may arguably save a person's life. These cases would arguably also satisfy criteria for involuntary psychiatric hospitalisation in that they suffer from drug-induced mental disorders (e.g. delirium or psychosis). But many mental health acts specifically exclude persons with alcohol and drug dependence from provisions for involuntary psychiatric treatment. Even if these persons can be legally treated, psychiatric services are often reluctant to accept them because of the challenges in managing them in the same settings as persons with psychotic disorders.

Another contentious issue is what forms of addiction treatment can be ethically used under legal compulsion. The acute symptoms of intoxication and delirium can be safely and effectively treated over a period of days to weeks (Mattick and Hall, 1996). But longer-term treatment is required to sustain abstinence. Compelling patients to accept longer-term treatment, especially if it involves drugs, is regarded as ethically more problematic (Janssens et al., 2004). Some drug treatments benefit a substantial proportion of addicted persons who receive them, such as methadone and buprenorphine maintenance for opioid dependence, and acamprosate, disulfiram and naltrexone for alcohol dependence (Lingford-Hughes et al., 2004). Nonetheless, in recent parliamentary inquiries, very few persons have argued that it is ethically acceptable to compel patients to receive these treatments (see chapter 6 NSW Parliament Legislative Council Standing Committee on Social Issues, 2004).

One ethicist who has advocated for the compulsory drug treatment of addiction is Caplan (2006). He has argued for the compulsory use of the opioid antagonist naltrexone to treat heroin-dependent people. Caplan argues that heroin-dependent persons should be compelled to receive implantable naltrexone because it will restore the autonomy that has been undermined by their addiction. The drug will do this by reducing cravings and blocking the euphoric effects of heroin, if they succumb to temptation (Caplan, 2006). We have elsewhere pointed out several problems with Caplan's view (Hall et al., 2008).

First, as argued above, heroin addicts are not always incapable of making autonomous decisions. Caplan's proposal to force these patients to have naltrexone implants assumes that they have some capacities of choice (even if he wants to limit these choices to those he thinks are valid). In fact, he would ignore addicted persons' residual autonomy in order to create autonomy for up to six months.

Second, there is weak evidence for the long-term efficacy and safety of naltrexone implants in uncoerced heroin-addicted patients. It is a plausible hypothesis that implantable naltrexone will improve on the poor efficacy and safety of oral naltrexone by improving adherence, but this needs to be tested in controlled clinical trials. To date there have been too few trials of sufficient size and duration to evaluate the efficacy of implantable naltrexone. There is therefore a very weak basis for the claim that coerced naltrexone implants will be safe and effective when used under legal coercion.

The lack of evidence for the safety and efficacy is a more general problem shared by all forms of paternalistically motivated coerced addiction treatment. There are no randomised controlled trials in which large groups of addicted persons have been randomly assigned either to receive compulsory treatment or not. We thus do not have any evidence that the compulsorily treated group has higher rates of abstinence, or more realistically, reduced rates of hospitalisation, premature mortality and morbidity caused by their drug dependence (Broadstock et al., 2008; New South Wales Standing Committee on Social Issues, 2004). There are no observational studies that compare the outcomes of addicted persons treated involuntarily with those of addicted persons who were not. Most of the evidence on coerced addiction treatment comes from studies of offenders who have received addiction treatment under legal coercion (as summarised above). It is not clear how relevant this literature is to compulsory treatment for the patient's own good. The evidence typically cited for the efficacy of involuntary paternalistic treatment of addicted persons is weak, small case series of patients treated in this way (see reviews in Broadstock et al., 2008; New South Wales Standing Committee on Social Issues, 2004).

The historical experience with paternalistic coerced addiction treatment does not inspire confidence in its efficacy (Gostin, 1991). Legal provisions allowing civil commitment for addiction have largely fallen into disuse in Australia, the USA and other countries that permit it. In the absence of detailed historical analyses of the reasons for this, we offer the following hypotheses based on Hall's personal observations of compulsory treatment under the Inebriates legislation in NSW in the early 1970s and the evidence presented to a recent NSW Parliamentary review of this Act. Judicial oversight of the Act was perfunctory, with applications routinely accepted as authorising compulsory treatment for the maximum six months. Treatment was largely custodial and provided in rural areas in hospitals that were unattractive places to work. The level of security required to prevent patients from absconding made these settings more like gaols than hospitals.

Conclusions

The major evidence offered for the claim that addiction is a brain disease comprises the following: the chronicity of treated addiction; animal models that reveal persistent changes in brain circuitry produced by the chronic use of drugs of addiction; human neuroimaging studies suggesting that similar processes are at work in human addiction; and evidence that genetics plays a role in the risk of developing addiction. Critics of the brain disease model have countered that addictive drug use is more responsive to its consequences than the brain disease model would allow. This implies that most persons with any form of addiction recover without treatment, and that the drug use of persons treated for addiction can be reduced by providing small incentives for abstinence.

The competing moral and medical views of addiction have very different implications for addicted persons' responsibility for criminal acts. However, the justice system in many countries operates on a compromise between these views. It seems to be generally agreed that addicted persons find it difficult to resist compulsions to use drugs when undergoing withdrawal. Yet these compulsions are not generally seen as sufficiently strong to exculpate addicted persons for committing criminal acts to obtain and use drugs. It also seems to be accepted that addicted persons are not fully responsible for their actions in that their decision-making capacity is impaired, but not to the degree sufficient to exculpate them. This approach results in addicted persons being treated as responsible for their criminal acts while addiction is accepted as a reason for mitigation in setting penalties. The criminal courts often offer treatment to addicted offenders instead of imprisonment, with imprisonment reserved for those who fail to comply with treatment. This approach is best justified by a consequentialist theory of punishment in that coerced treatment is a more effective and less expensive way of reducing drug use and crime than imprisonment. There is reasonable evidence that this approach is effective in reducing re-offending by addicted offenders.

Compulsory treatment of addiction for paternalistic reasons presupposes severe impairment of autonomy in severely addicted persons, very much like that implied by the strongest form of the brain disease model of addiction. This type of compulsory addiction treatment was adopted a century ago in Australia and the USA but has largely fallen into disuse. It is now being revived using a rationale similar to that provided for involuntary psychiatric treatment. It is not clear how compelling this rationale is, and there is no evidence that this is an effective and cost-effective approach to dealing with such individuals. Compulsory addiction treatment requires a stronger justification than it has received to date, and any such treatment that is introduced should be rigorously evaluated.

REFERENCES

Agrawal, A., Verweij, K. J. H., Gillespie, N. A., Heath, A. C., Lessov-Schlaggar, C. N., et al. (2012). The genetics of addiction: a translational perspective. *Translational Psychiatry*, **2**, e140.

Ambermoon, P., Carter, A., Hall, W., Dissanayaka, N. N. W. and O'Sullivan, J. D. (2011). Impulse control disorders in patients with Parkinson's disease receiving dopamine replacement therapy: evidence and implications for the addictions field. *Addiction*, **106**, 283–93.

American Psychiatric Association (1994). *Diagnostic and Statistical Manual of Mental Disorders: DSM-IV*. Washington, DC: American Psychiatric Association.

Aos, S., Miller, M. and Drake, E. (2006). *Evidence-Based Public Policy Options to Reduce Future Prison Construction, Criminal Justice Costs, and Crime Rates*. Olympia, WA: Washington State Institute for Public Policy.

Bachman, J. G., Wadsworth, K. N., O'Malley, P. M., Johnston, L. D. and Schulenberg, J. (1997). *Smoking, Drinking, and Drug Use in Young Adulthood: The Impacts of New Freedoms and New Responsibilities*. Mahwah, NJ: Lawrence Erlbaum.

Belenko, S. (2002). The challenges of conducting research in drug treatment court settings. *Substance Use & Misuse*, **37**, 1635–64.

Bonnie, R. J. (2002). Responsibility for addiction. *Journal of the American Academy of Psychiatry and the Law*, **30**, 405–13.

Brecht, M. L., Anglin, M. D. and Wang, J. C. (1993). Treatment effectiveness for legally coerced versus voluntary methadone maintenance clients. *American Journal of Drug and Alcohol Abuse*, **19**, 89–106.

Broadstock, M., Brinson, D. and Weston, A. (2008). *The Effectiveness of Compulsory, Residential Treatment of Chronic Alcohol or Drug Addiction in Non-offenders: A Systematic Review of the Literature: Health Services Assessment Collaboration (HSAC)*, University of Canterbury.

Burns, T. and Dawson, J. (2009). Community treatment orders: how ethical without experimental evidence? *Psychological Medicine*, **39**, 1583–6.

Caplan, A. (2006). Ethical issues surrounding forced, mandated, or coerced treatment. *Journal of Substance Abuse Treatment*, **31**, 117–20.

Carter, A. and Hall, W. (2012). *Addiction Neuroethics: The Promises and Perils of Neuroscience Research on Addiction*. London: Cambridge University Press.

Chandler, R. K., Fletcher, B. W. and Volkow, N. D. (2009). Treating drug abuse and addiction in the criminal justice system: improving public health and safety. *JAMA*, **301**, 183–90.

Charland, L. C. (2002). Cynthia's dilemma: consenting to heroin prescription. *American Journal of Bioethics*, **2**, 37–47.

Courtwright, D. (2010). The NIDA brain-disease paradigm: history, resistance, and spinoffs. *BioSocieties*, **5**, 137–47.

Degenhardt, L. and Hall, W. (2012). Extent of illicit drug use and dependence, and their contribution to the global burden of disease. *The Lancet*, **379**, 55–70.

Dolan, K. (1991). Prisons and AIDS: a review of the VIIth International Conference on AIDS. *International Journal of Drug Policy*, **2**, 23–6.

Fergusson, D. M., Boden, J. M. and Horwood, L. J. (2008). The developmental antecedents of illicit drug use: evidence from a 25-year longitudinal study. *Drug and Alcohol Dependence*, **96**, 165–77.

Foddy, B. and Savulescu, J. (2006). Addiction and autonomy: can addicted people consent to the prescription of their drug of addiction? *Bioethics*, **20**, 1–15.

Gordon, M. S., Kinlock, T. W., Schwartz, R. P. and O'Grady, K. E. (2008). A randomized clinical trial of methadone maintenance for prisoners: findings at 6 months post-release. *Addiction*, **103**, 1333–42.

Gostin, L. O. (1991). Compulsory treatment for drug-dependent persons: Justifications for a public health approach to drug dependency. *The Milbank Quarterly*, 561–93.

Grichting, E., Uchtenhagen, A. and Rehm, J. (2002). Modes and impact of coercive inpatient treatment for drug-related conditions in Switzerland. *European Addiction Research*, **8**, 78–83.

Hall, W. (1996). *Methadone Maintenance Treatment as a Crime Control Measure*. Sydney: NSW Bureau of Crime Statistics and Research.

Hall, W., Capps, B. and Carter, A. (2008). The use of depot naltrexone under legal coercion: the case for caution. *Addiction*, **103**, 1922–4.

Hall, W. and Lucke, J. (2010). Legally coerced treatment for drug using offenders: ethical and policy issues. *Crime and Justice Bulletin*, **144**, 1–12.

Heyman, G. (2009). *Addiction: A Disorder of Choice.* Cambridge, MA: Harvard University Press.

Higgins, S. T., Bernstein, I. M., Washio, Y., Heil, S. H., Badger, G. J. et al. (2010). Effects of smoking cessation with voucher-based contingency management on birth outcomes. *Addiction*, **105**, 2023–30.

Hubbard, R. L. (1989). *Drug Abuse Treatment: A National Study of Effectiveness.* London: University of North Carolina Press.

Hyman, S. E. (2007). The neurobiology of addiction: implications for voluntary control of behavior. *American Journal of Bioethics*, **7**, 8–11.

Janssens, M., Van Rooij, M., ten Have, H., Kortmann, F. A. M. and Van Wijmen, F. C. B. (2004). Pressure and coercion in the care for the addicted: ethical perspectives. *Journal of Medical Ethics*, **30**, 453–8.

Kendler, K. S., Chen, X., Dick, D., Maes, H., Gillespie, N. et al. (2012). Recent advances in the genetic epidemiology and molec.ular genetics of substance use disorders. *Nature Neuroscience*, **15**, 181–9.

Kincaid, H. and Sullivan, J. A. (2010). Medical models of addiction. In D. Ross, H. Kincaid, D. Spurrett and P. Collins (eds.), *What Is addiction?* (pp. 353–73). Cambridge, MA: MIT Press.

Koob, G. F. and Le Moal, M. (2006). *Neurobiology of Addiction.* New York: Academic Press.

Koob, G. F. and Volkow, N. D. (2010). Neurocircuitry of addiction. *Neuropsychopharmacology*, **35**, 217–38.

Leshner, A. I. (1997). Addiction is a brain disease, and it matters. *Science*, **278**, 45–7.

Levy, N. (2012). Autonomy, responsibility and the oscillation of preference. In A. Carter, J. Illes and W. Hall (eds.), *Addiction Neuroethics: The Ethics of Addiction Research and Treatment* (pp. 139–52). New York: Elsevier.

Lewis, M. J. (1992). The early alcoholism treatment movement in Australia, 1859–1939. *Drug and Alcohol Review*, **11**, 75–84.

Lingford-Hughes, A., Welch, S. and Nutt, D. (2004). Evidence-based guidelines for the pharmacological management of substance misuse, addiction and comorbidity: recommendations from the British Association for Psychopharmacology. *Journal of Psychopharmacology*, **18**, 293–335.

Mattick, R. P. and Hall, W. (1996). Are detoxification programmes effective? *Lancet*, **347**, 97–100.

McLellan, A. T., Lewis, D. C., O'Brien, C. P. and Kleber, H. D. (2000). Drug dependence, a chronic medical illness: implications for treatment, insurance, and outcomes evaluation. *JAMA*, **284**, 1689–95.

McMillan, J. A. (2007). Mental illness and compulsory treatment. In R. E. Ashcroft and R. Gillon (eds.), *Principles of Health Care ethics* (2nd edn., pp. 443–8). Chichester: John Wiley & Sons.

Moore, T. J., Ritter, A. and Caulkins, J. P. (2007). The costs and consequences of three policy options for reducing heroin dependency. *Drug and Alcohol Review*, **26**, 369–78.

Morse, S. J. (2004). Medicine and morals, craving and compulsion. *Substance Use & Misuse*, **39**, 437–60.

New South Wales Standing Committee on Social Issues (2004). *Report on Inebriates Act 1912*. Sydney: New South Wales Parliament.

NSW Parliament Legislative Council Standing Committee on Social issues (2004). *Report on the Inebriates Act 1912*. Sydney: The Committee. Report 33. Available at: www.parliament.nsw.gov.au/Prod/parlment/committee.nsf/0/2578557b574b0450ca256f000000123b/$FILE/01%20Inebriates%20Report%20-%20Introduction.pdf (Accessed 25 July 2012).

Palm, J. and Stenius, K. (2002). Sweden: integrated compulsory treatment. *European Addiction Research*, **8**, 69–77.

Porter, L., Arif, A. and Curran, W. J. (1986). *The Law and the Treatment of Drug- and Alcohol-Dependent Persons: A Comparative Study of Existing Legislation*. Geneva: World Health Organization.

Prinsen, E. and Van Delden, J. (2009). Can we justify eliminating coercive measures in psychiatry? *Journal of Medical Ethics*, **35**, 69–73.

Robins, L. (1974). *The Vietnam Drug User Returns* (Special Action Office Monograph, Series A, No. 2). Washington, DC: US Government Printing Office.

Robins, L. N. (1993). Vietnam veterans' rapid recovery from heroin addiction: a fluke or normal expectation? *Addiction*, **88**, 1041–54.

Ross, D., Sharp, C., Vuchinich, R. and Spurrett, D. (2008). *Midbrain Mutiny: The Picoeconomics and Neuroeconomics of Disordered Gambling*. Cambridge, MA: MIT Press.

Satel, S. (1998). For addicts, force is the best medicine. *Wall Street Journal*.

(2001). Is drug addiction a brain disease? In P. Heymann and W. Brownsberger (eds.), *Drug Addiction and Drug Policy: The Struggle to Control Dependence* (pp. 118–43). Cambridge, MA: Harvard University Press.

Sheehan, K. A. (2009). Compulsory treatment in psychiatry. *Current Opinion in Psychiatry*, **22**, 582–6.

Simpson, D. and Friend, H. (1988). Legal status and long-term outcomes for addicts in the DARP Followup Project. In C. Leukefeld and F.M. Tims (eds.), *Compulsory Treatment of Drug Abuse: Research and Clinical Practice* (pp. 81–98). Rockville, MD: NIDA.

Sutherland, W. J., Bellingan, L., Bellingham, J. R., Blackstock, J. J., Bloomfield, R. M. et al. (2012). A collaboratively-derived science-policy research agenda. *PLoS ONE*, **7**, e31824.

Swift, W., Coffey, C., Carlin, J. B., Degenhardt, L. and Patton, G. C. (2008). Adolescent cannabis users at 24 years: trajectories to regular weekly use and dependence in young adulthood. *Addiction*, **103**, 1361–70.

Szasz, T. S. (1975). *Ceremonial Chemistry: The Ritual Persecution of Drugs, Addicts, and Pushers*. London: Routledge.

Vaillant, G. (2001). If addiction is involuntary, how can punishment help? In P. B. Heymann and W. N. Brownsberger (eds.), *Drug Addiction and Drug Policy: The Struggle to Control Dependence* (pp. 144–67). Cambridge, MA: Harvard University Press.

Volkow, N., Fowler, J. S., Wang, G. J., Teland, F. and Baler, R. (2010). Imaging dopamine's role in drug abuse and addiction. In I. L. S. Iversen, S. Dunnett and A. Bjorklund (eds.), *Dopamine Handbook* (pp. 407–17): Oxford University Press.

Volkow, N. D. and Li, T. K. (2004). Drug addiction: the neurobiology of behaviour gone awry. *Nature Reviews. Neuroscience*, **5**, 963–70.

Webb, M. B. (2003). Compulsory alcoholism treatment in New South Wales. *Medicine and Law*, **22**, 311–27.

Weintraub, D., Koester, J., Potenza, M. N., Siderowf, A. D. and Stacy, M. et al. (2010). Impulse control disorders in Parkinson disease: a cross-sectional study of 3090 patients. *Archives of Neurology*, **67**, 589–95.

Wild, T. C., Wolfe, J. and Hyshka, E. (2012). Consent and coercion in addiction treatment. In A. Carter, J. Illes and W. Hall (eds.), *Addiction Neuroethics: The Ethics of Addiction Research and Treatment* (pp. 153–74). New York: Elsevier.

Yaffe, G. (2001). Recent work on addiction and responsible agency. *Philosophy and Public Affairs*, **30**, 178–221.

9 Assessment and modification of free will via scientific techniques: two challenges

Nicole A Vincent

ABSTRACT

This chapter highlights two challenges for the broadly compatibilist idea that cognitive neuroscience and behavioural genetics might one day assist in the assessment, restoration and enhancement of free will by developing techniques to measure and modify people's mental capacities. First, I argue that it is still far from clear precisely how the notion of 'capacity' that lies at the core of the compatibilist approach should be understood in order to fulfil its normative function. Second, some mental incapacities can be equally re-described as character flaws, which makes it ambiguous whether particular neurological or genetic features should diminish guilt, mitigate, and perhaps even excuse, or condemn and aggravate, and whether it would be appropriate to offer, coerce or compel affected parties to undergo medical treatments. I highlight these challenges not to undermine compatibilism but to strengthen it by discussing its weaknesses, and I relate my discussion of these weaknesses to some of the claims made by other authors in this volume.

The shifting conceptual foundations of neurolaw

Hard determinism

Early scholarship in the field of neurolaw that dealt with the topic of responsibility often presupposed a hard determinist theoretical foundation. For instance, in their much-cited and discussed paper Joshua Greene and Jonathan Cohen argue:

> New neuroscience will change the law, not by undermining its current assumptions, but by transforming people's moral intuitions about free will and responsibility. This change in moral outlook will result not from the discovery of crucial new facts or clever new arguments, but from a new appreciation of old arguments, bolstered by vivid new illustrations provided by cognitive neuroscience. We foresee, and recommend, a shift away from punishment

aimed at retribution in favour of a more progressive, consequentialist approach to the criminal law. (2004:1775)

Similarly, in a more recent article Anthony Cashmore argues:

> Many discussions about human behavior center around the relative importance of genes and environment, a topic often discussed in terms of nature versus nurture. In concentrating on this question of the relative importance of genes and environment, a crucial component of the debate is often missed: an individual cannot be held responsible for either his genes or his environment. From this simple analysis, surely it follows that individuals cannot logically be held responsible for their behavior. Yet a basic tenet of the judicial system and the way that we govern society is that we hold individuals accountable (we consider them at fault) on the assumption that people can make choices that do not simply reflect a summation of their genetic and environmental history. As de Duve has written, 'If ... neuronal events in the brain determine behavior, irrespective of whether they are conscious or unconscious, it is hard to find room for free will. But if free will does not exist, there can be no responsibility, and the structure of human societies must be revised.' (2010:4499)

Subsequent reflection on the role that genetics, the environment and stochasticism play in shaping human behaviour leads Cashmore to assert that 'we are mechanical forces of nature [which] have evolved the phenomenon of consciousness, which [in turn] has conferred upon us the illusion of responsibility', and thus he concludes that 'it is time for the legal system to confront [t]he reality [that] not only do we have no more free will than a fly or a bacterium, in actuality we have no more free will than a bowl of sugar. The laws of nature are uniform throughout, and these laws do not accommodate the concept of free will' (2010:4503).

In this hard determinism inspired picture, scientific findings are claimed to show that everyone's actions are consequences of factors such as the laws of nature over which they never had, nor could they be expected to have had, any control. This, in turn, is taken to entail that nobody is responsible for what they do, since everyone does the only thing that they ever could have done. Hard determinism rules out free will by ruling out alternative possibilities of action, and responsibility for action on this view presupposes free will. That then leads adherents of this position to claim that backward-looking aims of punishment like retribution should be abandoned and replaced with forward-looking aims like prediction, prevention and reform.

However, even if we set aside questions about such matters as whether scientific experiments can confirm the truth of metaphysical theses like determinism, or whether the truth of determinism would indeed necessitate the pursuit of those particular forward-looking aims, a more basic problem is that these arguments simply ignore an approach according to which determinism does not challenge responsibility.

Compatibilism and its capacitarian core

Predicating responsibility not on the universe's metaphysics but on people's psychology, *compatibilists* suggest that people are responsible for what they do only if at the time of acting they possessed a sufficient quantity of the right kinds of mental capacities. John Fischer and Mark Ravizza (1998) re-deploy this idea, though they give mental capacities physical form since on their account we are responsible for those actions that issue from our own *moderately reasons-responsive mechanisms*. Roughly speaking, in Fischer and Ravizza's framework moderately reasons-responsive mechanisms implement, embody or instantiate mental capacities which are required for moral agency. They also emphasize two further points: (1) that incapacities for which we are responsible do not exculpate (the *tracing* condition); and (2) that those mental capacities must be our own (the *ownership* condition). But at the core of their account lies the same familiar *capacitarian* idea that responsibility tracks mental capacity.

Various considerations might be cited to explain why the last decade has seen a gradual shift away from hard determinism towards compatibilism in neurolaw research and scholarship. For instance, much lay and legal mileage is undoubtedly gained by moving away from the view that responsibility hinges on the universe's metaphysics and towards the view that responsibility hinges on people's psychology; this is, after all, a very intuitive picture of what matters for responsibility. Relatedly, because compatibilism takes the law's commitment to responsibility seriously, this makes it easier for the law to reciprocate by taking science seriously. The law's staple diet consists of a generous serving of responsibility talk and practices, and a theoretical approach like hard determinism which eliminates responsibility is not one that could ever be expected to be taken seriously by the law. But, in my opinion, the reason why Fischer and Ravizza's particular approach has been so prominent in much of the recent compatibilist-inspired neurolaw scholarship is because of the *mechanistic* way in which they render the notion of 'mental capacity', since this in principle opens up a wealth of opportunities for the scientific community to study responsibility. For instance, scientists might study what mechanisms paradigmatically fully responsible agents possess and how those mechanisms operate. They might work on developing techniques to more individually, accurately and less subjectively inspect people's mechanisms to gauge their true mental capacities. They might study how youth, advanced age and mental disorders affect these mechanisms. Or they might indeed even attempt to develop interventions to create, restore and enhance the function of these mechanisms in order to create, restore and enhance people's responsibility-relevant mental capacities.

If we adopt an approach according to which a person's responsibility hinges on the degree to which they possess the right kinds of mental capacities which are in turn embodied in physical mechanisms – for instance, though not necessarily, in brain mechanisms[1] – then scientists will have a role to play in contributing to our understanding of free will and to improving our responsibility practices by developing techniques to illuminate and modify those mechanisms.

The two challenges

A similar range of ideas about the contribution that science can make to our understanding of free will and responsibility and to our moral and legal responsibility practices is also reflected in some of this volume's other chapters.

For instance, adopting an approach that explicitly re-deploys John Martin Fischer and Mark Ravizza's reasons-responsive compatibilism, Farah Focquaert, Andrea L. Glenn and Adrian Raine write that empirical findings reveal that psychopaths have affective and cognitive deficits – i.e. impaired mental capacities of a moral responsibility relevant sort – that either partially or fully diminish their guilt (see Chapter 6 of this volume). They argue that we should divert such individuals away from the criminal justice system and focus instead on developing and deploying medical treatments to restore/enhance these capacities. Gerben Meynen's piece analyses the impact that mental disorders have on (free) will in terms of the mental disorder's impact on the mental capacities involved in behavioural option generation, selection and translation into action. His characterization of drug addiction-related free will impairments as impairments of the brain's free will circuits again reflects a strong capacitarian and mechanistic approach. Although he puts his suggestions about interventions in terms of treatments for disorders, in effect the aim is to repair impaired circuits in order to restore or create the constituent capacities that make up the mental capacities required for behavioural option generation, selection and translation into action (see Chapter 7 of this volume). Finally, Maartje Schermer's discussion of how various neuromodulation techniques might reduce, restore or enhance autonomy is explicitly and thoroughly capacitarian (see Chapter 11 of this volume). For instance, in the context of talking about a conception of autonomy as a capacity for self-governance, she writes that this 'is a psychological capacity that depends on certain mental abilities [a synonym for "capacities"], like the abilities to understand information, to hold certain goals and values, to reflect on them, to reason and to make rational choices, and to act on those choices' (p. 207). She explains that '[a]ltering brain structure or functioning can obviously affect mental capacities, including those ... that are crucial for autonomy' (p. 206). The notion that responsibility and free will hinge critically on mental capacities is central to each of these authors' analyses.

Nevertheless, despite having advanced a similar range of suggestions as these and other authors elsewhere (e.g. Vincent 2010), below I highlight two challenges which in my view have yet to be tackled in order to secure a sound conceptual foundation for scholarly and empirical research in this field, namely: (1) how to understand the notion of capacity so that it does the normative work that it was intended to do; and (2) how to distinguish mental capacity deficits which typically excuse/mitigate from character flaws which typically condemn/aggravate.

Mental capacity, *you say?*

Compatibilism was meant to provide an account of how responsibility is possible without making reference to notions that do not fit a deterministic picture of the universe – e.g. without requiring access to genuine alternative possibilities. However, keeping in mind the centrality of the concept of capacity to the compatibilist approach, I worry that the senses in which a deterministic universe can accommodate capacities are not obviously senses that can ground responsibility.

Consider how Fischer and Ravizza attempt to capture the notion of capacity. On their account mental capacities are meant to be embodied in moderately reasons-responsive mechanisms. We are told that for a mechanism to be moderately reasons-responsive it has to be *regularly receptive* to reasons (this just means that the mechanism has to be sensitive to reasons in a non-irregular or rationally defensible manner) and *weakly reactive* to those reasons to which it is receptive (which on their account requires that in at least some possible world that mechanism will react to those reasons even if in this world it does not). The notion of 'moderateness' is crucial to their account because it is meant to capture the idea that mechanisms might have capacities rather than just determinate ways of operating and, importantly, that people might be blameworthy when they do not use those capacities, when they are weak-willed. However, my worry is that in a given scenario any particular mechanism will either *respond* or *not respond* to the reasons to which it was receptive — there is no in-between and thus apparently no moderateness. I am stuck in the here-and-now of this world with no ability to hop across into other possible worlds. Thus, I cannot see how drawing attention to how a mechanism from which my action issued in this world might operate in *other* possible worlds is meant to soften the blow of the deterministic challenge to responsibility.

Neil Levy argues that Fischer and Ravizza's analysis of 'capacity' and 'moderateness' in terms of what happens in other possible worlds is not problematic on account of the sort of reason which I highlight because they are not proposing an account of conditions under which mechanisms are moderately reasons-responsive and thus under which people possess capacities. Rather, they are only offering an analysis of how to understand the notions of moderateness and capacity (Levy 2008:227–8). Here is how John Fischer puts this point elsewhere:

> Given that one can *make sense* of modal or dispositional properties (at least in part) in terms of non-actual possible worlds, on my favored approach to moral responsibility non-actual possible worlds (or hypothetical scenarios of certain sorts) are pertinent to moral responsibility, but not in virtue of indicating genuine metaphysical access; rather, they help to specify the sorts of properties that must be exemplified by the actual-sequence mechanism that issues in the behavior in question. [T]he *purpose* of the assessment of alternative scenarios makes the crucial difference. If the point or purpose of the invocation of alternative scenarios [had been] to establish that one has genuine metaphysical access to alternative possibilities, then I grant that only ... scenarios with the same past and laws as the actual world [would have been] relevant ... But this is not the purpose or 'use' to which I put alternative scenarios in my approach to moral responsibility; rather, the purpose of the assessment of ranges of non-actual possibilities is to establish the nature of the properties that are in fact (actually) exemplified in the sequence of events leading to the behavior under consideration. (Fischer 2005:147–8, my emphasis)

However, although I appreciate the subtlety of their strategy – that they merely attempt to provide an analysis of what we mean by the notion of capacity, not to suggest that anyone has metaphysical access to other possible worlds – my problem with this kind of reply is that it seems like a proposed analysis of capacity should surely satisfy at least two conditions. Not only should it capture a plausible meaning of the word *capacity* in which anyone who ever turned out to have (sufficient) capacity in that sense could be deemed responsible for what they do (let us call this the *relevance* condition). This sense should also be one that can find implementation within a deterministic universe, for otherwise nobody will ever actually have capacity in that sense in a deterministic universe (let us call this the *implementability* condition). Viewed against a backdrop of these two conditions, what the worry I express above amounts to is that while Fischer and Ravizza's analysis of capacity satisfies the first of these conditions – i.e. it yields a plausible sense of capacity that could, at least in principle, warrant practices like blame and retributive punishment – it does not satisfy the second condition, since without access to other possible worlds nobody would ever actually have capacities.

For precisely the same sorts of reasons why the incompatibilist *alternative possibilities* sense of capacity does not warrant blame or retributive punishment in the eyes of those non-compatibilists who believe that determinism is true – that is, in the eyes of hard determinists; namely, because nobody would actually have alternative possibilities – so too the fact that nobody can hop across into other possible worlds also means that Fischer and Ravizza's analysis of capacity cannot warrant such things as blame and retributive punishment. The mere fact that this (the possible worlds analysis) is what Fischer and Ravizza mean when they use the word *capacity* no more justifies holding people responsible than does the fact that what libertarians mean by *can* is something like 'genuine alternative possibilities'. What people mean by the words that they utter has little normative force if what they mean cannot be realized in the world in which we live.

To be clear, my point is not that a deterministic world has no room for capacities. For instance, consider briefly the following six senses of capacity. There is a sense in which things that have not yet happened, but which will happen as the future unfolds, have the capacity to happen. We might call this the *unfolding* sense of capacity. Then, as I recently suggest elsewhere:

> [w]e might have a *dispositional* sense of capacity in mind when we say that wine glasses are fragile since they will probably break if they are exposed to a sufficiently forceful shock (e.g. see Levy 2008:227–8). There is a sense in which I have the capacity to lift a 40 kilogram box but not an 80 kilogram box given my musculature — we might call this the *strength* sense. A bridge might have capacities in the *stress* sense in which in virtue of the tensile properties of the materials from which it is built it can withstand a particular load. In the *volumetric* sense containers of different dimensions have the capacity to hold different amounts of stuff. And given my ability to speak English, Polish and some Dutch, we might also recognize an *ability* sense of capacity. The world clearly has capacities in all of these senses. In a deterministic universe the future would presumably indeed unfold as time rolled on, glasses would usually break when dropped, some people would be stronger than others, bridges would collapse under too much stress, containers of varying sizes would hold different volumes of stuff, and some people would speak more languages than others. (Vincent 2013a:183)

I enumerate these senses of capacity and point out that deterministic worlds would have capacities in all of these senses in part to ensure that I am not misinterpreted as suggesting that a deterministic universe simply cannot accommodate capacities. It can. However, my point is that it is still very far from clear how Fischer and Ravizza's sense of capacity – a sense which they analyse in terms of what a given mechanism does in other possible worlds – (or any of these other senses for that matter) is meant to address the problem which it was meant to address: namely, to explain how responsibility can be reconciled with determinism while keeping in mind that nobody would have access to genuine alternative possibilities.[2] My unease can be stated in another and more general way. I worry that compatibilism may not yet have delivered on its promise of providing an account of responsibility that does not predicate responsibility on the existence of alternative possibilities. It may rather have merely swapped one set of modal ideas for another set of modal ideas. Instead of talking about alternative possibilities as we once did, these days we talk about capacities. However the considerations that I raise above lead me to worry that this is merely a terminological rather than a substantive change.

The chief compatibilist innovation, and indeed its most appealing feature, is its capacitarian core. However, what we still need is a better account of what we mean by *capacity*, and of why having (sufficient) capacity in that sense might at least sometimes justify paradigm cases of responsibility practices such as blame and genuinely retributive punishment.

Why not character flaws?

In recent years, the capacitarian idea that *mental incapacities excuse* and that sufficiently impaired mental capacities diminish guilt which lies at the core of the compatibilist approach has played a prominent role in what various people have said about the moral and legal responsibility of psychopaths. Naturally, this idea is much more broadly accepted than just in debates about the responsibility of psychopaths, and so this section's discussion of psychopathy should be treated as illustrative of the broader problem that I am attempting to highlight – namely, an uncritical acceptance of the capacitarian interpretation of data (with a corresponding set of moral and legal implications in regards to responsibility) that could equally be interpreted in a charactarian manner (that has radically different moral and legal implications).

According to those who endorse the currently prominent compatibilist approach to free will and responsibility, empirical studies suggest that affect also plays an important role in moral judgment (e.g. see the special issue edited by Gerrans and Kennett 2006; especially Prinz 2006) alongside reason, and that psychopaths have deficits in both affective and rational mental capacities (Blair 2008; Hare and Neumann 2010; Kennett 2010). These deficits appear to be congenital with at least a partial genetic and neurophysiological basis (Harenski et al. 2010). They are not something for which psychopaths can be straightforwardly blamed. Hence compatibilist-inspired scholars have argued that psychopaths should be at least partly excused for what they do, or that their sentences should be partly mitigated (Fine and Kennett 2004; Levy 2007; Haji 2010). Those who endorse this *mental incapacity account* usually characterize psychopathy as a kind of insanity or moral madness, as a deficit, disorder or mental illness/disease. For instance, they talk about psychopaths being significantly less able than non-psychopaths to do certain things which moral agents must be capable of doing, and about them having neurocognitive deficiencies which they compare to blindness and disability. This approach and related terminology depict psychopaths as victims of mental disease, not dissimilar to criminally insane individuals. On this view psychopaths labour under the weight of a mental disorder which is the true cause of their strange, harmful, illegal and immoral behaviour through the mental incapacities that it creates.

However, under another description psychopaths have serious character flaws. In contrast to the mental incapacity account, those who endorse the *character flaw account* view psychopaths as agents whose actions express their truly rotten character/personality and corrupt values. Accordingly, on this view, they ought to be condemned for the evils that they inflict. Heidi Maibom has conveyed this point particularly clearly and forcefully. 'To put it colloquially,' she says, 'the psychopath is more bad than mad. In fact, unless we think that bad people must also be mad, there is little reason to think of [them] as mad' (2008:179). She argues that 'part of what we think makes bad people bad is exactly their moral beliefs. It is, in part, their beliefs about the moral value of Jews that makes Nazis so culpable. Another way to put the same point is to say... that allowing moral ignorance to be an excusing condition would be to rule out the possibility of there being evil people' (2008:180). For these reasons Maibom urges that 'both the disorder that psychopaths experience and the sorts of murders they perpetrate are better examples of badness than madness. Psychopathy is a moral disorder, and psychopaths' actions are the results of their being bad more than of their being mad. 'Consequently', she concludes, 'being a psychopath does not count as an excuse since it would contravene the entire point of our legal system to exculpate the bad' (2008:182).

Maibom's position seems to gain further weight when we consider how the revised version of the psychopathy checklist (PCL-R) describes psychopaths. Among other features, psychopaths are described as being emotionally cold, shallow, superficial, insincere, deceitful, manipulative, predatory, parasitic, selfish, callous, aggressive, sadistic, domineering, opinionated, cocky, arrogant, narcissistic, boastful, shameless, short-tempered, impulsive, impatient, stimulation-seeking, careless, lacking forethought, unreflective, irresponsible and unremorseful. This list does not read like a typical clinical description of the aetiology or symptomatology of a genuine mental disease or illness. Rather, it seems to testify to psychopaths' many nasty and condemnable personality or character traits. And given these character traits, it is hardly surprising that psychopaths commit some of the most horrendous crimes imaginable.

It would therefore appear that before we can decide whether to excuse or to condemn psychopaths, we must first ascertain whether to classify them as *bad* or as *mad* (Kröber and Lau 2000). However, the badness/madness distinction is just as slippery and elusive as the character flaw/mental incapacity distinction. Admittedly, there are some cases where a madness or disease interpretation suggests itself more readily. Two examples are the famous case of Phineas Gage and the more recent case of Burns and Swerdlow's (2003) forty-year-old patient who developed paedophilic urges when a tumour developed that pressed on the orbitofrontal region of his brain. He lost those urges when the tumour was resected, and then regained and subsequently lost them yet again as the tumour regrew and was again removed. Both of these examples involve trauma, sufficiently sudden changes and visually identifiable causal factors that we intuitively view as 'damage' and 'disease'. Consequently, it feels more appropriate to attribute the observed changes in such a person's behaviour to disease rather than to them. The person, we might suppose, lies buried beneath the disease, or maybe they no longer even exist because they were obliterated or transformed into a very different person by the disease or damage. However, what should we say about cases in which slowly and gradually developing congenital brain differences result in behaviour similar to that exhibited by Burns and Swerdlow's patient? Should the behaviour of such 'natural-born paedophiles' – i.e. people who have always had brains that function in a similar way to Burns and Swerdlow's patient's brain when it was compressed by the tumour – be attributed to disease even though their brains may have always been like that? Or should their behaviour be attributed to them? Alternatively, how about people who develop certain brain features early in life – either because of their terrible upbringing (perhaps people like Robert Alton Harris (see Watson 1987) and Susan Wolf's (1987) fictional JoJo character), or due to genetic factors combined with environmental influences (Caspi et al. 2002) – and those brain features now predispose them to committing atrocities? Would their behaviour be an expression of a disease of their minds? Or would it be an expression of their evil selves? Whether we classify psychopaths' mental condition as madness or as badness is not likely to be something that might, for instance, be discovered under a microscope by a pathologist in a lab, or during a health check-up with your physician. The physical facts underdetermine our characterization (Reimer 2008; Vincent 2011a:90). Thus, the mad/bad distinction is unlikely to settle how character flaws can be distinguished from mental incapacities.

Traditional psychiatric techniques based on behavioural observations are also unlikely to settle this matter because behavioural data – e.g. the fact that someone has always been nasty – is compatible with either a character flaw or a mental incapacity description. For instance, suppose that behavioural observations revealed that a particular individual always made the wrong moral judgments. Such data might indicate only that they do not rather than that they cannot make the right moral judgments. Alternatively, suppose that behavioural observations revealed that this same individual has seldom or never controlled his or her angry outbursts. This too might establish only that they do not rather than that they cannot control themselves. As Bernadette McSherry points out, 'it is impossible to devise an objectively verifiable test to determine when an accused could not control him or herself and when he or she merely would not' (2004:188). Robert Sapolsky also draws attention to the difficulties associated with 'distinguishing between an irresistible impulse and one that is to any extent resistible but which was not resisted' (2004:1790). The fact that someone has rarely or maybe even never done something such as acting in a morally appropriate manner does not by itself establish that they cannot do it. It might just be that they are lazy or that they do not want to do it. Behavioural observations cannot settle this matter because, conceptually speaking, a modal fallacy is committed when conclusions about what cannot occur are derived purely from observations about what does not occur (Vincent 2011b).

Furthermore, even if neuroimaging scans identified brain-based correlates of psychopathy, this would not settle the matter either because it would still be unclear whether such images would have revealed the neurophysiological bases of psychopaths' mental incapacities or the implementation of their character flaws (Reimer 2008; Sadler 2008). Without a clear empirical basis for distinguishing those features of brain structure or function which correlate with character from those features which correlate with mental capacities, there would be no particular reason to suppose that what such scans would have identified would support either the mental incapacity account or the character flaw account. However, given the ease with which one can shift back and forth between viewing something in one moment as a mental incapacity and in the next moment as a character flaw, and given that at the conceptual level it is not clear how to distinguish one from the other, there is little hope that empirical investigations of brain structure and function can settle this.

Finally, some have tried to get around this problem by suggesting that there is nothing here that needs to be resolved, because the content for which psychopaths are condemned (i.e. their bad character) is different from the content for which they are excused (i.e. their actions) (Levy 2007; Vincent 2011a). There is actually no contradiction in allowing the same evidence to both excuse and condemn. However, the limitations of this response manifest themselves when we consider possible future medical treatments that would, for instance, make psychopaths more empathic. Although such treatments sound attractive when they are conceptualized as aiding in the creation, restoration or enhancement of a mental capacity (Bublitz and Merkel 2009; Merkel et al. 2007) – after all, who could object to giving psychopaths a (better) mental tool with which to reason morally[3] – these medical treatments begin to sound troubling and even sinister when they are re-described as attempts to modify psychopaths' character (Greely 2008; Lewis 1963). In his book *A Clockwork Orange*, Anthony Burgess put this worry as follows: 'Does God want woodness or the choice of goodness? Is a man who chooses the bad perhaps in some way better than a man who has the good imposed upon him?' (2000). The central idea, if I understand Burgess correctly, is that humans are not things to be modified and fiddled with at the state's discretion. We are not like broken toys that can be tinkered with and fixed like mere objects. Rather, to respect our dignity, we must be engaged with as agents *via* our capacity for reason and reflection. From this perspective, it would be thoroughly undignified to impose on anyone an utter inflexibility (hence Burgess's reference to 'woodness') in virtue of which they could do no other than to do (what we say is) good, and some (Duff 2005) have argued that respect for this dignity requires punishment not treatment.[4] My point, which I borrow from Lewis (cited above), is that while the medicalization of criminal behaviour and talk of 'treating' afflicted individuals with medical procedures to 'cure' them of their 'mental incapacities' initially sounds humane, compassionate and progressive in comparison to punishment, if what such treatments would alter – perhaps against their wishes and protests – is people's character, then they may in fact be the ultimate examples of state brutality. Even if we set aside concerns about the efficacy and side effects of such treatments, at a conceptual and normative level we may object to modifying people's character because it is one thing to punish someone for what they do or to imprison them for who we think they are and thus what we think they might do if set free, but it is quite another to change them and to deny them the right to think what they want to think and to be who they want to be (Shaw 2014; Vincent 2014).

The above discussion highlights a tension between two equally plausible but mutually incompatible views of psychopathy. This tension which can be captured by employing a variety of different but related dichotomies:[5]

Mental incapacity	—	Character flaw
Cannot	—	Does not
Mad	—	Bad
Disease	—	Person
Illness	—	Depravity
Disorder	—	Difference
Has	—	Is

Do psychopaths have mental incapacities or character flaws? Is it that they cannot understand what they ought to do and to control their actions in light of that understanding, or that they just do not exercise their cognitive and volitional capacities? Are psychopaths mad or are they bad? Is their behaviour the expression of a mental disease, or is it just them doing what they want to do? Are they mentally ill or simply depraved? Are psychopaths' brains disordered or merely different?[6] Do these individuals have psychopathy, or is it rather that some people are psychopaths?

The distinction between character (flaws) and mental (in)capacities plays a pivotal role within courtrooms and in important social debates. On the capacitarian account mental incapacities (of the right kind and degree) excuse or mitigate, but character flaws do not. If anything, character flaws condemn and aggravate. But given what I have said above, precisely how are we meant to determine whether something should be classified as a mental capacity deficit or as a character flaw, whether the person who exhibits the related physical symptoms should be excused or condemned, whether at sentencing their punishment should be mitigated or aggravated, and whether they should be treated or punished? I worry that at present we have no principled way of distinguishing mental (in)capacities from character (flaws).

I concede that it is conceivable that the notion of 'character' is past its use-by date. Perhaps we should simply dispense with it rather than trying to find ways of integrating this old and perhaps confused pre-scientific idea into present-day theoretical frameworks.[7] And perhaps we indeed ought to do that. However, my main point then would be that if we really wish to reject the idea of character, and the related idea that character assessments might play a role in how we treat people, then we should do this mindfully and explicitly. We should not do this by adopting a conceptual framework that simply reinterprets all things that could otherwise be described as character flaws as mental incapacities. This would surreptitiously carve away a sizeable chunk of our moral landscape by blinding us to competing interpretations of the same data. The fact that the authors cited at the top of this subsection all interpret the findings from the range of empirical studies of psychopathy as evidence of psychopaths' diminished mental capacities, and that the character flaw interpretation and its radically different consequences seldom get a mention in the compatibilist literature, is in my view ample evidence that capacitarianism has shielded many excellent researchers from noticing a competing interpretation of the data that they cite.

Discussion

In section 1 I argued that a gradual shift away from hard determinism towards compatibilism underpins contemporary claims about the role that cognitive neuroscience and behavioural genetics can play in the study of free will and responsibility. These are claims to the effect that these sciences may one day help us to assess, restore and enhance free will by developing techniques and technologies to measure and modify people's mental capacities. But in the second section, I highlighted two problems with the capacitarian core of this compatibilist approach. First, I argued that we are yet to arrive at a way of understanding the notion of capacity and the central role it plays in compatibilist theory in such a way that it can do the normative work that it was intended to do without surreptitiously helping ourselves to incompatibilist ideas about what matters for responsibility. Second, I also argued that it is far from clear why we should think that the various cited empirical findings are indeed evidence for mental capacity deficits which typically excuse/mitigate, when there exists an alternative interpretation which is equally compatible with this empirical data, namely that it highlights character flaws which typically condemn/aggravate.

But what of it? Why should anyone care about these challenges? To answer these 'So what?' questions, in what follows I return to some of the claims which other authors in this volume make, to point out how the issues that I raise above create complications for what they say.

A couple of points are salient with regard to Focquaert, Glenn and Raine's chapter. First, it would be helpful for them to spell out with greater precision exactly how the empirical data that they cite support their claims about what psychopaths can and cannot do rather than what they do and do not do. After all, in large part functional neuroimaging reveals merely what does or does not happen in the brain, not what can or cannot happen (Vincent 2008). And while it is not implausible to suggest that a sustained pattern of (non-)activation might indeed be explained by the lack of a capacity for another pattern of activation, this cannot merely be assumed as a foregone conclusion. Admittedly, Focquaert, Glenn and Raine also cite a mountain of behavioural as well as structural neuroimaging data to bolster their claims about psychopaths' impaired capacities. However, as I argue in the above-cited paper (Vincent 2008), behavioural data face precisely the same problem as functional neuroimaging data – they only establish what is and is not done rather than what can and cannot be done – and while it is easier to see how structural data can support claims about impaired capacities – no mechanism or the wrong kind of mechanism, thus no functionality or the wrong kind of functionality – even setting aside multiple-realizability, this just leads us to the other problem.

Second, why should we interpret those structural features as evidence of impaired capacity rather than as evidence of character flaws? Focquaert, Glenn and Raine repeatedly characterize the significance of empirical findings using the language of deficit and disorder. We are told about psychopaths having deficits, disorders, impairments, damaged mechanisms, inabilities and limited abilities; a kaleidoscope of concepts that ring of pathology and connect this with the notions of impaired capacity and incapacity. However, my worry is that this only reveals their firm capacitarian theoretical leanings – their preference for a capacitarian over a charactarian interpretation of the data. Yet they do not explain why they are entitled to set aside the competing charactarian interpretations of the same data. The question is why should we view these data as signs of pathology, disease, impairment (and a whole range of other value-laden incapacity-like concepts that tip our intuitions towards diminished guilt and treatment instead of punishment) rather than viewing them, rather unsurprisingly (unsurprisingly, that is, since as materialists we must assume that everything has an implementation of some sort, often but not necessarily within the brain) as the physical instantiations or implementations of bad people or of people with bad values or something similar. Relatedly, this theoretical leaning leads them to endorse a move towards treatment rather than punishment, but while this view seems charitable and humane when we conceptualize psychopathy as an illness – after all, who wouldn't endorse treating someone with an illness – before psychopathy is pathologized and we proceed with medical treatment, we really should consider the charactarian interpretation and the related question of how comfortable we feel about changing people – changing their values, commitments, preferences, their selves – when the changes are not characterized through the biasing lens of the language of pathology, disease and disorder.

In part because of its explicit focus on '[h]ow mental disorders can compromise the will', Gerben Meynen's chapter is particularly prone to this latter kind of criticism too. For instance, he writes (p. 139):

> Although a patient has alternative possibilities, and although his or her actions are motivated by reasons, we may feel that, due to a mental disorder, the patient is not 'him- or herself'... the person is 'different' from who he or she used to be. If this is the case, we may feel that the disorder is bringing about the behavior. Consequently, ... we may not blame the person.

The implication is that we may not blame the patient because the disease is to blame. The disease 'dunnit', as it were. But there are at least three problems here. (1) The use of the terminology of 'patients' and 'disorders' is question-begging against the charactarian presupposition, because it expresses rather than establishes through argument that what is observed is an impaired capacity rather than a character flaw. (2) This terminology as well as other locutions about people who '*suffer* from kleptomania' (Meynen, my emphasis) bias our judgment in favour of imposing medical treatments, sometimes even coercively, which we may not have otherwise considered if the charactarian description had been adopted. (3) It posits pathology and disease as things that stand apart from the person – as conditions that inflict themselves upon their will, or that diminish or perhaps warp their mental capacities – without recognizing the problematic nature of the relationship between people and their (allegedly pathological) states. In cases like anti-social personality disorder and psychopathy where the alleged pathology is something that was always there, rather than something which developed perhaps because of a traumatic injury, this problem is particularly vivid. It seems difficult to explain why some feature that makes up that person should be thought of as a pathology (rather than as a difference, an instance of their badness) and why it is legitimate to view it as something that stands apart from them and inflicts itself on them rather than it being just a part of who they are.

These three points, as well as the second point I made while commenting on Focquaert, Glenn and Raine's chapter, apply equally to Maartje Schermer's chapter, which is thoroughly capacitarian in its approach. For instance, Schermer writes that '[n]euromodulation can ... restore autonomy, as it does in cases when patients are successfully treated for conditions that have a negative impact on autonomy' (p. 216). The conditions that she cites to demonstrate her point are Alzheimer's disease, obsessive-compulsive disorder, drug addiction, and attention deficit and hyperactivity disorder. The central idea here is not dissimilar to Meynen's. Treatments for disorders can restore autonomy not just qua ameliorating the disorder itself, but qua resolving the mental incapacities that constitute that disorder. It's the mental capacities that allegedly ultimately matter, not whether we call it a disorder. However, although Schermer is to be commended for distancing herself from the distorting effects that employing the terminology of disease, disorder and pathology in general can have on our thinking, the problem is that talk of incapacities, inabilities and deficits has precisely the same effects.

Lastly, because the two points that I raise in this chapter – i.e. that there are problems with the notion of capacity employed by compatibilists and that it is not clear how to distinguish mental incapacities from character flaws – have been misinterpreted by some as an expression of a general disgruntlement with compatibilism, I will end this chapter with the following disclaimer. I highlight these challenges not to undermine compatibilism, but to ultimately strengthen it through open discussion of features which may be viewed by some as weaknesses. My conviction is that both problems can be adequately addressed, and that is indeed the focus of my own on-going project as a compatibilist which I describe elsewhere (Vincent 2013a, b). However, I do not believe that we have developed the necessary solutions yet, and for this reason we ought to be charitable to incompatibilists, to libertarians, and to anyone else who expresses doubts about compatibilism. We should take their doubts seriously. This, and not an expression of disgruntlement with compatibilism or even giving up on the compatibilist project, is what this chapter has tried to accomplish.

NOTES

1 There are compelling reasons to suppose that the mind is embodied and extended (Glannon 2011). Hence, compatibilists should not assume that the mechanisms in virtue of which some people are responsible for what they do must of necessity reside in people's brains.

2 See Vincent (2013b) for a much more detailed and nuanced discussion.

3 Some might object if psychopaths were to be coerced or compelled to undergo such treatments. But suppose that the only reason why some psychopaths might resist such treatments is that they just do not know any better – perhaps because their very lack of this mental tool is what prevents them from seeing how important this tool really is – whereas we do know better. Assuming that we are right, this would, I believe, diminish the strength of such an objection.

4 Two clarifications. One, the claim about punishment can naturally only be sustained if psychopaths are indeed responsible for their behaviour. However, unless we assume from the outset that psychopaths' mental features such as flat affect (and others which are commonly cited by capacitarians) diminish their guilt *by depriving them of an important responsibility-relevant mental capacity* – a capacitarian assumption of the very sort that this section aims to highlight – then we will not yet have reason to suppose that their responsibility would be compromised. Two, [missing text]

5 This table and the following paragraph are borrowed with minor modifications from Vincent (2014:38–9).

6 A point here requires emphasis. Conceivably, one might reply to this rhetorical question that empirical evidence surely indicates that their brains are *disordered*, and that the critical question is whether or to what extent the disorder is of such a degree that it impairs their capacity for moral reasoning. While I acknowledge that this reply might be forthcoming, what I wish to emphasize is that technically what the empirical evidence indicates is that their brains are different, but whether we refer to that difference as something that is disordered depends on taking an ultimately contestable normative stance. I agree that psychopaths don't reason like we do, and there can also be differences between our and their volition (greater impulsivity), but in my view one must presuppose certain normative commitments (which, for methodological reasons, I wish to resist presupposing) to get to the claim that empirical evidence indicates that their brains are disordered. More importantly, the point of drawing attention to these dichotomies is precisely to bring out the fact that a range of conceptual and normative commitments come along for the ride whenever we call someone (e.g.) mad rather than bad, or ill rather than depraved. And I do this to highlight that our thinking is swayed by these conceptual and normative commitments, not by some natural or innate or necessary categorization of various conditions into either one or the other category. And doing this is important because I would like to make readers aware of how their conceptual and normative commitments predispose them to reach certain judgments.

7 A less radical response to my worry is the suggestion that character is just a bundle of mental capacities. However, I cannot see how this can address my concerns since if that is what character is – just a bundle of mental capacities – and mental incapacities of the right sort and degree excuse, then why should a bundle of incapacities – i.e. more incapacities – condemn rather than excuse? If the notion of character and its place in the moral landscape is to be taken seriously, then this requires accommodating it in a way that recognizes that bad character condemns rather than excuses, but the bundle theory of character cannot do this.

REFERENCES

Blair, R. J. R. (2008). 'The cognitive neuroscience of psychopathy and implications for judgments of responsibility'. *Neuroethics* **1**(2): 149–57.

Bublitz, J. C. and R. Merkel (2009). 'Autonomy and authenticity of enhanced personality traits'. *Bioethics* **23**(6): 360–74.

Burgess, A. (2000). *A Clockwork Orange (with an Introduction by Blake Morrison)*. London: Penguin Books.

Burns, J. M. and R. H. Swerdlow (2003). 'Right orbitogrontal tumor with pedophilia symptom and constructional apraxia sign'. *Archives of Neurology* **60**: 437–40.

Cashmore, A. R. (2010). 'The Lucretial swerve: the biological basis of human behavior and the criminal justice system'. *Proceedings of the National Academy of Sciences of the United States of America* **107**(10): 4499–504.

Caspi, A., J. McClay, T. E. Moffitt, J. Mill, J. Martin et al. (2002). 'Role of genotype in the cycle of violence in maltreated children'. *Science* **297**: 851.

Duff, R. A. (2005). 'Punishment, dignity and degradation'. *Oxford Journal of Legal Studies* **25**(1): 141–55.

Fine, C. and J. Kennett (2004). 'Mental impairment, moral understanding and criminal responsibility: psychopathy and the purposes of punishment'. *International Journal of Law and Psychiatry* **27**(5): 425–43.

Fischer, J. M. (2005). 'Reply: the free will revolution'. *Philosophical Explorations* **8**(2): 145–56.

Fischer, J. M. and M. Ravizza (1998). *Responsibility and Control: A Theory of Moral Responsibility*. Cambridge University Press.

Gerrans, P. and J. Kennett (2006). 'Introduction: is cognitive penetrability the mark of the moral?' *Philosophical Explorations* **9**(1): 3–12.

Glannon, W. (2011). *Brain, Body, and Mind: Neuroethics with a Human Face*. New York: Oxford University Press.

Greely, H. T. (2008). 'Neuroscience and criminal justice: not responsibility but treatment'. *University of Kansas Law Review* **56**: 1103–38.

Greene, J. and J. D. Cohen (2004). 'For the law, neuroscience changes nothing and everything'. *Philosophical Transactions of the Royal Society of London*: 1775–85.

Haji, I. (2010). 'Psychopathy, ethical perception, and moral culpability'. *Neuroethics* **3**(2): 135–50.

Hare, R. D. and C. S. Neumann (2010). 'Psychopathy: assessment and forensic implications'. *Responsibility and Psychopathy: Interfacing Law, Psychiatry, and Philosophy*. L. Malatesti and J. McMillan (eds.). Oxford University Press: 93–123.

Harenski, C. L., R. D. Hare and Kiehl, Kent A. (2010). 'Neuroimaging, genetics, and psychopathy: implications for the legal system'. *Responsibility and Psychopathy: Interfacing Law, Psychiatry, and Philosophy*. L. Malatesti and J. McMillan (eds.). Oxford University Press: 125–54.

Kennett, J. (2010). 'Reasons, emotion and the psychopath'. *Responsibility and Psychopathy: Interfacing Law, Psychiatry, and Philosophy*. L. Malatesti and J. McMillan (eds.). Oxford University Press: 243–59.

Kröber, H. L. and S. Lau (2000). 'Bad or mad? Personality disorders and legal responsibility: the German situation'. *Behavioral Sciences and the Law* **18**: 679–90.

Levy, N. (2007). 'The responsibility of the psychopath revisited'. *Philosophy, Psychiatry & Psychology* **14**(2): 129–38.

(2008). 'Counterfactual intervention and agents' capacities'. *The Journal of Philosophy* **CV**(5): 223–39.

Lewis, C. S. (1963). 'The humanitarian theory of punishment'. *Res Judicatae* **6**: 224–30.

Maibom, H. L. (2008). 'The mad, the bad, and the psychopath'. *Neuroethics* **1**(3): 167–84.

McSherry, B. (2004). 'Criminal responsibility, "fleeting" states of mental impairment, and the power of self-control'. *International Journal of Law and Psychiatry* **27**: 224–57.

Merkel, R., G. Boer, J. M. Fegert, T. Galert, D. Hartmann et al. (2007). *Intervening in the Brain: Changing Psyche and Society*. Berlin: Springer.

Prinz, J. (2006). 'The emotional basis of moral judgments'. *Philosophical Explorations* **9**(1): 29–43.

Reimer, M. (2008). 'Psychopathy without (the language of) disorder'. *Neuroethics* **1**(3): 185–98.

Sadler, J. Z. (2008). 'Vice and the diagnostic classification of mental disorders: a philosophical case conference'. *Philosophy, Psychiatry & Psychology* **15**(1): 1–17.

Sapolsky, R. M. (2004). 'The frontal cortex and the criminal justice system'. *Philosophical Transactions of the Royal Society of London* **359**: 1787–96.

Shaw, E. (2014). 'Direct brain interventions and responsibility enhancement'. *Criminal Law and Philosophy* 8(1): 1–20. Doi: 10.1007/s11572-012-9152–2: 20 pages.

Vincent, N. (2008). 'Responsibility, dysfunction and capacity'. *Neuroethics* **1**(3): 199–204.

(2010). "On the relevance of neuroscience to criminal responsibility." *Criminal Law and Philosophy* **4**(1): 77–98. Doi: 10.1007/s11572-009-9087–4.

(2011a). 'Madness, badness and neuroimaging-based responsibility assessments'. *Law and Neuroscience, Current Legal Issues,* Vol. XIII. M. Freeman (ed.). Oxford University Press: 79–95.

(2011b). 'Neuroimaging and responsibility Assessments'. *Neuroethics* **4**(1): 35–49. Doi: 10.1007/s12152-008-9030–8.

(2013a). 'Blame, desert and compatibilist capacity: a diachronic account of moderateness in regards to reasons-responsiveness'. *Philosophical Explorations* 6(2): 178–194. Doi: 10.1080/13869795.2013.787443.

(2013b). 'A compatibilist theory of legal responsibility'. *Criminal Law and Philosophy*. OnlineFirst. Doi: 10.1007/s11572-013-9249–2).

(2014). 'Restoring responsibility: promoting justice, therapy and reform through direct brain interventions'. *Criminal Law and Philosophy* **8**(1): 21–42. OnlineFirst. Doi: 10.1007/s11572-012-9156-y.

Watson, G. (1987). 'Responsibility and the limits of evil: variations on a Strawsonian theme'. *Responsibility, Character, and the Emotions*. F. Schoeman (ed.). Cambridge University Press: 256–86.

Wolf, S. (1987). 'Sanity and the metaphysics of responsibility'. *Responsibility, Character and the Emotions: New Essays in Moral Psychology*. F. Shoeman (ed.). New York: Cambridge University Press: 46–62.

Part IV

Neural circuitry and modification of the will

10 Implications of functional neurosurgery and deep-brain stimulation for free will and decision-making

Nir Lipsman and Andres M. Lozano

ABSTRACT

This chapter describes the contributions that functional neurosurgery for disorders of motor and mind function can make to understanding the nature of free will in human behavior. It has become increasingly clear that voluntary decision-making is governed by a heterogeneous set of cortical and subcortical structures whose actions, on a timescale of milliseconds, have far-reaching implications. We outline advances in the field that are helping define what it means to make free and voluntary decisions and how brain implants, such as deep-brain stimulation (DBS), can help us to understand the anatomy underlying these decisions. When properly functioning, the brain's decision-making apparatus allows us to navigate the world and make choices that are in our perceived best interests. A dysfunctional apparatus underlies many psychiatric and neurologic disorders, from addiction and depression, to Parkinson's and Alzheimer's disease. In Parkinson's disease, for example, brain implants and dopaminergic therapy can help restore motion function and improve ambulation. Both, however, can also lead to impulsive decision-making and disinhibition. It is apparent, then, from studies of surgical treatment in psychiatry and neurology, that structures with prominent autonomic/affective projections play key roles in these disorders and may influence patient decision-making beyond conscious awareness. As a result, and given its privileged access to the human brain, functional neurosurgery can provide unique insight into brain dysfunction, and restoration through modulation can inform our conception of free will.

Introduction

Neurosurgeons, with few exceptions, rarely enter into discussions surrounding free will and volition, traditionally the purview of philosophers. This is a valuable missed opportunity, for several reasons.

First, notwithstanding the complexity of operationalizing these concepts, they are doubtless "brain-based," and our understanding of them will, at least in part, come from a better understanding of brain function. Second, both neurologic and psychiatric disease and its treatment can alter what are traditionally considered the components of free will and action, namely, motivation, intentions, desires, as well as more basic motor and sensory functions. Finally, unique access to the brain allows neurosurgeons to trace human behavior from individual cells, to overt, observable actions, providing a comprehensive framework for the empirical study of motivated action (Mukamel & Fried 2012). The extent to which knowledge of brain *pathology* informs knowledge of *normal* brain function is, however, controversial and an important limitation of current research. Indeed, our knowledge of the neural mechanisms underlying normal human behavior has remained largely indirect and limited to non-invasive imaging and brain recordings (e.g. with functional neuroimaging, electroencephalography or magnetoencephalography) and naturalistic or experimental observations of behavior (e.g. Kostelecki et al. 2012). This is, however, beginning to change. The last twenty years in particular have seen a renaissance in brain science with technical advances in recording and stimulation informing both the neural mechanisms underlying willed action and the subjective experience of decision-making.

We now understand that brain circuits comprised of mono- and polysynaptically connected structures provide reciprocal feedback, redundancy, and control, and govern most if not all human behavior. As a result, common brain disorders, including Parkinson's disease (PD), major depressive disorder (MDD), obsessive-compulsive disorder (OCD) and Alzheimer's disease (AD), are increasingly being understood as "circuit disorders." Different types of circuit pathology can include over- or underactivity of critical nodes in the circuit, as well as abnormal firing rates, patterns, and coherence within and between anatomic structures (Lozano et al. 2002; Eusebio & Brown 2007; Mayberg 1997). Such circuit dysfunction leads to clinical symptoms, with the goals of treatment being the restoration of circuit integrity (Johansen-Berg et al. 2008; Kuhn et al. 2008). Functional neurosurgery is a subdiscipline of neurosurgery, whose broad aims include restoration of circuit function through ablation or stimulation of neural targets involved in motor, seizure, and psychiatric disorders, among others. Here, we describe the anatomy and circuitry relevant to free will and decision-making, and what the surgical treatment of these disorders, can tell us about these constructs.

Anatomy and circuitry of decision-making

At the level of observed behavior, free will is a necessary but not sufficient component of human decision-making. Other critical factors include desires, values, and the integrity of a sensory-motor system. Free will, at the level of subjective experience, can be defined as the feeling associated with ownership of one's actions, or the feeling that one makes choices independent of external influences. This experience ensures that one's decisions and actions are consistent with one's own desires, and therefore congruent with how one wants to behave. The ability to "freely choose" ensures that the responsibility for the choice, and its consequences, lies with the individual. Critically, the failure of free choice implies that neither the choice nor its consequences can be attributed to the individual; they are not responsible, because the choice was not theirs. What does free will look like at a neuroanatomic, structural level, or at the individual neuron or even neurotransmitter level? These are much more difficult questions that current neurosurgical techniques have nevertheless attempted to address. First, however, a better understanding of the involved anatomy and the concepts underlying this research is required.

Decision-making is complex and entails several components including judgment, predicting consequences of actions, and weighing the merits of alternative choices and scenarios. In addition, decision-making involves both a motor and motivational component, underscoring the intimate relationship between structures that govern both functions. Several cortical and subcortical structures participate in decision-making, but here we focus on those structures that provide higher-level inputs informing motor actions when deciding between alternative choices, namely the prefrontal cortex (PFC) and limbic basal ganglia.

The contributions of the PFC to both personality and decision-making have been known for well over a century, given the infamous case of Phineas Gage, a railroad worker who suffered a traumatic brain injury. Miraculously, Gage not only survived the railroad spike that penetrated his brain at high velocity, but went on to have a well-documented recovery. Despite this, however, friends and relatives concluded that "Gage was no longer Gage," with something of his previously personality forever changed. Image reconstruction performed in 2004 using Gage's own skull, provided evidence that the spike had caused severe damage to Gage's left frontal lobes, entering the brain at the orbitofrontal cortex (OFC) and sparing the superior sagittal sinus, thus saving his life (Ratiu & Talos 2004). The OFC is a component of the larger, and anatomically complex, prefrontal cortex. In general terms, the PFC comprises orbital, medial, and dorsal components (Clark et al. 2005). The orbital (OFC) and medial (ventral and dorsomedial prefrontal cortex) components have traditionally been considered critical to personality, motivation, and higher-order contributions to mood and affective regulation. These regions receive diffuse inputs from across the cortex, including the medial temporal lobe, anterior cingulate, parietal lobe, and components of the basal ganglia. As a result, the PFC is optimally positioned to generate "guided behavior," or decisions and actions that are guided by external (i.e. environmental) and internal (i.e. "self-generated") stimuli. It is also generally assumed that different afferent projections to the PFC are responsible for different components of behavior. Specifically, these projections determine temporal sequencing and overall integration of behavior as well as object identification, wherein affective tone, emotions, and memories are embedded in (and extracted from) objects and people (Clark et al. 2005).

Much of what we know about OFC function has come from the lesion and trauma literature, where the region has been rendered dysfunctional. For example, OFC lesions have been associated with symptoms such as disinhibition (failure to prevent inappropriate or antisocial actions), emotional lability, impulsivity, and irrational decision-making. This implies that the OFC plays a role in regulating emotion-guided behavior, and decision-making that is in one's best interests (Rolls 2004). Frontotemporal dementia (FTD) is a neurodegenerative disease that preferentially targets those regions of the brain. In contrast to the more common Alzheimer's disease, FTD has an earlier age of onset, typically in the 50s, and is associated with more prominent disturbances in behavior and decision-making (Viskontas et al. 2007). Patients are emotionally labile, impulsive, and less concerned about sociocultural standards and norms. Judgment is impaired and behavior inappropriate, leading to significant functional impairment and ultimately institutionalization secondary to lack of insight and progressive decline.

The lack of insight in FTD and AD, which is a hallmark of both illnesses, raises important points related to free will and the brain. Here, we can distinguish between two types of "free will disturbance": primary and secondary. With primary disorders, individuals either literally attribute their actions and decisions to external influences (e.g. hallucinations and delusion in schizophrenia) or report an absolute absence of intention, or knowledge, to move or decide (e.g. alien hand syndrome). Dementia and its associated lack of insight would fit into primary disturbances. In all of these conditions, either patients do not attribute their actions to themselves (See Chapter 4 in this volume), or if they do, they fail to recognize that, as a result of an underlying pathologic process, their aberrant behavior is incongruent with either personal or societal norms. In contrast, secondary disorders of free will are those where patients do not doubt that the source of their actions is their own but instead may report a loss of control over their actions. Examples here include patients with OCD, who know their actions are excessive and disproportionate but who continue to engage in them "despite themselves" or despite "knowing better." In other words, they recognize the correct course of action but fail to take it. This distinction is important because it may be easier to treat secondary disorders of free will, where structures are intact but may be "hijacked" by a dysfunctional process. The principle attribution of actions to oneself, even if one cannot execute them, may portend a better prognosis.

Imaging studies have shown that the vmPFC is critical for reward-and/ or reinforcement-driven behavior. This region generally receives diffuse input from cortical and subcortical regions. Especially important is the fact that it receives large afferent projections from brainstem dopaminergic structures, such as the ventral tegmental area (VTA), thus underscoring its role in learning and reward. Its role in autonomic pathways, through its hypothalamic, insular, and amygdalar projections, also means it participates in more basic vegetative, or "bottom-up" processes responsible for the physiological responses to stimuli. As a result of its diverse functions, the vmPFC has been implicated in many neuropsychiatric conditions, most notably major depression (Mayberg 1997; Mayberg et al. 2005). Activity within vmPFC, and more specifically in regions anterior and inferior to the corpus callosum, is increased in individuals thinking of sad events (Mayberg 1999). Further, hyperactivity in this area normalizes compared to healthy controls, when depressed patients recover, whether with pharmacology, psychotherapy or deep-brain stimulation (Kennedy et al. 2001; Mayberg et al. 2005). The significance and meaning of vmPFC hyperactivity remains unclear and is likely related to the ability, or lack thereof, of structures such as the amygdala and ventral striatum, to impose a type of "emotional homeostasis" (Giacobbe et al. 2009). Although the mechanisms of treatments such as DBS are unknown, it may be that focal disruption within this region may lead to a resetting of activity and restoration of circuit integrity. In some ways, major depression is a prototypical secondary disorder of free will. Patients often know and can recognize what would be the "correct" course of action, but feel they cannot execute these actions, secondary to an emotional paralysis.

The basal ganglia are a collection of subcortical nuclei that play critical roles in generating voluntary movements. Structures such as the globus pallidus, caudate, putamen, and subthalamic nucleus are important nodes in the motor circuit. They participate in action selection, and the integration of both bottom-up (unconscious, e.g. brain stem, spinal cord) and top-down (conscious, e.g. motor cortex, supplementary motor area) influences on behavior. Several lines of evidence, however, point to a broader role for these structures that extends beyond their involvement in purely motor circuitry. They include: (i) high levels of comorbidity between neurologic (e.g. Tourette's syndrome) and psychiatric disorders (e.g. obsessive-compulsive disorder) (Como et al. 2005); (ii) the anxiolytic effect noted with surgical procedures on "motor structures" (e.g. subthalmic nucleus [STN] DBS for PD and comorbid OCD leads to improvement in OCD [Chabardès et al. 2012]), and (iii) imaging studies that have implicated similar structures in movement and psychiatric disorders (Ballanger et al. 2009). Nowhere are these principles better exemplified than in the STN. The STN is a 5 mm-wide structure that nevertheless can be subdivided according to unique afferent/efferent projections subserving motor, associative, and limbic functions. As a result, the STN, which previously had been considered predominantly a motor structure, has been recast as a key structure in psychiatric conditions, particularly those where there is a prominent *motor* component, such as OCD. At the level of the brain, therefore, neurological and psychiatric disorders are literally fused together. Thus, many now describe these as "neuropsychiatric" disorders. It is not surprising, then, that various treatments for these disorders, whether antipsychotics in schizophrenia, or DBS and dopaminergic medications in PD, can be associated with both motor and limbic effects.

The STN's "multiple personalities" underscore one of the unifying principles of the neuroanatomic basis of behavior, namely that virtually all behavior, whether normal or pathologic, is governed by the activity of neural circuits. Although such circuits have been known for over half a century, and have been classically described as parallel and segregated "loops," more recent evidence, such as the case of STN, suggests that there is more overlap in the system than previously thought (Alexander et al. 1986; Ballanger et al. 2009). The power of circuit-based descriptions of behavior is that individual nodes within the circuits can be studied and used to explain behavioral pathology. For example, pathological firing of neurons in the motor subcircuit of STN in the beta frequency range is associated with PD's motor symptoms, while firing of neurons in the ventral intermediate (Vim) nucleus of the thalamus in essential tremor (ET) is entrained to the frequency of the tremor (Eusebio & Brown 2007). In both instances, DBS at these targets (STN in PD and Vim in ET) abolishes the neurophysiological pathological signature of the condition and leads to symptom improvement.

Although we do not have similar neurophysiological signatures in psychiatric disorders, a robust imaging literature points at several key structures, or critical nodes, that make up the unique circuits believed to underlie symptoms.

Each of the above-described regions plays an integral role in decision-making and the execution of voluntary movements under motivational guidance. Also, each has been implicated in behavioral pathology, wherein decision-making is at least partially, if not primarily, affected. We next turn to the role that neurosurgery, with brain mapping and DBS in particular, has played in elucidating the roles of these structures in decision-making, and how altering decision-making deficits in some psychiatric conditions can inform our conceptions of free will.

Functional neurosurgery and deep-brain stimulation

Functional neurosurgery has approached the study of decision-making and hence free will, in two ways: by actually treating disorders of decision-making dysfunction, with ablative or stimulation-based treatments; and by exploring the neural mechanisms underlying voluntary decision-making and volition. The latter has applied techniques inside and outside of the operating room, sometimes involving direct recording from putatively involved anatomic structures. We discuss each in turn.

Modulating decision-making pathology

We have described the anatomy of decision-making and how anatomic structures have been putatively linked to disorders where decision-making is hijacked or dysfunctional. Further, neuroanatomic structures exist as critical nodes within circuits, or loops, where node dysfunction is transmitted throughout the circuit. In this way, relatively localized disturbances can have network-wide influences, helping to explain why in some neuropsychiatric disorders: (i) imaging studies identify a diverse set of anatomic abnormalities; (ii) coherence, in both neuronal firing rates and patterns, between remote anatomic structures is critical to disease maintenance; (iii) the clinical picture is often diverse, involving cognitive, affective, and perceptual disturbances; and (iv) focal disruption, by surgical ablation or stimulation, can lead to remote effects on the entire circuit, which correspond to the intervention's clinical effect.

DBS is a surgical procedure that involves the implantation of unilateral (or bilateral) electrodes into the deep brain under stereotactic guidance. Electricity, which is generated from an implanted "pacemaker"-type battery, is used to interfere with neural activity locally, thereby influencing activity remotely in mono- and poly-synaptically connected structures. Functional imaging studies, using positron emission tomography (PET), combined with DBS, have shown that brain metabolism in key, disease-relevant, structures change significantly with chronic stimulation (Mayberg et al. 2005; Lozano et al. 2008). DBS has been applied to several disorders where decision-making is either partially or primarily affected, influencing several disease circuits, including motor (Parkinson's disease), mood (major depression), "mixed" (obsessive-compulsive disorder, anorexia nervosa), and cognitive (Alzheimer's disease). What does DBS in these disorders tell us about the circuitry and nature of decision-making and free will?

Motor circuit

DBS is highly effective in treating motor circuit dysfunction. Currently, both the FDA and Health Canada approve DBS for the management of Parkinson's disease and essential tremor. The FDA also provides a humanitarian device exemption use of DBS in dystonia (Collins et al. 2010). The most common indication is PD, where DBS is associated with significant improvements in tremor and rigidity. These motor effects have translated into substantial improvement in quality of life, related to both a reduction in disabling symptoms and reductions in medication doses with subsequent improvements in medication-related adverse events. DBS enables patients to do things that they otherwise would not be able to do, as a result of their previously disabling motor symptoms. In this way the procedure can be considered a "prosthetic of the will," that enhances freedom and decision-making, rather than replaces it (Lipsman & Glannon 2013).

DBS in PD has also been associated with limbic side effects, such as increased impulsivity, as well as mood and personality changes (Hälbig et al. 2009; Schneider et al. 2010). Interestingly, treatment of PD's motor symptoms with dopaminergic medications has also been associated with similar symptoms in some patients, suggesting a common underlying pathogenesis and mechanism (Weintraub et al. 2010). As DBS is a focal therapy, unlike medications, it suggests that activity within the STN, which is the most common DBS target for PD and which plays a role in both motor and limbic pathways, may be partly responsible for these symptoms. DBS in PD has a dual role, then. It can enhance voluntary decision-making by treating motor symptoms, but it may also be associated with impulsive and potentially pathological decision-making. The STN emerges as a key anatomic structure for action selection, wherein the motivational and limbic influences on decision-making interact and overlap with more basic motor functions. Physiological investigations of free will, which have typically focused on cortical structures, should therefore also focus on this critical structure as well.

Mood and anxiety circuits

The success of DBS in diseases of motor circuitry has led to its assessment in other circuit-based conditions, such as major depression and obsessive-compulsive disorder (see Anderson et al. 2012 and Holtzheimer & Mayberg 2011 for review of clinical results). Although the decision-making obstacles in these conditions are not necessarily physical, the principles underlying the clinical efficacy of DBS are similar in motor and non-motor circuitry. For example, in PD, one's tremor, rigidity, and akinesia may lead to a shying away from typically enjoyable activities and a withdrawal from social interactions. In depression, one's mood, anhedonia, and low energy may have similar consequences. Just as DBS in PD leads to a "release" of these symptoms, DBS in depression may have a similar effect, thus enhancing and enabling, rather than replacing, the patient's own decision-making abilities.

The targets most commonly used in DBS for major depression are the subcallosal cingulate (SCC) and the nucleus accumbens (Nacc), both prominent nodes in mood and affective regulation circuitry. In OCD, common targets include the ventral caudate/striatum (Nacc), and, interestingly, the STN. The STN's appearance here should come as no surprise. We have already seen that it is directly implicated in primary motor disorders, and further that its "multiple personalities" allow it to participate in different circuits, including limbic circuitry. OCD is marked by both a thought (anxiety-generating obsessions) and a motor component (anxiolytic compulsions). Critically, DBS for OCD aims to reduce anxiety, by targeting limbic structures, rather than addressing the action components of the condition by targeting motor structures. A reduced *drive* to engage in time-consuming and disabling compulsions, which the patient realizes are disproportionate, is the desired outcome. If patients feel unable to control their compulsions secondary to paralyzing anxiety that *compels* them to act in a pathological fashion, DBS provides them with control by inhibiting their anxiety. Here too, as in PD and depression, the ability to act in accordance with one's wishes is enhanced by DBS.

Probing decision-making circuitry

The neural mechanisms underlying voluntary decision-making are currently under active investigation. Much of this work has been aided by the ability to probe the brain directly and record activity from single or multiple neurons in response to various tasks. Such work is revealing interesting insights, and also posing many new questions. One group has recorded activity from neurons in the supplementary motor area (SMA) in patients with epilepsy who are undergoing neural recording to identify the focus of seizure activity (Fried et al. 2011). Researchers found that 1.5 seconds prior to the decision to voluntarily move their fingers, patients had significant neuronal recruitment in their SMA. The group argued that a specific firing-rate threshold needed to be surpassed by SMA neurons prior to the sense of volition being consciously appreciated by patients. The SMA plays a critical role in planning motor movement, and its electrical stimulation in awake patients undergoing neurosurgery has been linked to the "urge" to move, even in the absence of overt voluntary movements (Fried et al. 1991). Though unlikely the seat of volition in the brain, the identification of a neural "signal" related to volition in the SMA, prior to conscious awareness, that in addition predicts subsequent urges to move, suggests that it is intimately associated with the *will to act*.

As with all brain functions, volition and will are likely broadly distributed and hardly limited to a single cortical structure. One group employed awake brain mapping of the cortex in patients undergoing tumor resections, attempting to dissociate the will to move from actual movement. Focusing on the inferior parietal and pre-motor areas, they found that stimulation of the inferior parietal lobule led to subjective desires to move the contralateral limbs (Desmurget et al. 2009). Interestingly, increasing the intensity of the stimulation never elicited an actual movement, but rather a consistent "will" to engage in *any* sort of movement. The authors further note that this broad "will to move" was in contrast to that seen with SMA stimulation, where there was an urge to execute more specific types of movements (e.g. turning leg in, etc.). Such results suggest a broadly distributed volitional network, wherein the motivation or desire to move (Parietal Lobe) may be dissociated in space from more specific cortical instructions, or plans, to move (SMA) (Desmurget & Sirigu 2012).

Although these results are exciting, it may be too soon to suggest that the mechanisms underlying volition and decision-making have been uncovered. Results from single-neuron studies, for example, will not adequately capture the behavior of broad-scale neural networks, and how different regions of the brain communicate with each other. Volition is too complex a topic to ascribe to a single anatomic location, or circuit, and indeed it may be the distributed action of virtually the entire brain that allows the sensation of voluntary action to emerge as a seemingly cohesive and seamless experience.

DBS as a "third party"

As a neuropsychiatric intervention, DBS is unique in several respects. First, it interfaces directly and focally with an anatomic structure believed to underlie or sustain a given set of symptoms. This is different from a medication which has broad effects on the entire brain or neurotransmitter system. The DBS electrodes are intermediaries between anatomic structure and function, and as a result DBS becomes a "third party" in the free will and behavior debate (Lipsman & Glannon 2013). Exactly how DBS achieves its effect remains unknown, although it is clear that its effects extend well beyond the stimulated target, and it is therefore in a position to influence a wide range of structures and behaviors.

A key principle of DBS therapy, and another feature that distinguishes it from other forms of treatment, is that the patient need not *do* anything for the therapy to work. Stimulation is automated and externally controlled; there are no pills to take or therapy in which to engage. To the extent that DBS is influencing cortical-subcortical circuitry, therefore, it is change that is occurring without the knowledge or assistance of the patient. Although subjectively, it may appear that DBS is influencing voluntary decision-making, we have argued that DBS achieves this effect by reducing obstacles to healthy choices, or those choices that are congruent with the patient's wishes. In PD, it reduces motor symptoms, in depression, it reduces incapacitating sadness and anhedonia, and in OCD, it reduces paralyzing anxiety.

Conclusion

In this chapter we have reviewed the neural anatomy and circuitry of decision-making, and how that knowledge has translated into new potential therapies for some neuropsychiatric conditions. Neurosurgical technology has allowed researchers, for the first time, to obtain direct measures of the mechanisms underlying free and voluntary decisions, and DBS is allowing some patients to reclaim freedom over their actions. Although it is true that neurosurgeons rarely venture into discussions of free will, agency, and volition, it was indeed a neurosurgeon, Wilder Penfield, who was among the first to empirically study these concepts. Penfield's brain mapping of awake patients, beginning in the 1940s, contributed substantially to our understanding of the generation of language, individual percepts, as well as the will to voluntary action (Rasmussen & Penfield 1947; Penfield 1958, 1968). Although much has changed since Penfield's work, much has remained the same, including the potential contributions that neurosurgeons, with their privileged access to the living brain, can make to understanding human behavior and its neural origins.

REFERENCES

Alexander, G. E., DeLong, M. R., and Strick, P. L. (1986). Parallel organization of functionally segregated circuits linking basal ganglia and cortex. *Annual Review of Neuroscience* 9:357–81.

Anderson, R. J., Frye, M. A., Abulseoud, O. A., Lee, K. H., McGillivray, J. A., Berk, M., and Tye, S. J. (2012). Deep brain stimulation for treatment-resistant depression: efficacy, safety and mechanisms of action. *Neuroscience & Biobehavioural Reviews* 36(8):1920–33.

Ballanger, B., van Eimeren, T., Moro, E., Lozano, A. M., Hamani, C., Boulinguez, P., Pellecchia, G., Houle, S., Poon, Y. Y., Lang, A. E., and Strafella, A. P. (2009). Stimulation of the subthalamic nucleus and impulsivity: release your horses. *Annals of Neurology* 66(6):817–24.

Chabardès, S., Polosan, M., Krack, P., Bastin, J., Krainik, A., David, O., Bougerol, T., and Benabid, A. L. (2012). Deep Brain Stimulation for Obsessive-Compulsive Disorder: Subthalamic Nucleus Target. *World Neurosurg.* Mar 30 [Epub ahead of print].

Clark, D. L., Boutros, N. N., and Mendez, M. F. (2005). *The Brain and Behavior.* 2nd edn. Cambridge University Press.

Collins, K. L., Lehmann, E. M., and Patil, P. G. (2010). Deep brain stimulation for movement disorders. *Neurobiology of Disease* 38(3):338–45.

Como, P. G., LaMarsh, J., and O'Brien, K. A. (2005). Obsessive-compulsive disorder in Tourette's syndrome. *Advances in Neurology* 96:249–61.

Desmurget, M., Reilly, K. T., Richard, N., Szathmari, A,, Mottolese, C., and Sirigu, A. (2009). Movement intention after parietal cortex stimulation in humans. *Science* 324(5928):811–13.

Desmurget, M., and Sirigu, A. (2012). Conscious motor intention emerges in the inferior parietal lobule. *Current Opinion in Neurobiology* 22(6): 1004–11.

Eusebio, A., and Brown, P. (2007). Oscillatory activity in the basal ganglia. Parkinsonism & Related Disorders *13 Suppl* 3:S434–36.

Fried, I., Katz, A., McCarthy, G., Sass, K. J., Williamson, P., Spencer, S. S., and Spencer, D. D. (1991). Functional organization of human supplementary motor cortex studied by electrical stimulation. *Journal of Neuroscience* 11(11):3656–66.

Fried, I., Mukamel, R., and Kreiman, G. (2011). Internally generated preactivation of single neurons in human medial frontal cortex predicts volition. *Neuron* 69(3):548–62.

Giacobbe, P., Mayberg, H. S., and Lozano, A. M. (2009). Treatment resistant depression as a failure of brain homeostatic mechanisms: implications for deep brain stimulation. *Experimental Neurology* 219(1):44–52.

Hälbig, T. D., Tse, W., Frisina, P. G., Baker, B. R., Hollander, E., Shapiro, H., Tagliati, M., Koller, W. C., and Olanow, C .W. (2000). Subthalamic deep brain stimulation and impulse control in Parkinson's disease. *European Journal of Neurology* 16(4):493–97.

Holtzheimer, P. E., and Mayberg, H. S. (2011). Deep brain stimulation for psychiatric disorders. *Annual Review of Neuroscience* 34:289–307.

Johansen-Berg H., Gutman, D. A., Behrens, T. E., Matthews, P. M., Rushworth, M. F., Katz, E., Lozano, A. M., and Mayberg, H. S. (2008). Anatomical connectivity of the subgenual cingulate region targeted with deep brain stimulation for treatment-resistant depression. *Cerebral Cortex* 18(6):1374–83.

Kennedy, S. H., Evans, K. R., Krüger, S., Mayberg, H. S., Meyer, J. H., McCann, S., Arifuzzman, A. I., Houle, S., and Vaccarino, F. J. (2001). Changes in regional brain glucose metabolism measured with positron emission tomography after paroxetine treatment of major depression. *American Journal of Psychiatry* 158(6):899–905.

Kostelecki, W., Mei, Y., Garcia Dominguez, L., and Pérez Velázquez, J. L. (2012). Patterns of brain activity distinguishing free and forced actions: contribution from sensory cortices. *Frontiers in Integrative Neuroscience* 6:84.

Kühn, A. A., Kempf, F., Brücke, C., Gaynor Doyle, L., Martinez-Torres, I., Pogosyan, A., Trottenberg, T., Kupsch, A., Schneider, G. H., Hariz, M. I., Vandenberghe, W., Nuttin, B., and Brown P. (2008). High-frequency stimulation of the subthalamic nucleus suppresses oscillatory beta activity in patients with Parkinson's disease in parallel with improvement in motor performance. *Journal of Neuroscience* 28(24):6165–73.

Lipsman, N., and Glannon, W. (2013). Brain, mind and machine: what are the implications of deep brain stimulation for perceptions of personal identity, agency and free will? *Bioethics* 27: 465–470.

Lozano, A. M., Dostrovsky, J., Chen, R., and Ashby, P. (2002). Deep brain stimulation for Parkinson's disease: disrupting the disruption. *Lancet Neurology* 1(4):225–31.

Lozano, A. M., Mayberg, H. S., Giacobbe, P., Hamani, C., Craddock, R. C., and Kennedy, S. H. (2008). Subcallosal cingulate gyrus deep brain stimulation for treatment-resistant depression. *Biological Psychiatry* 64(6):461–67.

Mayberg, H. S. (1997). Limbic-cortical dysregulation: a proposed model of depression. *Journal of Neuropsychiatry and Clinical Neuroscience* 9(3):471–81.

Mayberg, H. S., Liotti, M., Brannan, S. K., McGinnis, S., Mahurin, R. K., Jerabek, P. A., Silva, J. A., Tekell, J. L., Martin, C. C., Lancaster, J. L., and Fox, P. T. (1999). Reciprocal limbic-cortical function and negative mood: converging PET findings in depression and normal sadness. *American Journal of Psychiatry* 156(5):675–82.

Mayberg, H. S., Lozano, A. M., Voon, V., McNeely, H. E., Seminowicz, D., Hamani, C., Schwalb, J. M., and Kennedy, S. H. (2005). Deep brain stimulation for treatment-resistant depression. *Neuron* 45(5):651–60.

Mukamel, R., and Fried, I. (2012). Human intracranial recordings and cognitive neuroscience. *Annual Review of Psychology* 10(63):511–37.

Penfield, W. (1958). Some mechanisms of consciousness discovered during electrical stimulation of the brain. *Proceedings of the National Academy of Sciences USA* 44(2):51–66.

(1968). Engrams in the human brain: mechanisms of memory. *Proceedings of the Royal Society of Medicine* 61(8):831–40.

Rasmussen, T., and Penfield, W. (1947). The human sensorimotor cortex as studied by electrical stimulation. *Federation Proceedings* 6(1 Pt 2):184.

Ratiu, P., and Talos, I. F. (2004). Images in clinical medicine: the tale of Phineas Gage, digitally remastered. *New England Journal of Medicine* 351(23):e21.

Rolls, E. T. (2004). The functions of the orbitofrontal cortex. *Brain and Cognition* 55(1):11–29.

Schneider, F., Reske, M., Finkelmeyer, A., Wojtecki, L., Timmermann, L., Brosig, T., Backes, V., Amir-Manavi, A., Sturm, V., Habel, U., and Schnitzler, A. (2010). Predicting acute affective symptoms after deep brain stimulation surgery in Parkinson's disease. *Stereotactic Functional Neurosurgery* 88(6):367–73.

Viskontas, I. V., Possin, K. L., and Miller, B. L. (2007). Symptoms of frontotemporal dementia provide insights into orbitofrontal cortex function and social behavior. *Annals of the New York Academy of Sciences* 1121:528–45.

Weintraub, D., Koester, J., Potenza, M. N., Siderowf, A. D., Stacy, M., Voon, V., Whetteckey, J., Wunderlich, G. R., and Lang, A. E. (2010). Impulse control disorders in Parkinson disease: a cross-sectional study of 3090 patients. *Archives of Neurology* 67(5):589–95.

11 Reducing, restoring, or enhancing autonomy with neuromodulation techniques

Maartje Schermer

ABSTRACT

This chapter focuses on the question of how deep brain stimulation (DBS) and other new and emerging neuromodulation techniques such as transcranial magnetic stimulation (TMS), transcranial direct current stimulation (tDCS), and neurofeedback can influence our autonomy, that is, our capacity to govern ourselves. First, the concept of autonomy is clarified and related to concepts like authenticity or free will. Distinctions are made between autonomy as capacity and as condition, local and global autonomy, autonomous choice and executive autonomy.

Next, a brief overview of the main existing and emerging neuromodulation techniques is given. It is then argued that neuromodulation techniques can impact on autonomy in various ways. Neurodmodulation can reduce autonomy by impeding the capacities needed for autonomous choice, or by affecting a person's values and preferences. However, if the person endorsed these changes, his global autonomy can remain intact. Furthermore, it is argued, neuromodulation can also restore or even enhance capacities necessary for autonomy. Finally, it is argued that differences between techniques have consequences for their impact on autonomy. "Passive" techniques like DBS are more prone to abuse and to disrupting autonomy than techniques – like neurofeedback – that require active participation.

Introduction

"The advent of new modes of behavioral technology raises important issues for our understanding of human nature and our moral views about how people ought to influence one another." With these words Gerald Dworkin opened his 1976 article about autonomy and behavior control. At the time, the advent of new behavior-modifying techniques like psychotropic drugs, neurosurgery, and subliminal suggestion was cause for philosophical reflection on how to understand important concepts like freedom of the will and autonomy. Behaviorist psychology was putting its mark on views about human nature and was claiming there was no place for notions like free will and autonomy. Dworkin's words are still relevant today. With new techniques like deep brain stimulation (DBS), neuroscience is increasingly putting pressure on received ideas about how the mind works, in a way that again raises philosophical questions about free will, autonomy, and related concepts.

This chapter focuses on the question of how DBS and other new and emerging neuromodulation techniques such as transcranial magnetic stimulation (TMS), transcranial direct current stimulation (tDCS), and neurofeedback can influence our autonomy, that is, our capacity to govern ourselves. The fact that these techniques interfere directly with our brains and thus appear to "short-circuit" our own rational and volitional capacities is the most pressing reason for concern. Altering brain structure or functioning can obviously affect mental capacities, including those mental capacities and states that are crucial for autonomy. We may therefore fear that technology will take over, that it will annihilate our free will, change our personal identity, or turn us into some kind of robot. We may also fear that others will abuse the power of these techniques. Such fear led the European Group on Ethics and New Technologies (EGE) to make firm recommendations that "the use of ICT [Information and Communication Technology] implants to obtain remote control over the will of people should be strictly prohibited" (EGE 2005). On a less alarmist but equally important note, we may ask whether these techniques might also help us restore or enhance autonomy, and how they might change our understanding of ourselves and our relationship to ourselves.

In what follows, I define the concept of autonomy and give a brief overview of the main existing and emerging neuromodulation techniques. I argue that neuromodulation techniques have the potential to reduce, restore or even enhance autonomy. In addition, I will discuss how the differences between techniques reflect on their impact on autonomy; especially the way in which the active participation required for neurofeedback makes this technique different from the passive receipt of DBS.

The concept of autonomy

Autonomy is one of the most complex and most discussed concepts in moral philosophy. There is considerable overlap between the concept of autonomy and freedom of the will, liberty, and freedom of thought and action. Moreover, autonomy is also closely related to concepts of authenticity and personal identity. There are many different theories and conceptions of autonomy, and different approaches to the notion of autonomy are taken in the various sub-fields of ethics and philosophy. In medical ethics, for example, respect for patient autonomy is interpreted as the right of patients to make their own treatment choices and is intended to protect them from paternalistic interventions by doctors. It is operationalized in the doctrine of informed consent. In moral and political philosophy more generally, the notion of autonomy refers to self-governance, to "being one's own person, directed by considerations, desires, conditions, and characteristics that are not simply imposed externally on one, but are part of what can somehow be considered one's authentic self" (Christman and Anderson 2005: 3).

Feinberg (1986) distinguishes between autonomy as a *right* to sovereign authority, a *character ideal*, a *capacity* for self-government, and an *actual condition*. The *right* to *sovereign authority* grounds a negative right to self-determination, and much discussion has been devoted to questions about the preconditions and limits of this right (Schermer 2002). Respect for autonomy in this sense entails that persons cannot be subjected to neuromodulating experiments or treatments against their will but need to give a free and informed consent. However, the specific concern I want to raise here about autonomy in the context of neuromodulation is not primarily a concern about forced treatments or involuntary application of these techniques. This concern can be addressed by fairly standard approaches already included in laws and guidelines. In the context of neuromodulation, the notions of autonomy as a capacity and as a condition are of more interest.

The *capacity* for self-government is a psychological capacity that depends on certain mental abilities, like the abilities to understand information, to hold certain goals and values, to reflect on them, to reason and to make rational choices, and to act on those choices. These abilities can be possessed to different degrees by different people, or by the same person in different situations or points in time. These psychological capacities can be affected by interventions in the brain, such as neuromodulation.

The *actual condition* of autonomy is the condition of being in charge of one's life, being in the broadest sense a self-governing individual. The condition of self-governance is understood by Feinberg in terms of a set of global properties or virtues of persons, united by family resemblance; these include properties such as authenticity, self-determination, and self-possession. In my interpretation, it means being an authentic person who makes his own choices and leads his life in accordance with his own goals and values. Autonomy in this sense is a *global* property of persons; persons can be more or less autonomous in this sense. It is important to distinguish this global property of persons from the autonomy of specific isolated desires, choices, or actions. The latter is called *local autonomy* (Christman and Anderson 2005; Taylor 2005).

In most contemporary theories of autonomy, the condition of authenticity is central. The core idea is that in order to be called autonomous, a person must be "really him- or herself." In the influential theory of Dworkin, desires or preferences of a person can be called autonomous (i.e. "really his or hers") when the person identifies with them, and the process of identification was free of subverting influences such as manipulation or coercion. Dworkin referred to this latter point as "procedural independence." Dworkin developed his theory in the 1970s when behaviorist psychology was at its peak and new psychological techniques to influence behavior of people, such as subliminal suggestion and operant conditioning, were discovered and applied. It was against this background that he spoke of "subverting influences." We may wonder whether neuromodulation techniques such as DBS or TMS can also influence preference formation, or the process of second-order identification with one's first-order preferences in ways that are subverting and render them inauthentic.

Later adaptations of Dworkin's theory shifted the emphasis from local autonomy of preferences to autonomy as a global property of persons and stressed the importance of the capacity to reflect upon one's motivational structure and make changes in that structure: "autonomy is conceived of as a second-order capacity of persons to reflect critically upon their first-order preferences, desires, wishes and so forth and the capacity to accept or attempt to change these in light of higher-order preferences and values" (Dworkin 1988: 20). John Christman and others have further developed a historical notion of autonomy in which the genesis of preferences, values, and goals is important. The formation of preferences and the like should not be influenced by factors the person himself resists (or would have resisted to if he were aware of them) (Christman and Anderson 2005; Taylor 2005). As DeGrazia formulates it, preference formation and identification should not result from "influences that [the person] would, on careful reflection, consider alienating" (2005: 102). Critical reflection and identification or endorsement are thus necessary for authenticity and hence autonomy.

Being autonomous means leading one's life in accordance with one's own choices, that is, choices based on one's authentic values and goals, which in turn implies a capacity to reflect upon and endorse or reject the factors that influence one's beliefs and behaviors. This does not necessarily imply that for global autonomy one must reflect upon every choice or action, but it does mean that important values and preferences that make up one's practical identity need to be reflectively endorsed at some point in one's life. As George Agich has argued, even habits and routines can be authentic if they "spring from a developed identity" (1993).

It has recently been argued that the notion of autonomy as used in (medical) ethics has focused one-sidedly at making choices or decisions, and has neglected the equally important dimension of being able to translate ones autonomous choices into effective action (Naik et al. 2009).

Therefore autonomy, understood as a global property of persons, should also be taken to include the ability to make one's choices effective in one's life. This can be referred to as *executive autonomy*. It requires, for example, the ability to make plans and to actually follow up on them. Akrasia, weakness of will, is an example of a situation where executive autonomy fails. One has the capacity for autonomous choice, but fails to actually execute this choice.

Autonomy and neuroscience

Recent advances in neuroscience and cognitive science challenge our naive view of ourselves as fully rational and autonomous beings, as always reasonable originators of our own choices and actions (Sie and Wouters 2010). Research shows that many if not most of our actions are automatically and unconsciously initiated and that only some of our actions are deliberate and consciously based on reasons. According to the thesis of the adaptive unconscious (Wilson 2002), most of the reasons we believe we have and that we believe steer our actions are actually only constructions made up after the fact. According to this view, most of our behavior and actions are actually directed by unconscious processes and influences (Bargh and Chartrand 1999).

However, while these recent insights from behavioral and cognitive neuroscience show that our decisions and behaviors are less rational and reason-driven than we ourselves presume, this does not take away the capacity to step back and reflect that is central to autonomy. As Felsen and Reiner state: "Neurobiology does not exclude the possibility that decisions can be made autonomously. [. . .] with enough time and effort, an agent is capable of employing deliberative, well-considered, and rational processes" (2011:10).

Although some of the assumptions and beliefs underlying the traditional discourse on autonomy may have to be revised or reinterpreted in light of neuroscientific evidence, this does not mean that we should abandon the whole idea of autonomy altogether. On the contrary, new neuroscientific knowledge challenges us to rethink the ways in which or the degrees to which we are autonomous. It is against this background that we can also meaningfully inquire into the effects of new neurotechnologies on our capacity for autonomous choice and action, and, ultimately, on our global autonomy as persons.

Neuromodulation: influencing the mind by manipulating the brain

Neuromodulation refers to a set of relatively new technological methods of influencing the mind by direct intervention in the brain. There are various forms of neurostimulation, which need to be distinguished from neurofeedback. In order to understand the possible effects of these techniques on autonomy, some insight into what these techniques entail and how they function is necessary.

Invasive neurostimulation

Neurostimulation techniques can be subdivided into invasive and non-invasive techniques. The main invasive form of neurostimulation used today is deep brain stimulation (DBS).

DBS involves the surgical implantation of two or more electrodes of about 1.27 mm diameter into specific brain areas. These electrodes are connected to a pacemaker implanted beneath the collarbone, which sends electrical impulses to the brain. The stimulation can be adjusted for exact location and for amplitude of the current, and the device can be switched off. The treating physician sets and adjusts the stimulation parameters. In motor disorders such as Parkinson's disease, the patient can control the device by turning it on or off, though in psychiatric disorders the physician typically controls it. The exact mechanism by which this electrical brain stimulation has its therapeutic effect is not fully understood yet. Nevertheless, DBS has been used successfully in the treatment of neurological illnesses such as Parkinson's disease, tremor, and dystonia, and is currently being investigated for a wide variety of psychiatric and other conditions, such as obsessive-compulsive disorder (OCD), major depression (MD), addiction, obesity, and Alzheimer's disease. Moreover, it may prove possible to use it for enhancement of cognitive functions, mood, or other mental functions in healthy subjects, a prospect that raises significant ethical controversy (Synofzik and Schlaepfer 2008; Pacholczyk 2011). Well-known side effects of DBS include personality changes associated with behavior and mood.

Non-invasive brain stimulation

Non-invasive brain stimulation (NIBS) includes transcranial electrical stimulation, the most frequently used form of which is transcranial direct current stimulation (tDCS); and transcranial magnetic stimulation or TMS. tDCS involves the placement of two surface electrodes on the scalp, through which small electrical currents are applied for the duration of about 20 minutes; this needs to be repeated in several sessions for effects to take hold. TDCS can increase or decrease cortical excitability depending on the direction of the current; these direct effects may last from minutes to hours and can translate into physiological and behavioral modifications, especially in combination with training. The exact working mechanisms are not yet fully understood (Zimerman and Hummel 2010). It is used as an investigative tool, but increasingly also as potential treatment for neurological conditions and in rehabilitation, e.g. after stroke (Tanaka et al. 2011). It also holds promise for the enhancement of cognitive and other brain functions in healthy subjects (Zimerman and Hummel 2010; Hamilton et al. 2011; Cohen Kadosh et al. 2012). For example, tDCS might improve planning ability, or facilitate the learning of new motor tasks or a new language, by transient improvement of the activity and neuroplasticity in the associated brain areas. The long-term effects of training sessions with tDCS can last up to a year (Dockery et al. 2009). tDCS appears to be well-tolerated, easy to use, and less expensive than other techniques.

TMS is a technique involving the application of magnetic fields to the brain, by holding a coil of wire over the head of the subject. The rapid time-varying magnetic field induces small currents in the brain causing hyper- or hypo-polarization of the neurons. Repetitive application of a series of fast pulses (rTMS) can produce increased or decreased cortical excitability, thus turning certain brain areas "on" or "off." A number of sessions are necessary to attain longer lasting effects. TMS is used as a research tool and is FDA approved for the treatment of depression; clinical trials are being performed to test it for treatment of other neuropsychiatric conditions, such as aphasia and motor rehabilitation after stroke, negative symptoms of schizophrenia, Alzheimer's, disease, tinnitus, and tic disorders like Tourette's syndrome (Rossi et al. 2009). It has also been reported to stimulate creativity and to give subjects savant-like abilities (Osborne 2003). Like tDCS, it can be combined with training and may enhance neuroplasticity and specific brain functions (Steven and Pascual-Leone 2006); it is therefore frequently mentioned as a potential tool for (cognitive) enhancement (Hamilton et al. 2011; Cohen Kadosh et al. 2012). Compared to tDCS, rTMS can be focused more precisely, but it is less easy to use, more expensive, and holds a risk of inducing seizures. The currents in tDCS are too small to induce seizures, but (repeated) application of strong magnetic fields can have that effect in some subjects.

Neurofeedback

Neurofeedback is a different neuromodulation technique. It does not work via invasive or non-invasive external stimulation of the brain, but through the subject's own mental activity. The subject can see a real-time representation of his own brain activity as recorded by either EEG or fMRI on a screen and can learn to find the mental activity that influences that brain activity. By performing this mental activity (e.g. thinking of a certain experience, or activity) the subject can influence his brain activity, and this is fed back to him directly in the form of changing patterns or pictures on the screen. For example, an animation of a thermometer can be used, and the subject be asked to keep the temperature at a certain level, using his brain activity (see Linden et al. 2012). In this way, specific brain areas and activity patterns can be trained in a number of sessions; the effects may last up to months or even years after the training sessions (Angelakis et al. 2007). Feedback using fMRI has a considerable higher spatial precision than that using EEG and will therefore probably be better suited to influence specific mental states or functions (Johnston et al. 2009). Neurofeedback can thus be used to train individuals to regulate activity patterns in specific brain areas. According to Hammond: "the process is a little like exercising or doing physical therapy with the brain, enhancing cognitive flexibility and control" (2011: 306). EEG-neurofeedback is used for attention deficit hyperactivity disorder (ADHD), anxiety, and addictions, and might in principle be used for cognitive enhancement (Angelakis et al. 2007; Rabipur and Raz 2012). fMRI-neurofeedback has been proposed as potential treatment for disorders such as phobias, depression (Linden et al. 2012), and pedophilia (Renaud et al. 2011).

In sum, all these techniques have the potential to alter brain activity, physiology, and perhaps structure and thereby influence associated mental abilities and mental states. They can all have longer-lasting effects, although the duration of effects of non-invasive neuromodulation and neurofeedback is not yet clear. While the effects of DBS are mostly reversible when the stimulation is turned off, Synofzik and Schlaepfer state that "it has to be questioned whether DBS-induced changes to volitional behaviour and decisional preferences are indeed reversible in all DBS subjects" (2012: 34). These techniques can alter mood, cognitive capacities, motivations, desires, and behavior and thus appear to affect autonomy. In the next section, it will be argued that actual effects on autonomy can differ depending on the situation and circumstances.

Reducing, restoring, and enhancing autonomy

Since neuromodulation can affect many of the capacities relevant to autonomy, and can influence mood and behavior, it makes sense to ask whether neuromodulation techniques infringe on autonomy. This could provide a reason for governments or professional guidelines to restrict the range of its application, or a reason for subjects to reject it. The influence of neuromodulation on autonomy is much more complex than this question presumes, however. Neuromodulation can reduce, restore, or enhance autonomy, or leave it unaffected. Obviously, it matters here which aspect or interpretation of autonomy we are talking about. I distinguish between autonomy as an actual global condition of persons (encompassing authentic decision-making and executive autonomy); autonomy as a "local" property of specific choices and actions; and capacities necessary for autonomy such as self-reflection, rational decision-making, or executive powers.

Reducing autonomy

The most obvious way in which neuromodulation can lead to non-autonomous action is when behavior or movements are induced in a way that bypasses or undermines the agent's voluntary control of them. For example, electrical stimulation of a certain brain area will cause laughter, without anything funny being said or done. TMS can cause a person's hand to move involuntarily. In these cases behavior is induced by neuromodulation in a way that clearly makes it non-autonomous. However, it appears that such examples are limited to relatively simple actions. It does not seem realistic (at least not for the near future) to believe that more complex behaviors can be induced directly. The fear expressed by the EGE, that such techniques might be used to obtain "control over the will of people" and turn them into some kind of remote-controlled robots seems unwarranted.

Neuromodulation can also reduce autonomy by disturbing the capacities necessary for autonomous decision-making. For example, DBS may affect the cognitive and affective capacities that are necessary for rational choice and sound judgment, and thereby negatively influence the competence to decide. The case of a Dutch Parkinson's patient who became manic after DBS treatment and lost his decisional capacities is a good example of this (Leentjes et al. 2004; Glannon 2009; Schermer 2009). Although this case may be extreme, the occurrence of manic symptoms is a well-known potential side effect of DBS that can negatively affect competence to decide. In the context of medical treatment, such an infringement on capacities will never be intentional, but it can be an unintended side effect.

The most difficult cases to judge are those in which neuromodulation affects the person's deep-seated values, preferences, and character traits – his or her personal narrative identity or practical identity. Here the core of personal autonomy, the person's authenticity, is at stake. This reflects on autonomy both as a global property of persons ánd as a local property of choices and actions. Can a person still be called "really himself" or "really herself" when important aspects of who the person is are altered by neuromodulation? Can the behavior and actions stemming from these changes be really one's own?

There has been some discussion in the literature about this question (e.g. Bublitz and Merkel 2009; Schermer 2011; Lipsman and Glannon 2012), and there are a number of reports about changes in people's behavior, inclinations, and preferences after DBS. Moreover, there are some suggestions about how certain traits of persons might by changed by neuromodulation. Examples of such changes are:

- the emergence of a strong inclination or (first-order) desire to gamble in persons who did not care for gambling before their DBS treatment;
- increase in sexual desire, thoughts, and behavior ("hypersexuality") in some patients treated with DBS;
- decrease in a (specific type of) sexual desire or preference, as would be intended in treatment of pedophiles;
- becoming more short-tempered, as reported by the spouse of a patient treated with DBS: "He is not like he was before. He gets annoyed over the smallest things. He is almost aggressive towards me sometimes" (Gisquet 2008: 1849);
- becoming more laissez-faire: "after the surgery I became very lazy, previously I was not at all like that. I would drop a handkerchief and not bother to pick it up" (Gisquet 2008: 1849);
- becoming less impulsive and more self-controlled, as is the aim in neuromodulation-based treatments for ADHD or addiction.

The important question here is: does neuromodulation influence preference formation, or the process of second-order identification with one's preferences, in ways that are subverting and render them inauthentic?

Does it influence the formation of new desires or traits in a way that the person him- or herself would resist, or find alienating?

DeGrazia's theory of personal identity is roughly in line with the theories of autonomy of Dworkin and Christman outlined earlier. He has argued extensively that changes in narrative identity, e.g. changes in internal psychological style, intelligence, or personality, brought about by medication or other technology can be autonomous (DeGrazia 2005). He does not explicitly refer to neuromodulation, but we can follow the same line of thought. This implies that whether the new traits, preferences, or values listed above are authentic or not depends on two things: whether the person identifies with his or her new traits or desires; and whether he or she identifies with their genesis. This latter condition asks whether the person would, on reflection, consider the influence of the neuromodulation on the process of preference formation and of identification to be a subverting or alienating influence.

Recall the case of the manic Parkinson's patient. He probably did not really identify (on a higher level of reflection) with his new desires to buy expensive cars and make sexual advances to nurses. He definitely lacked the capacity to reflect on the genesis of these desires, since he had anosognosia and denied that anything about him had changed at all. The capacity to reflect on his motivational structure, necessary for autonomy, was lost completely due to the DBS.

Suppose that the "lazy" patient would, on reflection, not like his "new self." Suppose he would become annoyed by his own carelessness and lethargy and would resist it as alien to himself. In that case he would be less autonomous than he was before. Or suppose that the "short-tempered husband" would at first identify with his new behavior but then, on reflection, realize that his behavior was different from before and probably caused by the DBS. Suppose he did not like the idea of being influenced so much by this device and considered it an illegitimate interference with his thoughts and feelings. In that case his new traits and behavior would not be autonomous either.

One can also imagine, however, that changes induced by neuromodulation could be perfectly autonomous on this account. Pedophiles who do not identify with their sexual desires and want to get rid of them might welcome the opportunity to change their preferences with neuromodulation. If they consider this trait as alien to themselves, they may decide to change it, or have it changed. If, on reflection, they consider neuromodulation to be a good and acceptable means to this end, the changes brought about can be considered authentic. Changes in traits or preferences induced by neuromodulation can thus be deemed autonomous if the individuals themselves endorse their new traits, that is are positive about the changes in their personality or views, *and* are aware of the way in which they have come about and approve of this. So, they must not resist these new traits or the neuromodulation that brought them about, nor must they be unknowingly manipulated into these new traits. This implies that in principle a person's retrospective judgment of changes in his or her preferences or traits is authoritative, not his or her prospective judgment. Merkel et al. (2007) have argued that personality changes can only be authentic if patients approve of them before the changes take place. But this would imply that unintended and unforeseen changes in a person's traits or preferences could never become authentically his or her own. Even more problematic, it would imply that the unintended changes in our preferences, goals, or values, as shaped by our upbringing or experience, would never be authentic because we would not have approved of them before the fact. Therefore, retrospective reflective endorsement of preferences or traits and their genesis suffices to consider new preferences or traits authentic, and choices and actions based on them autonomous.

Restoring autonomy

Neuromodulation can also restore autonomy, as it does in cases when patients are successfully treated for conditions that have a negative impact on autonomy. The autonomy of people with compromised cognitive functions, e.g. because of brain damage or Alzheimer's disease could be (partly) restored if neuromodulation would live up to its promises of cognition improvement.

Other cases are a bit more complex. Take, for example, obsessive-compulsive disorder or addiction, both paradigmatic examples of disorders that negatively affect autonomy. Actions performed by a patient with OCD, like repetitive hand washing or checking the locks, are not autonomous since they stem from urges or strong desires – compulsions – which the patient does not identify with. In most cases, the compulsions are experienced as alien, and the patient can appreciate the irrationality of the resulting behavior, but can nevertheless not resist. His or her higher-order cognitive control over his or her behavior fails. Successful treatment of this disorder, e.g. with DBS, can restore autonomy. Instead of acting on compulsions (first-order preferences), one can again act on one's second-order volitions, or, put differently, in line with one's own self-identity and according to the values and goals one identifies with. A similar argument can apply in cases of addiction.

Because OCD, addiction, and probably some other psychiatric conditions too impair a person's autonomy and render much of his or her behavior non-autonomous, successful treatment of these conditions can be said to restore autonomy. In such cases one may call the DBS an "internal prosthesis for the will" (Ford and Kubu 2007). I mean to use the word prosthesis here in a positive sense, as a support, something that helps to restore lost functions, in this case: autonomous control over one's actions, being able to act in accordance with one's authentic preferences. One might consider a prosthesis to be something alien, something external to oneself and therefore problematic when it comes to restoring autonomy. It might be argued that the "auto" or self cannot be restored by something that is external to it (see Lipsman and Glannon 2012). However, it appears that many people who use some sort of prosthesis like a limb-prosthesis or cochlear implant – which are brain–computer interfaces, just like DBS – quite easily adapt to these and incorporate the prosthesis into their self-image and body scheme. It is not clear why one could not do the same with prostheses for impaired or damaged brain functions. Philosophical support for the position that such a prosthesis can be considered a true part of the self can be found in Clark and Chalmers' extended mind hypothesis (Clark and Chalmers 1998; cf. Anderson 2008). As discussed in the previous section, when considering the influence on autonomy the judgment on whether the influence of a prosthesis is "alien" to the person or not should be made by that person alone.

Another example of restoration of autonomy with the aid of neuromodulation concerns treatment of ADHD. When treated successfully, for example with neurofeedback, the patients' capacities for concentration and impulse-control increase, and this enables them to act more in accordance with the goals and values they identify with. As some ADHD patients successfully treated with psychopharmaceuticals claim, they are even "more themselves" with medication than without, because the medication enables them to do things they truly want and value (Bolt and Schermer 2009). The same can be said for treatment with neurofeedback, tDCS, or TMS. The difference with DBS would be that there is no prosthesis involved here (and no "chemical support" as with the use of psychopharmaceuticals). Instead, the brain might be "rewired" without leaving any permanent foreign objects in place. Whether this is a relevant difference will be further discussed below.

In sum, all treatments with neuromodulation that successfully treat symptoms of diseases or disorders that reduce autonomy in any way can be said to restore autonomy. They can do this on different levels, for example by strengthening the patient's cognitive capacities required for rational decision-making; by improving impulse control and cognitive control over one's own behavior; or by restoring the affective and motivational capacities essential for autonomy. Neuromodulation can help persons to be "more themselves," to act on desires and choices that are truly their own and in line with their authentic values and goals.

Enhancing autonomy

It may even be possible to enhance autonomy through neuromodulation. The distinction between the treatment of neuropsychiatric disorders and the enhancement of normal traits is not sharp but fluent (Schermer and Bolt 2011). When treatment is taken to refer to restoring to normal and enhancement to improving over and above normal, it becomes clear that the dividing line between the two concepts is normality. Yet normality is very difficult to define when it comes to the kinds of capacities we are concerned with here. Treating concentration disorders fades into enhancing normal concentration; restoring self-control in addiction fades into strengthening self-control in the everyday akratic person; treating cognitive disorders fades into improving cognition in the intellectually intact (Greely et al. 2008). As noted, capacities relevant to autonomy, such as cognitive capacities, can be influenced and sometimes improved by neuromodulation. So in theory as well as practice restoring autonomy might fade into enhancing autonomy.

Neuro-enhancement – also referred to as "cosmetic neurology" (Chatterjee 2006) – can be consistent with autonomy when it involves adapting one's preferences and traits to one's authentic values and goals. Just as unintended changes in preferences or traits can become authentic through reflective endorsement, so too can intentionally sought adaptations in the self make one more authentic (DeGrazia 2005; Bolt and Schermer 2009; Levy 2011). Another aspect of autonomy that might arguably be enhanced through neuromodulation is one's executive autonomy: by increasing one's willpower and enhancing one's capacity to resist temptation and weakness of will, it might be possible to bring one's actual behavior more in line with one's authentic preferences and choices.

An interesting philosophical question that presents itself here is whether autonomy can in theory be enhanced indefinitely, or whether there is an optimal state of autonomy. It seems that the ideal of autonomy would count as such an optimal state; but it is by no means clear what the ideal of autonomy entails exactly. We may agree that enhancing the cognitive and affective capacities necessary for rational decision-making would increase our ability for autonomous decision-making. Strengthening our willpower, or our capacity for self-control, for planning, and for the actual execution of plans would strengthen executive autonomy. If neurofeedback could help us to avoid or decrease incidents of akrasia, or could help decrease ego-depletion, then this would contribute to the capacity to act autonomously and consequently to autonomy as a global property of the person. Persons who are more "in control" of themselves due to TMS or neurofeedback training may be said to have enhanced their autonomy. But it appears that one could be too much in control; if one always acted completely in accordance with the values and goals one deeply identifies with, would there be any room left to change and develop these goals and values? Would it be possible to fully exercise freedom of choice and develop one's personal identity? If we were always to make completely rational decisions and act accordingly, wouldone not lose the capacity to be surprised, to learn from mistakes, or to accidentally stumble upon new interests or values? Would this not make one rigid and overly rationalistic? We could even take this thought experiment one step further. What would it mean if the "self" were to become completely malleable? Would persons come to see those aspects of themselves they did not like (their impulsive/depressed/compulsive/impatient/sentimental self) as completely split off from their "real" self if they could use neuromodulation techniques to fix or control the parts they found alien? Would such extreme self-creation make one the ideal example of an authentic and autonomous person? But who would be the "self" doing the creating?

Since there are no realistic prospects yet for such extreme enhancements and self-modulations, trying to answer these questions falls outside the scope of this contribution. However, they do point to important questions for theories of autonomy and authenticity. Moreover, they show us that neuromodulation technologies, especially if they were to become more powerful and widespread, are likely to contribute to changes in our self-understanding and our relationship with ourselves.

How differences between techniques matter

In this final section we will turn to the question of how the difference between techniques that influence the brain and mind reflects on their impact on autonomy. In his 1976 article, Dworkin claims that "we prefer methods of influence which work through the cognitive and affective structure of the agent, which require active participation of the agent in producing the change, to those which short-circuit the desires and beliefs of the agent and make him a passive recipient of the change" (1976: 28). This intuition is echoed in many contemporary writings on influencing the brain (e.g. Freedman 1998; Manninen 2006; Levy 2007).

Direct or indirect

A first distinction that is frequently made is that between direct and indirect modes of influencing the mind, correlating roughly with physical and mental influences. The idea that direct brain modulation is somehow more threatening to our self or to our autonomy than more traditional forms of influencing the mind – like education, training, or psychotherapy – may have more to do with the unfamiliarity of these new techniques than with sound argument, however. Neuroscientific research has made it clear that at the molecular and neuronal levels, the effects on the brain of either talk-therapy or psychopharmaceuticals can be the same. Likewise, practice and training can lead to structural anatomical changes in the brain as the famous example of London taxi drivers shows. The size of their hippocampus correlates with the amount of time spent driving and navigating (Maguire et al. 2000). These findings problematize the intuitive distinction between direct and indirect modulation of the brain.

tDCS and TMS in combination with training sessions are examples of techniques that blur the line between direct and indirect, physical and mental. TDCS or TMS may facilitate learning, but do not fundamentally change the mechanisms of normal learning. They require the same type of training, effort and exercise. The learning capacity of the brain (neuroplasticity) is enhanced by direct brain stimulation, but the actual changes associated with learning are brought about indirectly. Likewise, neurofeedback can be thought of as "a holistic approach that overcomes bio-psychological dualisms" (Linden at al. 2012: 9). Even though here there is no direct physical influence exerted on the brain, the technique vividly illustrates the intimate connection of brain and mind. Neurofeedback can be understood as mind-induced brain modulation.

Next to being difficult to uphold, the direct/indirect distinction is also not in itself sufficient reason to claim a difference in impact on the subject's autonomy. As discussed above, changed traits, desires, and values can be authentic and autonomous, even if they are brought about by directly modulating the brain, as long as the person in question identifies with them and their formation process. At the same time, changes brought about through more indirect influences may be non-autonomous, as cases of hypnosis and brainwashing show. It seems possible that a rather indirect technique like neurofeedback could produce non-autonomous behavior or traits. Suppose, for example, that the instructors of the neurofeedback gave false information to the subject, so that while the subject thought he or she was training for a more uplifted mood, he or she was in fact training his or her aggression or ruthlessness. Or suppose that the identification of the relevant brain areas was incorrect, due to some mistake or technical problem – this might also cause the subject in question to train the wrong abilities or traits: not those he or she expects and (autonomously) wants to train, but something he or she does not identify with. In such cases, the result would be non-autonomous because of non-identification and because the subject would not agree with the way in which these changes had come about. Still, for practical reasons, it appears that the potential to produce non-autonomous changes or behavior in people is greater with direct interventions like DBS than with more indirect interventions such as neurofeedback. With the former the subject has less control over the application once it has been implanted, and the effects on behavior are more outspoken.

Active or passive

A second distinction that intuitively matters is that between passive and active changes to the self or to one's traits, desires, and behavior. Whereas in DBS the subject is a passive recipient of the therapy and changes are induced without the active input of the subject him- or herself, in neurofeedback the active participation of the subject is indispensable to effectuate changes. Neurofeedback only works if the subject follows the instructions and exercises his or her own mental powers to influence his or her neuronal architecture. Although changes take place in the brain due to neurofeedback, these changes are not brought about by some force external to the subject – not by currents, magnetic fields, added neurotransmitters, or chemical substances – but by the subject's own mental power. This takes effort and exercise. The question is whether this active participation required for neurofeedback – and some applications of TMS and tDCS in combination with training – is relevantly different from the passive receipt of DBS, in terms of its impact on autonomy.

It can be argued on empirical grounds that techniques requiring active participation are more likely to support autonomy and less likely to reduce or disrupt it than passive techniques. First of all, the time and effort invested by subjects in neurofeedback training can be taken as a sign that they really want those changes; subjects reconfirm this every time they cooperate in the training. It is easier to stop the training and resist changes if one does not identify with them. Moreover, it may be easier for subjects to incorporate changes made through effort (tDCS training, neurofeedback) into their self-image and to make them their own. Unlike in DBS, there is no device, no "third element," that one can consider alien to oneself. Moreover, while DBS is in principle reversible and thus needs to be applied continuously to have effect, neurofeedback or tDCS may effectuate permanent changes, or at least changes that outlast the application of the technique. This may make such changes more likely to be considered one's own.

Another argument would be that effort invested in changing certain traits or adapting one's behavior would make these more truly one's own, in the sense that effort could be seen as conferring some sort of ownership. However, with regard to autonomy it is the process of identification and not the process of formation that is relevant. One might argue that certain traits require a certain genesis. Bublitz and Merkel (2009) follow Fischer and Ravizza in claiming that virtues are not truly virtues if they have been "implanted" through a device instead of acquired through exercise and education. This may be right, but it says nothing about the authenticity and autonomy of someone who has had virtues 'implanted as distinct from one who has become virtuous as a result of one's own effort.

Using or bypassing reason

A third and closely related distinction that is often made is that between mind-altering techniques that bypass reason and those that make use of reason, like psychotherapy. This is closely associated with the idea that we should regard persons (including ourselves) as rational, reasons-responsive beings, since this is a precondition for respecting them as beings with a potential for autonomy. By using techniques that do not appeal to reason or rational capacities to change traits, values, or preferences, we may regard persons in an overly mechanistic way. Using neuromodulation techniques like DBS implies, in a sense, that we treat ourselves as mere machines, and thus as non-autonomous. However, acknowledging that we are never completely "in control" of ourselves, that not all our actions and preferences are caused by our reasons, and that we indeed are, in certain respects, complex neurobiological machines (or mechanisms) does not imply that we cannot also be capable of autonomy. It is exactly the capacity that we have to step back and reflect on ourselves, including all the mechanisms that shape who we are, that lies at the heart of autonomy. The fact that we can relate to ourselves and effectuate changes in our motivational structure makes us autonomous. Even if the means we choose to do so bypass our rationality (like DBS), our choice to change ourselves in that way can still spring from our own rational and authentic preferences. In some cases, the traits or behaviors we want to change are themselves irrational, as in patients with phobias or OCD or in the case of "Lucy" described by Freeman (1998) and Levy (2007). It may be perfectly rational to use mechanistic means to effect changes in such cases, especially if they cannot be reached in other ways, or not without a disproportional amount of effort or hardship. Using our rationality and reasons-responsiveness and using mechanistic means need not be mutually exclusive but instead can be thought of as complementary.

It is not clear to what degree the objection of bypassing reason also holds for techniques that require mental activity and the participation of subjects themselves. In a sense, neurofeedback bypasses reason and makes one regard oneself in a mechanistic way. Traits or preferences must be understood as brain states or functions and the technique as a means of adapting brain activity. It is not "reasons" that cause changes in the brain, but the performance of mental tasks such as imagining a pleasant situation, or "rehearsing the aversive repercussions of the deviant sexual behaviour of the patient for himself" in cases of pedophilia (Renaud et al. 2011: 269). The goal of these mental tasks is to change brain activity in a specific area, and the patient must focus on the visual feedback in order to try to perform the right mental activity. He is not asked to focus on the reasons he might have for trying to change. Somehow "performing the right mental activity in order to adapt brain-activity in a specific area" sounds different from "rehearsing the reasons one has to control ones unwanted sexual impulses." However, it is not clear whether there is a real difference here, or whether these are just two different descriptions of the same situation. Does neurofeedback bypass reason here, or does it enhance the effect of reason? Is it a mechanistic way to control or govern oneself, or is it a reason-based way? I would say neurofeedback shows that these cannot be understood as mutually exclusive categories.

Conclusion

Neuromodulation can be effected by various existing and emerging techniques. Depending on the context, the exact effects, and the person in question, neuromodulation can have disrupting, restorative, or enhancing effects on autonomy. Neurodmodulation can sometimes impede the capacity for autonomy, as it does in cases of DBS-induced mental incompetence, for example. More difficult cases to judge are those in which the intervention affects the person's values and preferences, his or her practical identity. Changes in these values may be non-autonomous when they are induced involuntarily. However, if the person reflectively endorses the new preferences, values, or traits and the way in which they were formed, they can be considered autonomous. So, the global autonomy of the person subjected to neuromodulation can be disrupted, but this is not a necessity.

Neuromodulation can also restore capacities necessary for autonomy, as it does in cases when patients are successfully treated for obsessive-compulsive disorder or addiction, or other autonomy-compromising disorders. Last, but not least, it may even be possible to enhance autonomy through neuromodulation, for example by improving cognitive capacities or impulse control, or by helping the person to make desired changes in his or her motivational structure.

There are subtle but relevant differences between techniques. Some are more prone to abuse and to disrupting autonomy than others. Active mental involvement, such as required by neurofeedback (and in some applications of TMS and tDCS), makes it more likely that persons can identify with changes and make them their own.

Finally, the self-understanding and self-relationship that are implicitly promoted by these techniques deserve to be further investigated. We appear to be moving in the direction of a self-understanding in which we accept that we are not fully in rational control of ourselves and that we can understand ourselves to a certain degree as neuronal mechanisms. At the same time, we retain our mental capacity to step back and reflect on these mechanisms and our reasons, and to use neuromodulating techniques to steer ourselves in the direction that we desire and identify with. Thinking about neuromodulation techniques can help us gain a better understanding of ourselves and of the relationship between our brains and our minds.

REFERENCES

Agich, G. J. (1993) *Autonomy and Long-Term Care*. New York: Oxford University Press.

Anderson, J. (2008) Neuro-prosthetics, the extended mind and respect for persons with disability. In Düwell, M., Rehmann-Sutter, Chr., and Mieth, Dietman (eds.) *The Contingent Nature of Life: Bioethics and Limits of Human Existence*. Springer, pp. 259–274.

Angelakis, E., Stathopoulou, S., Frymiare, J. L., Green, D. L., Lubar J. F., et al. (2007) EEG Neurofeedback: a brief overview and an example of peak alpha frequency training for cognitive enhancement in the elderly. *The Clinical Neurpsychologist* 21, 1: 110–129.

Bargh, J. A. and Chartrand, T. L. (1999) The unbearable automaticity of being. *American Psychologist* 54, 7: 462–479.

Bolt, I. and Schermer, M. (2009) Psychopharmaceutical enhancers: enhancing identity? *Neuroethics* 2: 103–111.

Bublitz, J. C. and Merkel, R. (2009) Autonomy and authenticity of enhanced personality traits. *Bioethics* 23: 360–374.

Christman, J. and Anderson, J. (eds.) (2005) *Autonomy and the Challenges to Liberalism*. Cambridge University Press.

Clark, A. and Chalmers, D. (1998) The extended mind. *Analysis* 58: 7–19.

Chatterjee, A. (2006) The promise and predicament of cosmetic neurology. *Journal of Medical Ethics* 32: 110–113.

Cohen Kadosh, R. and Levy, N., O'Shea, J., Shea, N., and Savulescu, J. (2012) The neuroethics of non-invasive brain stimulation. *Current Biology* 22, 4: 108–111.

DeGrazia, D. (2005) *Human Identity and Bioethics*. New York: Cambridge University Press.

Dockery, C. A., Heuckel-Weng, R., O'Shea, J., Shea, N., and Savulescu, J. (2009) Enhancement of planning ability by transcranial direct current stimulation. *The Journal of Neuroscience* 29, 22: 7271–7277.

Dworkin, G. (1976) Autonomy and behaviour control. *Hastings Center Report*, vol. 6, no. 1, pp. 23–28.

(1988) *The Theory and Practice of Autonomy*. Cambridge University Press.

EGE – European Group on Ethics in Science and New Technologies (2005). *Ethical Aspects of ICT Implants in the Human Body*. Opinion no. 20. Retrieved from http://icaact.org/files/european-groups-ethics-ict-implants-opinion-20.pdf

Feinberg, J. (1986) *Harm to Self: The Moral Limits of the Criminal Law*. New York: Oxford University Press.

Felsen, G. and Reiner, P. (2011) How the neuroscience of decision-making informs our conception of autonomy. *AJOB Neuroscience* 2, 3: 3–14.

Ford, P. and Kubu, C. (2007) Ameliorating and exacerbating: surgical "prosthesis" in addiction. *American Journal of Bioethics* 7, 1: 29–32.

Freedman, C. (1998) Aspirin for the mind? Some ethical worries about psychopharmacology. In Parens, E. (ed.) *Enhancing Human Traits: Ethical and Social Implications*. Washington, DC: Georgetown University Press, pp. 135–150.

Gisquet, E. (2008) Cerebral implants and Parkinson's disease: a unique form of biographical disruption? *Social Science and Medicine* 67: 1847–1851.

Glannon, W. (2009) Stimulating brains, altering minds. *Journal of Medical Ethics* 35: 289–292.

Greely, H., Sahakian, B., Harris, J., Kessler, R. C., Gazzaniga, M., et al. (2008) Towards responsible use of cognitive enhancing drugs by the healthy. *Nature* 456: 702–705.

Hamilton, R., Messing, S., and Chatterjee, A. (2011) Rethinking the thinking cap: ethics of neural enhancement using noninvasive brain stimulation. *Neurology* 76: 187–193.

Hammond, D. C. (2011) What is neurofeedback: an update. *Journal of Neurotherapy* 15, 4: 305–336.

Johnston, S. J., Boehm, S .G., Healy, D., Goebal, R., and Linden, D. E. (2009) Neurofeedback: a promising tool for the self-regulation of emotion networks. *NeuroImage* Doi: 10.1016/j.neuroimage.2009.07.056.

Leentjes, A. F. G., Visser-Vanderwalle, V., Temel, Y., and Verhey, F. R. (2004) Manipuleerbare wilsbekwaamheid: een ethisch probleem bij elektrostimulatie van de nucleaus subthalamicus voor een ernstige ziekte van

Parkinson. *[Manipulable competence] Nederlands* Tijdschrift voor Geneeskunde 148: 1394–1397.

Levy, N. (2007) *Neuroethics: Challenges for the 21st Century*. Cambridge University Press.

(2011) Enhancing authenticity. *Journal of Applied Philosophy* 28, 3: 308–318.

Linden, D. E. J., Habes, I., Johnston, S. J., Linden, S., Tatineni, R., et al. (2012) Real-time self-regulation of emotion networks in patients with depression. *PLoS One* 7, 6: e38115.

Lipsman, N. and Glannon, W. (2012) Brain, mind and machine: what are the implications of deep brain stimulation for perceptions of personal identity, agency and free will? *Bioethics*, Doi: 10.1111/j.1467–8519.2012.01978.x.

Maguire, E. A., Gadian, G., Johnsrude, I. S., Good, C. D., Ashburner, J. et al. (2000) Navigation-related structural change in the hippocampi of taxi-drivers. *PNAS* 97 (8): 4389–4403.

Manninen, B. (2006) Medicating the mind: a Kantian analysis of overprescribing psychoactive drugs. *Journal of Medical Ethics* 32: 100–105.

Merkel, R., G. Boer, J. Fegert, Galert, T., Hartmann, D., et al. (2007) *Intervening in the Brain: Changing Psyche and Society*. Berlin: Springer-Verlag.

Naik, A. D., Dyer, C. B., Kunik, M. E., and McCullough, L.B. (2009) Patient autonomy for the management of chronic conditions: a two component re-conceptualization. *AJOB* 9, 2: 23–30.

Osborne, L. (2003) Savant for a day. *New York Times Magazine*, June 22.

Pacholczyk, A. (2011) DBS makes you feel good! *Frontiers in Integrative Neuroscience*, Doi 10.3389/fnint.2011.00014.

Rabipur, S. and Raz, A. (2012) Training the brain: fact and fad in cognitive and behavioural remediation. *Brain and Cognition* 79: 159–179.

Renaud, P., Joyal, C., Stoleru, S., Goyette, M., Weiskopf, N., et al. (2011) Real-time functional magnetic imaging, brain–computer interface and virtual reality: promising tools for the treatment of pedophilia. *Progress in Brain Research* 192: 263–272.

Rossi, S., Hallett, M., Rossini, P. M., Pascual-Leone, A., Avanzini, G., et al. (2009) Safety, ethical considerations, and application guidelines for the use of transcranial magnetic stimulation in clinical practice and research. *Clinical Neurophysiology* 120: 2008–2039.

Schermer, M. (2002) *The Different Faces of Autonomy*. Dordrecht: Kluwer Academic Publishers.

(2009) Changes in the self: the need for conceptual research next to empirical research. *AJOB* 9, 5: 45–47.

(2011) Health, happiness and human enhancement: dealing with unexpected effects of deep brain stimulation. *Neuroethics*, Doi: 10.1007/s12152-011-9097–5.

Schermer, M. and Bolt, I. (2011) What's in a name? ADHD and the grey area between treatment and enhancement. In Savulescu, J., ter Meulen, R., and Kahane, G. (eds.) *Enhancing Human Capacities*. Chichester: Wiley-Blackwell Publishers, pp. 179–193.

Sie, M. and Wouters, A. (2010) The BNC challenge to compatibilist free will and personal responsibility. *Neuroethics* 3: 121–133.

Steven, M. S. and Pascual-Leone, A. (2006) Transcranial magnetic stimulation and the human brain: an ethical evaluation. In Illes, J. (ed.) *Neuroethics: Defining the Issues in Theory, Practice and Policy*. Oxford University Press, pp. 201–212.

Synofzik, M. and T. E. Schlaepfer (2008) Stimulating personality: ethical criteria for deep brain stimulation in psychiatric patients for enhancement purposes. *Biotechnology Journal* 3: 1511–1520.

Synofzik, M., Schlaepfer, T. E., and Fins, J. J. (2012) How happy is too happy? *AJOB Neuroscience* 3, 1: 30–36.

Tanaka, S., Sandrini, M., and Cohen, L. G. (2011) Modulation of motor learning and memory formation by non-invasive cortical stimulation of the primary motor cortex. *Neuropsychological Rehabilitation: An International Journal* 21, 5: 650–675.

Taylor, J. S. (ed.) (2005) *Personal Autonomy: New Essays on Personal Autonomy and its Role in Contemporary Moral Philosophy*. Cambridge University Press.

Wilson, T. D. (2002) *Strangers to Ourselves: Discovering the Adaptive Unconscious*. Cambridge: Belknap Press.

Zimerman, M. and Hummel, F. C. (2010) Non-invasive brain stimulation: enhancing motor and cognitive functions in healthy old subjects. *Frontiers in Aging Neuroscience*, Doi 10.3389/fnagi.2010.00149

Part V

Legal implications of neuroscience

12 Neurobiology collides with moral and criminal responsibility: the result is double vision

Steven E. Hyman

ABSTRACT

Increasingly compelling, if not always mature, mechanistic descriptions of human decision making and action have kindled new interest in the question of free will. From my point of view as a skeptical practicing scientist, I briefly review the status of free will, and of compatibilist positions that find room for meaningful free will in a determinist universe. I argue against compatibilism, and in favor of an uncomfortable acceptance of the collision between scientifically supported determinism (plus chance) and our ineluctable intuitive sense of agency. Besides being more honest about scientific understandings of our intuitions, I argue that acceptance of this disjunction can yield productive debates with practical consequences in legislative bodies, policy circles, and criminal justice systems.

> We argue that neuroscience will probably have a transformative effect on the law . . . New neuroscience will change the law, not by undermining its current assumptions, but by transforming people's moral intuitions about free will and responsibility. (Greene and Cohen 2004)

> Brains do not commit crimes; people commit crimes. . . . advocates all too often make moral and legal claims that the new neuroscience does not entail and cannot sustain. (Morse 2006)

> Now give those kine a wide berth keep your thoughts intent on your course for home . . .
>
> But if you raid the beeves, I see destruction for ship and crew (Circe's warning to Odysseus to avoid the cattle of the sun god; Odyssey Bk. 12 lines 108–9, 111–112, Fitzgerald Translation)

Introduction: resurgent concerns about free will and responsibility

Why has there been resurgent interest in the problem of free will? After all, questions of whether human beings possess free will and how freedom relates to moral responsibility are truly ancient. The *Iliad* and *Odyssey*, composed between 1200 and 850 BC, which antedate evidence of formal philosophical inquiry, explore the complex relationship of free will to culpability. Gods intervene in human decisions and action, as in the episode of the cattle of the sun, but humans experience the consequences of their actions as if fully morally responsible. Early Christian thinkers such as Augustine of Hippo engaged in no small number of philosophical contortions to square the concept of an omnipotent and omniscient God with human free will and with the conundrum of how God could permit humans to do evil. In early modern times Descartes famously resorted to substance dualism in what now seems a desperate attempt to rescue human reason (although not human emotions) from the mechanistic worldview that he had himself played a significant role in promulgating.

New interest in free will and moral responsibility appears to have flowed from progress in human genetics (Sullivan et al. 2012) and more importantly in neuroscience and closely related branches of psychology. Together these have begun to flesh out mechanisms underlying diverse aspects of cognition and behavior, including insights into human decision making and action. In principle, these recent scientific discoveries do not raise substantially different obstacles to free will than much earlier views of a mechanistic universe from which Descartes (we should now say vainly) attempted to shield human reason. If anything the twentieth-century recognition of stochastic processes operating in physics and biology weakened eighteenth-century claims of essentially perfect predictive power conferred by determinist theories. It is not, however, abstract arguments about determinism, but salient results coming from modern genetics, neuroscience, and psychology that have rekindled interest in the problem of free will. Not only academic journals but also serious trade publications bear witness to reawakened anxieties and arguments concerning freedom and related issues such as moral and legal responsibility (Dennett 2003; Satel and Lilienfeld 2013). Roskies (2010) has pointed out that elucidation of neural mechanisms carry greater weight than metaphysical arguments in real-life settings such as courtrooms. A defense attorney might convincingly argue for mitigation of culpability by describing her client's receipt of harsh beatings as a child; she would produce only irritation and possibly derision in the court if she tried to get her client off the hook by arguing for determinism based on general physical principles. This is likely to be the case even though connections between childhood experience and specific adult criminal acts are tenuously probabilistic rather than convincingly causal, whereas the arguments from hard determinism could at least claim to address causality, even if only abstractly. Whether or not they are serving as jurors, people are generally concerned with intuitively comprehensible circumstances under which it would seem appropriate to hold others responsible rather than with philosophical arguments abstracted away from life experience (Wolf 1987).

There is growing recognition of the significant challenges confronting scientists who attempt to discover robust and replicable causal factors influencing cognition and behavior. Notwithstanding the publication of all too many poorly designed and non-replicable experiments (Ioannides et al. 2014), recent years have also seen significant and durable new insights into the underpinnings of human thought, emotion, and behavior. Many such advances in genetics and neuroscience have been made possible by the emergence of powerful new tools and technologies along with the steady progress in computation that has aided all of science. Thus, for example, the development of cheap and increasingly informative microarrays ("gene chips") along with more than a million-fold decrement in the cost of sequencing DNA during the last decade has made it possible to investigate the tens of thousands of individuals needed to draw conclusions about the influence of genes on behavior. As a result, after many years of frustration in which claims evaporated when more deeply probed (Duncan et al. 2014), the genetic analysis of schizophrenia, bipolar disorder, and autism are beginning to yield a stream of convincing and durable results (Sullivan et al. 2012; Ripke et al. 2014). That said, it will be the work of many years to turn these genetic findings into useful biological explanations given (1) the complexity of emerging genetic discoveries, e.g., that many hundreds or even thousands of small genetic influences act in different combinations to influence inter-individual differences in behavior, and (2) the many levels of biological organization intervening between genes and behavior. Nonetheless, in behavioral genetics, science is moving from vaporous reductive claims (Caspi et al. 2002) toward a far more solid, if sober, picture given recognition of the highly complex and probabilistic (rather than deterministic) actions of genes (McCarroll and Hyman 2013). Tools permitting the interrogation of such complex data sets include the ability to generate human neurons in vitro using stem cell technologies and related methods of cellular reprogramming along with new genome engineering technologies that make it increasingly easy to shuttle

DNA sequence variation of interest into and out of both cells and animal models (Wang et al. 2013).

At the level of systems and cognitive neuroscience, advances in brain imaging are being supplemented by the implementation of brain–machine interfaces (Tankus et al. 2013) and new forms of microscopy that can examine living brains. Optogenetics, a recent technology (Fenno et al. 2011), confers control over the firing of selected cells in the brain over a time course of milliseconds, thus permitting incisive investigations of brain circuits underlying specific behaviors in animal models. The result has been ever more compelling and detailed documentation of causal mechanisms that underlie such neural functions as learning and memory (Ramirez et al. 2013), valuation (Shultz et al. 1997; Montague et al. 2004), and decision making and action selection (Gold and Shadlen 2007; Kable and Glimcher 2009; Znamesnkiy and Zador 2013). Disagreements remain, of course; for example there are differing theories on how distributed neural circuits converge to select a particular action in response to stored information and sensory inputs (Cisek and Kalaska 2010). Such disagreements do not, however, represent scientific disarray, but rather competing hypotheses generated by vital fields of inquiry that are experimentally addressable. In short, unlike the grand but abstract theories of the seventeenth and eighteenth centuries, or abstract philosophical considerations, results emerging from contemporary genetics, neuroscience, and psychology are yielding, with increasing richness and detail, causal mechanisms that underlie cognition, emotion, motivation, and executive function. Despite occasionally desperate appeals, e.g., to quantum mechanics (Penrose 1989), there are no credible "Cartesian" loopholes for those beleaguered thinkers who still wish to affirm free will (Cashmore 2010).

Yet even if free will is illusory from the point of view of the causal mechanisms identified by science, it is no "mere illusion" in the sense of a mirage that quickly disappears as one approaches. Human social interactions are ineluctably grounded in mutual attributions of mental states and of freely formed intentions. Indeed attribution of such properties to self and others is a central component of mental health. Impairment in the ability to attribute mental states to others is a disabling core symptom of autism spectrum disorders for which genetic risk factors and neural substrates are currently being identified (Baron-Cohen and Belmonte 2005; Sullivan et al. 2012; Bernhardt et al. 2013). A sense that one's actions are being externally controlled, rather than free, is a highly disconcerting symptom of schizophrenia. An experience of lacking agency can produce maladaptive and dysphoric states (modeled by learned helplessness in animals) that activate stress responses, and that can prove damaging to overall health status (Singh-Manoux et al. 2003). It seems, in summary, that we human beings have developed dispassionate scientific explanations that falsify the intuitive understandings by which we, when healthy, experience ourselves, our interactions with others, and with the world (Wegner and Wheatley 1999; Wegner 2002). Moreover, the intuitive sense of free will and of authoring one's actions appears to be a universal characteristic of humanity except in severe disorders such as schizophrenia. Analytically, such shared cognitive mechanisms must be products of the structure and function of typical human brains. Many authors would, with justice, add that these mechanisms must also be products of evolution, indeed likely products of natural selection (Pinker 1997; Dennett 2003). While I assume this view is largely correct in doing so, we need not rely on such evolutionary hypotheses given evidence from the study of the human brain function in health and in illness.

The alluring pitfalls of introspection

Introspective experience (at least my experience) yields intuitively irresistible experiences of freedom and agency whether or not one is in possession of scientific knowledge to the contrary. I may hold a strong opinion, based on evidence (Wegner 2002; Custers and Aarts 2010), that introspection does not yield a veridical picture of how I make choices and initiate actions, but the contrary intuitions retain their power. Even when discussing this confounding state of affairs with my neurobiology students, my subjective sense of agency does not recede – until I become so absorbed in the interactions or in my fluent discourse that this aspect of subjectivity is submerged. (The ancient Greeks might at this point have invoked the Muses, a far older recognition than Freud's that important aspects of cognition and action are not attributable to conscious planning and effort.) In short, even when I hold in mind strong, scientifically grounded refutations of free will, I cannot think my way out of my sense of free, conscious agency – nor, in truth, does it seem particularly practical that I should do so beyond the transient thought experiment. I cannot imagine effectively negotiating the social or material world while working from a necessarily effortful cognitive framework that would deny free will. Indeed, lacking any deep intuition of what this would be like, I would hardly know what I would have to be thinking. Perhaps the closest human testimony to such a state would be the psychotic individual who feels externally controlled or who experiences thoughts being added to or deleted from his mind from the outside. To the listener, however, it would take an enormous leap of empathy and imagination to get even an approximation of what such an individual would actually be experiencing.

The concept of free will that I assume for the purposes of this chapter is will that can act independently of prior causes but is itself causally efficacious (contracausal freedom). Based on modern scientific views, contracausal freedom simply cannot obtain because the universe is governed by lawful causality combined with lawful stochastic effects – by lawful I mean stochastic effects explicable in terms of such frameworks as quantum mechanics, not magic, divine intervention, or other spooky processes. Laplace's classic formulation of determinism asserted that given knowledge of initial conditions (e.g., the position and momentum of every atom in the universe) at a point in time and of physical laws, all future states of the universe could be predicted. Laplacean determinism has been rendered incoherent by the recognition of stochastic effects introduced into the physical world by quantum mechanics, and by increasing appreciation of both stochastic effects and complexity in biology. Stochastic effects are well recognized in biology, e.g., apparently unpredictable occurrence of mutations in DNA sequences or differing patterns of gene expression within cells that seem otherwise identical. On this point, however, some circumspection is in order since what appears as chance at one level of observation might reflect deterministic processes at a lower level.

In any case, while chance and complexity undercut classical determinism by making the universe unpredictable, they do not, in any obvious way, confer meaningful freedom of will on human beings. Similarly, while cognition, emotion, executive function, and initiation of action represent complex emergent properties of activity in neural circuits, neither complexity nor stochasticity make room for uncaused causes – even if they eliminate the possibility of Laplacean prediction. While it is certainly not possible to predict the ultimate structure or functional properties of individual brains from their component atoms, molecules, cells, and synapses, there remains powerful evidence for "lawful" causality that operates in the building of brains. Notwithstanding the importance of individual differences in brains (and thus temperaments, capacities, vulnerabilities to disease, and the like) based on such factors as the initial shuffling and recombination of the parental genetic "card decks," mutations in DNA sequences at different stages of development, the location of epigenetic marks within the developing genome, and highly diverse environmental factors, brains develop structurally and functionally with a remarkable degree of similarity across all members of a species and even more similarly as individuals share a greater percentage of their DNA sequences with each other (Toga and

Thompson 2005). Remarkably, when a single human stem cell is cultured in a certain way, it can reliably be induced to produce a three-dimensional brain organoid that recapitulates important aspects of a miniature brain, including a partial cerebral cortex, and can model certain structural diseases (Lancaster et al. 2013). Genomes clearly contain the information needed to unfold in species-typical ways during development even if we are still profoundly ignorant of the language in which that information is written.

I judge myself a skeptical empiricist. I distrust sweeping theories as well as syncretic attempts to find explanatory unity in the face of contradictory evidence. Perhaps it is for this reason that I dislike the concept compatibilism, which denotes an acceptance of determinism (plus chance) as true, but at the same time a belief that humans still possess meaningful free will. The term that does the work in the previous sentence is "meaningful." Strawson's (1962) influential compatibilist analysis of free will was based on his observation of the universality of reactive attitudes toward other people in social interactions, attitudes based on the automatic attribution of freely formed intentions to others under most circumstances. From a perspective centered in human experience, Strawson's form of compatibilism gives primacy to the automatic ineluctable, intuitive framework of ordinary – we might now add neurotypical – human social cognition and emotion in attributing free will. In Strawson's essay (1962) the relationship of reactive attitudes to lawful causation remains murky from an epistemological perspective, perhaps, because human beings lack a deep intuitive sense of what it would mean to lack freedom and responsibility for one's actions.

Many versions of compatibilism come down to the claim that a deterministic universe (incorporating chance) need not drain our automatic (but non-veridical) intuitions of freedom and agency of significance – as we make choices and act in the world. To the contrary, it seems to me well worth recognizing the gulf between the causal scientific view of the world and the intuitive human view of freedom and agency. Instead of concocting mechanisms by which causal explanatory frameworks can be construed as consistent with the automatic intuitive framework of everyday life, it would seem more parsimonious and more truthful (insofar as we can understand these matters) to accept determinism as true, and the sense of freedom and agency as an automatic and involuntary product of human brains, and to shuttle cognitively between them as is appropriate to our cognitive state and the task at hand. Applying a causal scientific perspective to human action will often require effortful cognitive disengagement, and will yield explanations from an external perspective rather than an empathic, intuitive description. When engaged in the world, especially while interacting with other human beings (but not while interacting with robots), it would be generally adaptive to stand in the intuitive perspective of attributing agency. It is, however, important that we gain analytic clarity on the incompatibility of these understandings rather than eliding them, not only from the point of view of making truth claims but also from the point of view of utility. In place of compatibilism, I would argue for what I might call epistemic "double vision." Superficially this might be likened to the "particle-wave" duality of quantum physics. There are important differences, however: (1) The validity of describing light in terms of particles or waves depends only on the experimental context, whereas intuitions of freedom and agency are illusory from the point of view of science. (2) Outside the laboratory, the phenomenon of light is not well described either as particle or wave, but in ordinary human experience, nonveridical experiences of self as freely choosing agent seem quite real and salient, whereas mechanistic descriptions of one's behavior in terms of prior causation have little intuitive purchase. The "laboratories" in which the collision of the scientific-causal view of behavior and the intuitive-freedom-agency view is most often observable is in legislative bodies and courtrooms. As genetics, neuroscience, and psychology gain greater explanatory power, both lawmakers and courtroom adversaries are likely to press for changes in the current positions of equipoise between ascriptions of causal mechanisms, versus ascriptions of choices freely made with respect to relevant acts and behavioral tendencies. At the extremes, some may embrace premature scientific explanations, while others may resist explanations that are based on compelling data.

Moral responsibility and punishment

Moral responsibility is generally defined in operational terms: being in desert of praise or blame for an action. A broadly influential view in Western thought, beginning with Aristotle's Nicomachean ethics and extending to modern Anglo-American jurisprudence, holds that moral responsibility requires that the actor has freely formed an intention, acted in accord with it, and has not acted in ignorance of likely consequences. The freedom that is necessary to be deemed morally responsible has more recently been described as the ability to choose among genuinely open possibilities (Fischer 1999). In Anglo-American courts, a finding of guilt for most crimes requires not only commission of an illegal act but also *mens rea*, a guilty mind, appropriate to the crime. Criminal intent requires that the perpetrator was adequately rational at the time of the act to know what he or she was doing and not utterly incapable of controlling his or her behavior.

Punishment in essentially all systems of criminal justice involves some combination of retribution, representing society's moral outrage at the perpetrator and consequentialism, representing pragmatic attempts to decrease future crime, grounded historically in utilitarian theory (Bentham 1781). Typical consequentialist justifications for punishment include protection of society from dangerous individuals, deterrence of future criminal acts by setting an example, and rehabilitation of the criminal. While consequentialism is focused on the future (minimizing future crime), retributive justice essentially looks backward to the crime that occurred and sets out punishments that are fitting to (or proportionate to) the offense in the service of justice. Central to societal acceptance of retributive justice as practiced in Anglo-American courts is its congruence with human moral intuition, which takes the effects of actions into account but, more significantly, depends on intuitions of responsibility. Unless the law-breaker can be construed as morally responsible, retributivist responses to the crime are not seen as justified. It is, of course, too simplistic to posit an incomplete separation between retributive justice and consequentialism. Important rationales for retributive justice appeal to moral emotions such as making victims or society feel "whole," achieving a sense of catharsis and closure. However, the emotions that lie at the heart of retribution may also serve the consequentialist purpose of warning potential future criminals to desist from offending.

Recent empirical studies of moral intuition find that people assign blame to others based not only on the outcome of their action but also on inferences made about the mental state of the actor (Cushman 2008; Young and Saxe 2009). Economic games, often used in the laboratory to study cooperation, have also been employed to study attribution of mental states (McCabe et al. 2001; Fehr and Gachter 2002). In these settings punishment of free riders and individuals perceived as making unfair divisions of resources occurs ubiquitously and cross-culturally. In a commonly used two-person game, known as the ultimatum game, one player is assigned a sum of money and must propose a division. The second player must either accept the proposed division in which case both players keep their share, or refuse the division in which each player gets nothing. For the individual who receives a low proposal, refusal of monetary offers, no matter how small, appears irrational – it is better to get something rather than nothing. At the group level, however, refusal of small offers can be conceptualized as altruistic punishment, that is, at a cost to the punisher the unfair or uncooperative player may be "taught a lesson" by being denied payment. Altruistic punishment is powerfully influenced by attribution of mental states to opponents; it does not occur, for example, if the opponent is believed to be a mechanical device or computer. Unsurprisingly, punishment of unfairness or free riding is driven by emotion (typically anger), rather than rational calculation (Fehr and Gachter 2002).

Attribution of moral choices exhibits significant cross-cultural similarities (O'Neill and Petrinovich 1998), albeit with some differences (related, perhaps, to the influences of more individualist vs. more collectivist societies). There are also inter-individual differences in attribution of blame within a culture (Young and Saxe 2009) based on a person's temperament and prior experience (Bernhardt and Singer 2012). Inter-individual differences notwithstanding, moral judgments are deeply embedded in ordinary day-to-day human social interactions, and for that matter in interpretations of news stories, gossip, and fictional characters as well as appraisals of others made in more formal settings such as jury rooms. Moral intuition, like most fast, human cognition involves the automatic activation of cognitive heuristics and emotional responses unless specific measures are taken to encourage processes of deliberation (Kahneman and Tversky 1972) Such responses are deeply ingrained in human brains and thus human psychology (Glimcher and Rustichini 2004; Knoch et al. 2009). For the most part these permit efficient and successful navigation of a highly complex and shifting social landscape in which rapid judgments must often be made. Moral responses that involve attribution of mental states and choice to others are supported by typical human brain circuitry and are diminished among individuals with autism spectrum disorders (Moran et al. 2011).

Neurobiology in the courts

Arguments from genetics (Bernet et al. 2007) as well as neuroscience have entered the courtroom. Defense attorneys may try, especially at the time of sentencing, to demonstrate that some neural abnormality reduced the culpability of their clients; conversely prosecutors might argue that perpetrators with untreatable brain injuries should, based on their dangerousness, be incarcerated for a long time. Of possible relevance, not only for sentencing but also for parole decisions, attempts are underway to connect patterns of brain activity to risk of reoffending or rearrest (Aharoni et al. 2013).

While behavioral genetics, neuroscience, and psychology are making real progress in identifying general mechanisms that underlie decision making and behavior, there is a significant risk that both academics and courtroom adversaries will overreach in applications of scientific or medical evidence to the messy complexities of the real world. Advocates in the courtroom often fail to grasp (or admit to) the stark differences between laboratory studies that control as many variables as possible compared with the uncontrolled complexities of the real world where numerous causal influences impinge on a particular decision or act. Similarly, arguments made in the courtroom often fail to acknowledge the error of applying statistical averages derived from studies of groups to the situation of an individual actor in a particular context. Today's sometimes exuberantly excessive claims (Satel and Lillienfeld 2013) do not, however, negate real progress toward useful and valid mechanistic explanations. Over time, and applied with due care, science will likely have powerful implications for philosophical and jurisprudential considerations of human moral responsibility, criminal culpability, and punishment

Given their strongly articulated views, the arguments of Greene and Cohen (2004) and of Morse (2006) have frequently been starting points for discussions of whether neuroscience will or should alter current understandings of moral responsibility and attitudes toward punishment in the criminal justice system. Greene and Cohen (2004) foresee an evolution in understandings of moral and criminal responsibility as cognitive neuroscience-based explanations of human action progress and become disseminated. They argue that the eventual result will be a beneficial diminution in the role of retributive punishment, which they see as unenlightened and unfair – partly because moral blame is not warranted and partly because moral outrage often runs amuck leading to excessively harsh punishments.

Morse (2006, 2007), in contrast, argues that the upshot of advances in neuroscience for criminal justice will be almost nothing at all. This is because – assuming that the facts of a case demonstrate that the accused committed a criminal act – advanced systems of justice focus appropriately on the mental state of the accused at the time of the crime. The relevant information is in no way reliant on neuroscience-based explanations, but on psychological-level descriptions. Indeed, he notes that courts do not need neuroscience in order to consider mitigation of guilt when strong emotion or a brain disorder has influenced the rationality of the actor. New diagnostic technologies can be incorporated into existing legal frameworks once they have proven their worth, but as Morse argues, fully consistently with the current practice of Anglo-American courts, what matters is not a psychiatric or neurological diagnosis or findings from brain imaging, but the mental capacities of the defendant at the time of the criminal act. Where does consideration of these divergent views leave us?

The acceptance of modern scientific concepts entails rejection of contracausal freedom and thus moral responsibility in the sense that we have inherited from Aristotle – notwithstanding occasional arguments to the contrary based on tortured applications of stochasticity or complexity to the issue. Based on the kinds of technologies that I touched on briefly above, mechanistic understandings of human (and animal) decision making and behavioral control are growing in both explanatory power and credibility – although profound humility is in order given how much remains unknown. That caveat notwithstanding, over time such mechanistic explanations and even prediction will improve with respect to both species-typical and pathological cognitive and emotional states, and these will have real salience with respect to deliberative considerations of moral or criminal responsibility. Thus far it would seem that Greene and Cohen (2004) have their arguments right. Indeed they even recognize that intuitions of free will and attribution of moral choices and blameworthiness to others are automatic and ubiquitously human, likely explaining longstanding justifications for retribution, even if attitudes have been modified since Hammurabi and Genesis.

It seems foolhardy to argue overmuch about the degree to which science might produce a new framework for attribution of responsibility that will be widely accepted in some societies. Suffice it to say that Greene and Cohen (2004) believe that progress in cognitive neuroscience portends an evolving moral framework that will undercut traditional concepts of moral responsibility and thus vastly diminish the accepted role for retribution in civilized systems of justice. I am skeptical. Even if prosecutors, lawyers, judges, and legislators mustered the cognitive control to bracket their intuitive concepts of moral agency in favor of deterministic explanations of behavior, victims and societies at large might not. In the end, systems of laws and of justice have to be acceptable to wide swaths of their polities else a cadre of putatively enlightened determinists would not keep their positions for long. Given the power, and seeming necessity for mental health, of the human illusion of agency, both for self, and attributed to others, as Strawson (1962) observed, it is difficult to imagine a world in which scientifically based causal explanations come to dominate systems of justice. This surmise does not rule out the possibility that neuroscience will identify new species of incapacity that will be convincing in the courtroom. I would imagine, however, that in societies populated by *Homo sapiens* as they are, retribution will remain an important justification for punishment in a messy equilibrium with more utilitarian justifications such as deterrence, incapacitation of dangerous individuals, and rehabilitation.

My serious disagreement with Greene and Cohen (2004) is not, however, based on predicting whether scientifically inspired policies will supplant moral emotion and retributivism. Rather, I think it would be a mistake. Serious problems have long been recognized in schemes for basing laws, judgments of morality, and systems of punishment entirely on utilitarian principles. For example, it has been asked whether many parents would freely withhold food from their own children over an extended period or perhaps tuition to an excellent, but expensive school if those resources, wisely distributed, would create greater benefit for a large number of indigent children. Beyond the pragmatics, it is fair to ask whether such acts are morally superior or even justifiable. In terms of criminal responsibility, it has been pointed out that preventive detention for some repeat offenders could be deemed rational in consequentialist terms if its cost were less than the direct and indirect costs of the future crimes that might be prevented. What is newer than such critiques is that behavioral genetics, systems neuroscience, and cognitive neuroscience can reject the notion that humans possess nearly limitless plasticity that would permit widespread overwriting of automatic responses by new moral systems. Humans can indeed learn a great deal and espouse widely differing beliefs with great intensity, but it is also clear that our thoughts, emotions, and moral intuitions are, to a great degree undergirded and constrained by the structure and function of our brains. For a person committed to a scientific view, human moral intuition in all its variety is a product of human brains, not natural law.

Systems of law and of justice cannot accomplish their fundamental societal purpose of rendering justice (which includes a sense of closure and of putting things right) without resorting to concepts of moral responsibility and retribution. Of course, one cannot predict how, on specific matters, scientific discoveries and new technologies will reset the equipoise between the science of causal mechanisms and the human intuition of moral blame. This is particularly challenging since courts are far less concerned with a person's diagnosis or brain scan than with his mental capacities at the time a crime was committed. Given the power with which moral emotion acts in societies, I doubt that the balance will be reset as far toward causal explanations and consequentialist justifications as Greene and Cohen (2004) seem to predict and to advocate for.

Morse has good reason to defend an Anglo-American criminal justice system that has evolved over centuries, and that, in the main, functions well despite some miscarriages of justice. Moreover this approach to justice is generally well accepted by the societies in which it operates, an absolutely critical matter in democracies. However, in his defense of the status quo, Morse (2006) makes what I take to be a problematic claim. He argues that determination of the minimal rationality required to establish criminal intent is (1) compatible in a general sense with neuroscience, but at the same time (2) insulated from its mechanistic implications. In more detail, Morse notes that a finding of guilt and the application of retributive punishment is based jointly on commission of an illegal act and *mens rea*. He argues that the rationality required to establish *mens rea* is empirically discoverable at the level of psychology, as are mitigating circumstances such as strong emotion, e.g., rage or intense fear that a reasonable person might feel in the same circumstances, or else a mental defect resulting from disease or injury (Morse 2006, 2007). What matters is not a medical diagnosis or a spot on a brain scan, so much as whether the accused person had the necessary rationality for *mens rea* at the time of the crime. As a result, Morse argues, the law is insulated both from determinist metaphysics and fromthe causal theories of neuroscience. In his view neuroscience addresses itself to the wrong level of analysis. On Morse's epistemological views neuroscience might be able to do little more than gild the "Laplacean lily" (outside the courtroom door of course) since current neuroscience is only infrequently applicable to determinations of a defendant's mental states at the time of the criminal act.

My analysis of Morse's claim is that he has smuggled dualism (in compatibilist's clothing) into his arguments in order to render judicial determinations of *mens rea* as invulnerable as possible to the unwanted causal implications of neuroscience. Morse may be concerned that without an epistemological firewall, attempts to exploit mechanistic neural explanations might ultimately be permitted to erode human moral responsibility excessively. Indeed, Morse could read Greene and Cohen (2004) to say, given that the concept of contracausal free will is false, shouldn't criminal courts be replaced with centers for behavioral analysis and diagnosis, and shouldn't punishment be replaced with psychotherapy and skills training (and, of course for the incorrigibly dangerous, incarceration). This scenario would likely fail utterly as a social institution, if only because it would frustrate universal moral intuitions. Given the power with which moral emotion operates in human affairs, movement toward purely mechanistic explanations of crime would seem highly unlikely. (It is also frequently pointed out that the determination of effective consequentialist responses to criminal acts may be no more justified by truly relevant data than the determination of sentences based on retributive formulae based on law and culture.)

To return to Morse's published epistemic claims, his firewall against neurobiological mechanism requires artificially narrow rules for what qualifies as an explanation. True, psychological-level questions are often best answered with psychological-level explanations. Indeed, inappropriate reductionism is not only comically cumbersome, but also fails as explanation. It is hard to imagine a useful description of *mens rea* given in terms of molecules or neurons. However, there are circumstances in which explanations at one level of organization, e.g., psychological explanations, are poorly constrained within their level (i.e., leave too many plausible possibilities or seem tautologous). In such cases precision and utility can often be improved by referring to causes at the next "lower" level of complexity. For psychology this is likely to be neuroscience. In one hypothetical example, there might be many possible explanations for why a young adult might have failed to assert age-appropriate cognitive control over impulses that have resulted in an opportunistic crime. To provide just four common reasons: (1) longstanding habits that might have their basis in complex, interacting factors such as temperament, poor upbringing, or association with antisocial peer groups; (2) fatigue, stress, or other acute factors that might have sapped the needed resources for cognitive control over powerful impulses; (3) previously undiagnosed attention deficit hyperactivity disorder (ADHD); or (4) antisocial traits or antisocial personality disorder.

Morse might respond that given the present state of science, psychology would do as well or better than any brain studies in distinguishing among these possibilities. I suspect, however, that in coming years, examinations of brain structure and function will increasingly identify and constrain phenomenologically described mental states, tendencies, and behavioral syndromes. For example, an initial longitudinal structural magnetic resonance imaging (MRI) study of children and adolescents with ADHD found delayed maturation of their prefrontal cortex, a brain structure that plays the key role in cognitive control (Shaw et al. 2010). This is an initial study that needs replication and extension. What is significant, however, is both a broad scientific commitment to discovery of objective biomarkers for states now defined only descriptively and progress toward identifying underlying mechanisms that might subdivide today's lumped behavioral tendencies and syndromes.

Morse's argument will not stave off scientific and philosophical challenges to lawmakers and courts. A principled system of justice must, *inter alia*, accept the tested, mainstream science of its time, and our science is finding increasingly salient and applicable causal explanations of decision making and behavior. If our courts are to retain broad acceptance, they will have to take on the causal claims of neuroscience in multiple particular situations. Before I appear to align myself entirely with Greene and Cohen (2004), I should return to my view that the challenge for lawmakers and courts will not lie in jettisoning the intuitive human framework that takes freedom and moral blame as central to justice. Rather, lawmakers, policy makers, and courts will have to develop new ways to weigh and to articulate the significance of mechanistic neuroscience given the need to respect the overriding context of human moral intuition. Over long periods of time, public support for systems of justice requires that punishment be seen as fairly reflecting the degree of criminal responsibility. Analyses of particular crimes and just punishments that might change in light of scientific evidence will perforce be powerfully influenced by public opinion, politics, and social conditions. This is far from an exact and rational process, as evidenced by disproportionately severe penalties for nonviolent drug offenders promulgated in the United States in the late twentieth century.

It is not so easy to show, in a complex world of human beings, that redesigning criminal justice in consequentialist terms is either possible or necessarily superior to the admittedly flawed systems of justice that exist today even in democratic countries with strong institutions. Indeed, retributive and consequentialist justifications for punishment are often quite entangled. Thus, for example, retributivist expressions of moral outrage can serve as deterrents to potential offenders and can play a role in the rehabilitation of convicted criminals by serving as strong negative reinforcement. Alternatively, consequentialist justifications for punishments, such as protection of society, may easily be contaminated by moral emotion such as anger and disgust. Complex drivers, including moral outrage, would appear be at work in the prolonged civil commitment of child molesters who are considered still dangerous after completing their jail sentences, despite the good consequentialist goal of public safety. In contrast other potentially dangerous individuals who have committed crimes held less heinous by society might be released once they have served their sentence, that is, "paid their debt to society" to use a classic retributivist metaphor. In the case of drug-related crimes, it is particularly difficult to parse retribution, moral emotion, and consequentialist ideas related to deterrence, rehabilitation, and protection of society – including children.

Even nonviolent offenders convicted of drug trafficking have elicited particularly potent moral outrage in the United States during recent decades, but at the same time they have also been construed by policymakers and civic leaders as particularly dangerous vectors of social blight. The result has been a period of long mandatory minimum prison sentences that has produced high financial costs, has arguably been damaging to disadvantaged segments of society, and has produced large numbers of individuals with few skills and little ability to function outside of prisons. Proponents of consequentialist justice, beginning with

Bentham (1781), have seen the intuitive attributions of willful agency and the resulting moral emotions that underlie retributivism as untutored by advances in criminology and other social sciences, and tainted by idiosyncratic biases and crude affective reactions to perpetrators, such as excessive fear and intense anger that may run to blood lust. Such charges against retributivism have a good deal of justification, to be sure, but consequentialist approaches to justice almost invariably lack the data and methods to effectively minimize future crime (just as medicine generally lacks the data and methods to effectively prevent most diseases). Moreover, by attempting to eschew moral intuition and emotion, consequentialists risk undervaluing the moral emotions and hunger for justice that pervades most human societies in response to criminal acts, and thus risk the legitimacy of a society's institutions of justice.

I would argue that it follows from my incompatibilist view that it is healthy for legislative bodies and legal institutions to be increasingly aware of the collision between human moral intuition and the increasingly convincing and vivid evidence of involuntary causal mechanisms coming from diverse branches of science. It is healthy because, at least for now, there are no adequate theories with which to guide lawmaking, policy, or justice effectively, and moreover the balance between these opposing perspectives shifts depending on local history and culture and on the specific context in which transgressions occur.

REFERENCES

Aharoni, E., Vincent, G. M., Harenski, C. L., Calhoun, V. D., Sinnott-Armstrong, W., Gazzaniga, M. S., and Kiehl, K. A. 2013. Neuroprediction of future rearrest. *Proceedings of the National Academy of Sciences, USA* 110:6223–6228.

Baron-Cohen. S. and Belmonte, M. K. 2005. Autism: a window onto the development of the social and the analytic brain. *Annual Review of Neuroscience* 28:109–126.

Bentham, J. 1781. *An Introduction to Principles of Morals and Legislation*. Reprinted 1892. London: Methuen.

Bernet, W., Vnencak-Jones, C. L., Farahany, N., and Montgomery, S. A. 2007. Bad nature, bad nurture, and testimony regarding MAOA and SLC6A4 genotyping at murder trials. *Journal of Forensic Science* 52:1362–1371.

Bernhardt, B. C. and Singer, T. 2012. The neural basis of empathy. *Annual Review of Neuroscience* 35:1–23.

Bernhardt, B. C., Valk, S. L., Silani, G., Bird, G., Frith, U., and Singer, T. 2013. Selective disruption of sociocognitive structural brain networks in autism and alexithymia. *Cerebral Cortex*. July 17. Epub ahead of print.

Cashmore, A. 2010. The Lucretian swerve: the biological basis of human behavior and the criminal justice system. *Proceedings of the National Academy of Sciences, USA* 107:4499–4505.

Caspi, A., McClay, J., Moffitt, T.E., Mill, J, Martin, J., et al. 2002. Role of genotype in the cycle of violence in maltreated children. *Science* 297:851–854.

Ciske, P. and Kalaska. J. F. 2010. Neural mechanisms for interacting with a world full of action choices. *Annual Review of Neuroscience* 33:269–298.

Clark, A. 2007. What reaching teaches: consciousness, control, and the inner zombie. *British Journal for the Philosophy of Science* 58:563–594.

Cushman, F. 2008. Crime and punishment: distinguishing the roles of causal and intentional analysis in moral judgment. *Cognition* 108:353–380.

Custers, R. and Aarts, H. 2010. The unconscious will: how the pursuit of goals operates outside of conscious awareness. *Science* 329:47–50.

Dennett, D. C. 2003. *Freedom Evolves*. New York: Viking Penguin.

Duncan, L. E., Pollastri, A. R., and Smoller, J. W. 2014. Mind the gap: why many geneticists and psychological scientists have discrepant views about gene-environment interaction (GXE) research. *American Psychologist* 69:249–268.

Fehr, E. and Gachter, S. 2002. Altruistic punishment in humans. *Nature* 415:137–140

Fenno, L., Yizhar, O., and Deisseroth, K. 2011. The development and application of optogenetics. *Annual Review of Neuroscience* 34:389–412.

Fischer, J. M. 1999. Recent work on moral responsibility. *Ethics* 110:93–139.

Fitzgerald, R. (trans.) 1961. *The Odyssey of Homer*. New York: Doubleday & Co.

Gold, J. I. and Shadlen, M. N. 2007. The neural basis of decision making. *Annual Review of Neuroscience* 30:535–574.

Glimcher, P. W. and Rustichini, A. 2004. Neuroeconomics: the consilience of brain and decision. *Science* 306:447–452.

Greene J. and Cohen, J. 2004. For the law, neuroscience changes nothing and everything. *Philosophical Transactions of the Royal Society B. Biological Sciences* 359:1775–1785.

Haggard, P. 2008. Human volition: towards a neuroscience of will. *Nature Reviews Neuroscience* 9:934–946.

Ioannides, J. P. A., Munafo, M. R., Fusar-Poli, P., Nosek, B. A., and David, S. 2014. Publication and other reporting biases in cognitive sciences: detection, prevalence, and prevention. *Trends in Cognitive Sciences* 18:235–241.

Kable, J. W. and Glimcher, P. W. 2009. The neurobiology of decision: consensus and controversy. *Neuron* 24: 733–745.

Kahneman, D. 2011. *Thinking, Fast and Slow*. New York: Farrar, Straus, and Giroux

Kahneman, D. and Tversky, A. 1972. Subjective probability: a judgment of representativeness. *Cognitive Psychology* 3: 430-454. Repr. 1982 in D. Kahneman, P. Slovic, and A. Tversky (eds.), *Judgment under Uncertainty: Heuristics and Biases*. Cambridge University Press.

Koechlin, E. and Hyafil, A. 2007. Anterior prefrontal function and the limits of human decision-making. *Science* 318:594–598.

Knoch, D., Schneider, F., Schunk, D., Hohmann, M., and Fehr, E. 2009. Disrupting the prefrontal cortex diminishes the human ability to build a good reputation. *Proceedings of the National Academy of Sciences* 106: 20895–20899.

Lancaster, M. A., Renner, M., Martin, C.-A., Wenzel, D., Bicknell, L. S., et al. 2013. Cerebral organoids model human brain development and microcephaly. *Nature* 501:373–379.

Libet, B., Wright, E. W., and Gleason C. A. 1982. Readiness potentials preceding unrestricted "spontaneous" vs. pre-planned voluntary acts. *Electroencephalography and Clinical Neurophysiology* 54:322–335.

McCabe, K., Houser, D., Ryan, L, Smith, V., and Trouard, T. 2001. A functional imaging study of cooperation in two-person reciprocal exchange. *Proceedings of the National Academy of Science, USA* 98:832–835.

McCarroll, S. A. and Hyman, S. E. 2013. Progress in the genetics of polygenic brain disorders: significant new challenges for neurobiology. *Neuron* 80:579–587.

Montague, P. R., Hyman, S. E., and Cohen, J. D. 2004. Computational roles for dopamine in behavioural control. *Nature* 431:760–767.

Moran, J. M., Young, L. L, Saxe, R.,Lee, S. M., O'Young, D., Mavros, P. L., and Gabrieli, J. D. 2011. Impaired theory of mind for moral judgment in high-functioning autism. *Proceedings of the National Academy of Sciences, USA*. 108:2688–2692.

Morse, S. J. 2006. Brain overclaim syndrome. *Ohio State Journal of Criminal Law*. 3:397–412.

2007. Voluntary control of behavior and responsibility. *The American Journal of Bioethics* 7:12–14.

O'Neill, P. and Petrinovich, L. 1998. A preliminary cross-cultural study of moral intuitions. *Evolution and Human Behavior* 19:349–367.

Penrose, R. 1989. *The Emperor's New Mind*. Oxford University Press.

Pessiglione, M., Petrovic, P., Daunizeau, J., Palminteri, S., Dolan, R. J., and Frith, C. D. 2008. Subliminal instrumental conditioning demonstrated in the human brain. *Neuron* 59:561–567.

Pessiglione, M., Seymour, B., Flandin, G., Dolan, R. J., and Frith, C. D. 2006. Dopamine-dependent prediction errors underpin reward-seeking behavior in humans. *Nature* 442:1042–1045.

Pinker, S. 1997. *How the Mind Works*. New York: Norton.

Ramirez, S., Liu, X., Lin, P. A., Suh, J., Pignatelli, M., Redondo, R. L., Ryan, T. J., and Tonegawa S. 2013. Creating a false memory in the hippocampus. *Science* 341:387–391

Ripke, S., Neale, B. M., Corvin, A., Walters, James T. R., Farh, Kai, et al. 2014. Biological insights from 108 schizophrenia-associated genetic loci. *Nature*, 521:421–427.

Roskies, A. L. 2010. How does neuroscience affect our concept of volition? *Annual Review of Neuroscience* 33:109–130. 2013. Can neuroscience resolve issues about free will? In W. Sinnott-Armstrong (ed.), *Moral Psychology*, Vol. IV: *Free Will and Moral Responsibility*. Cambridge, MA: MIT Press, pp. 139–150.

Satel, S. and S. O. Lilienfeld. 2013. *Brainwashed: The Seductive Appeal of Mindless Neuroscience*. New York: Basic Books.

Schultz, W., Dayan, P., and Montague, P. R. 1997. A neural substrate of prediction and reward. *Science* 275:1593–1599.

Shaw, P., Gogtay, N., and Rapoport, J. 2010. Childhood psychiatric disorders as anomalies in neurodevelopmental trajectories. *Human Brain Mapping* 31:917–925.

Singh-Manoux, A., Adler, N. E., and Marmot, M. G. 2003. Subjective social status: its determinants and its association with measures of ill-health in the Whitehall II study. *Social Science & Medicine* 56:1321–1333.

Strawson, P. F. 1962. Freedom and resentment. *Proceedings of the British Academy* 48: 187–211. London: Oxford University Press. Repr. 1982 in G. Watson (ed.), *Free Will.* Oxford University Press, pp. 59–80.

Sullivan, P. F., Daly, M. J., and O'Donovan, M. 2012. Genetic architecture of psychiatric disorders: the emerging picture and its implications. *Nature Reviews Genetics* 13:537–551.

Tankus, A., Fried, I., and Shoham S. 2013. Cognitive-motor brain–machine interfaces. *Journal of Physiology Paris*. Doi:pii: S0928–4257(13)00035-1. Epub ahead of print.

Toga, A. W. and Thompson, P. M. 2005. Genetics of brain structure and intelligence. *Annual Review of Neuroscience* 28:1–23.

Wang, H., Yang, H., Shivalila, C. S., Dawlaty, M. M., Cheng, A. W., Zhang. F., and Jaenisch, R. 2013. One-step generation of mice carrying mutations in multiple genes by CRISPR/Cas-Mediated Genome Engineering. *Cell* 153:910–918.

Wegner, D. M. 2002. *The Illusion of Conscious Will.* Cambridge, MA: MIT Press.

Wegner, D. M. and Wheatley, T. 1999. Apparent mental causation: sources of experience of will. *American Psychologist* 54:480–491.

Wolf, S. 1987. Sanity and the metaphysics of responsibility. In F. Schoeman (ed.), *Responsibility, Character, and the Emotions: New Essays in Moral Psychology*. Cambridge University Press, pp. 46–62.

Young, L. and Saxe, R. 2009. Innocent intentions: a correlation between forgiveness for accidental harm and neural activity. *Neuropsychologia* 47(10):2065–2072.

Znamenskiy, P. and Zador, A. M. (2013) Corticostriatal neurons in auditory cortex drive decisions during auditory discrimination. *Nature* 497:482–485.

13 Neuroscience, free will, and criminal responsibility

Stephen J. Morse

ABSTRACT

This chapter argues that the folk-psychological model of the person and responsibility is not challenged by determinism in general or by neuro-determinism in particular. Until science conclusively demonstrates that human beings cannot be guided by reasons and that mental states play no role in explaining behavior, the folk-psychological model of responsibility is justified. This chapter discusses the motivations to turn to science to solve the hard normative problems the law addresses, as well as the law's psychology and its concepts of the person and responsibility. Then it considers the general relation of neuroscience to law, which I characterize as the issue of "translation." The limits of neurolaw are canvassed and the chapter argues that neurolaw poses no radical challenge to the concepts of the person and responsibility. The chapter is cautiously optimistic about the contribution that neuroscience may make to law in the near and intermediate term. The penultimate section examines some of the claims concerning responsibility made in other chapters in this volume followed by a brief conclusion.

Introduction

In a 2002 editorial published in *The Economist* (2002), the following warning was given: "Genetics may yet threaten privacy, kill autonomy, make society homogeneous and gut the concept of human nature. But neuroscience could do all of these things first." But neither genetics nor any other science that was predicted to revolutionize the law, including behavioral psychology, sociology, and psychodynamic psychology, to name but a few, has had this effect. This will also be true of neuroscience, which is simply the newest science on the block. Neuroscience is not going to do the terrible things *The Economist* fears, at least not in the foreseeable future. Neuroscience has many things to say, but not nearly as much as people who want to change the legal system would hope, especially in relation to criminal law.

In a series of articles and book chapters (Morse, 2004, 2006a, 2006b, 2007a, 2007b, 2011a, 2011b, 2011c, 2012, 2013a, 2013b, 2013c), I argue that the new cognitive, affective, and social neuroscience poses no fundamental challenge to the coherence of the doctrines and practices of criminal responsibility. Moreover, at present, the new neuroscience suggests no specific doctrinal reforms and has little role, if any, to play in the adjudication of criminal cases. At most, in the near to intermediate term, neuroscience may make modest contributions to legal policy and case adjudication. Although there have been major advances in neuroscience since I began the series, the conclusions I reached about the legal implications are entirely unchanged. Thus, there will inevitably be a great deal of overlap between this chapter and my previous writing on the topic because I have achieved a settled understanding about the relation between law and neuroscience. Until there are conceptual or scientific breakthroughs that will cast doubt on this understanding – and there well may be such breakthroughs – for now this is my story and I am sticking to it.

There is a problem about free will, but not in the law. The genuine problem of free will is metaphysical and often spawns confusion. Roughly, it refers to whether human beings possess the ability or power to act uncaused by anything other than themselves, which is referred to as libertarian freedom of the will. The importance of having this power or ability results from the controversial belief that it underwrites the possibility of holding people genuinely responsible. Solving the free will problem would have profound implications for responsibility doctrines and practices, but, at present, the problem plays no proper role in the law and neuroscience cannot solve it in any case. Criminal law addresses problems genuinely related to responsibility, including consciousness, the formation of mental states such as intention and knowledge, the capacity for rationality, and compulsion, but it never addresses the presence or absence of libertarian free will. Indeed, if criminal responsibility is properly understood, libertarian free will is not even foundational.

The new neuroscience has spawned a new generation of free will skeptics, not all of whom suffer from Brain Overclaim Syndrome (although most do), and most of whom wrongly believe that the discoveries of neuroscience entail consequentialism. Many of these claims suffer from confusions, however. Either the skeptics are preaching to the choir about libertarian freedom because almost no one believes that human beings possess such god-like powers, or they have failed sufficiently to respond to compatibilist accounts of responsibility that do not require libertarian freedom. Often, people in the latter group have not clearly identified what they mean by free will. In the words of the philosopher, Manuel Vargas (2013), the debate about free will has been bedeviled by "troubled, fragmented" thinking about the problem.

The central thesis of this chapter is that the folk-psychological model of the person that is central to our explanations of human behavior and to responsibility doctrines and practices is not challenged by determinism in general or by neurodeterminism in particular. Criminal responsibility doctrines and practices are fully compatible with the truth of determinism (or causal closure). Until science conclusively demonstrates that human beings are not responsive to and cannot be guided by reasons and that mental states do not play even a partial causal role in explaining behavior, the folk-psychological model of responsibility will endure as fully justified. Scientific findings, whether from neuroscience or other sciences, will be useful only if they help elucidate the law's folk-psychological criteria. This claim does not "wall off" the law's responsibility practices from science. Rather, it simply requires that the scientific data be translated into the law's folk-psychological criteria. As the eminent forensic psychiatrist Phillip Resnick says generally about legally relevant behavior: "You need to understand why. And you can't see why on an fMRI" (quoted in Doherty, 2007).

This chapter first addresses the law's motivation and the motivation of some advocates to turn to science to solve the very hard normative problems that law addresses. The next section discusses the law's psychology and its concepts of the person and responsibility. Then it considers the general relation of neuroscience to law, which I characterize as the issue of "translation." The following section canvasses various distractions that have bedeviled clear thinking about the relation of scientific, causal accounts of behavior to responsibility. Next, it examines the limits of neurolaw and considers why neurolaw does not pose a genuinely radical challenge to the law's concepts of the person and responsibility. The chapter then makes a case for cautious optimism about the contribution that neuroscience may make to law in the near and intermediate term. The penultimate section examines some of the claims concerning responsibility made by other chapters in this volume. A brief conclusion follows.

The source of neuroexuberance

Everyone understands that legal issues are normative, addressing how we should regulate our lives in a complex society. How do we live together?

What are the duties we owe each other? For violations of those duties, when is the state justified in imposing the most afflictive – but sometimes justified —– exercises of state power, criminal blame, and punishment? When should we do this, to whom, and how much?

Virtually every legal issue, including the criteria for criminal responsibility, is contested, and there is always room for debate about policy, doctrine, and adjudication. In a recent book, Professor Robin Feldman has argued that law lacks the courage forthrightly to address the difficult normative issues that it faces (2009). The law therefore adopts what Feldman terms an "internalizing" and an "externalizing" strategy for using science to try to avoid the difficulties. In the internalizing strategy, the law adopts scientific criteria as legal criteria. A futuristic example might be using neural criteria for criminal responsibility. In the externalizing strategy, the law turns to scientific or clinical experts to make the decision. An example would be using forensic clinicians to decide whether a criminal defendant is competent to stand trial and then simply rubberstamping the clinician's opinion. Neither strategy is successful because each avoids facing the hard questions and impedes legal evolution and progress. Professor Feldman concludes, and I agree, that the law does not err by using science too little, as is commonly claimed. Rather, it errs by using it too much because the law is too insecure about its resources and capacities to do justice.

A fascinating question is why so many enthusiasts seem to have extravagant expectations about the contribution of neuroscience to law, especially criminal law. Here is my speculation about the source. Many people intensely dislike the concept and practice of retributive justice, thinking that they are prescientific and harsh. Their hope is that the new neuroscience will convince the law at last that determinism is true, no offender is genuinely responsible, and the only logical conclusion is that the law should adopt a consequentially based prediction/prevention system of social control guided by the knowledge of the neuroscientist-kings who will finally have supplanted the platonic philosopher-kings (e.g., Greene & Cohen, 2006). On a more modest level, many advocates think that neuroscience may not revolutionize criminal justice, but neuroscience will demonstrate that many more offenders should be excused and do not deserve the harsh punishments imposed by the United States criminal justice system. Four decades ago, our criminal justice system would have been using psychodynamic psychology for the same purpose. More recently, genetics has been employed in a similar manner. The impulse, however, is clear: jettison desert, or at least mitigate judgments of desert. As will be shown below, however, these advocates often adopt an untenable theory of mitigation or an excuse that quickly collapses into the nihilistic conclusion that no one is really criminally responsible.

The law's psychology and concept of the person

Criminal law presupposes a "folk-psychological" view of the person and behavior. This psychological theory explains behavior *in part* by mental states such as desires, beliefs, intentions, willings, and plans. Biological and other psychological and sociological variables also play a causal role, but folk psychology considers mental states fundamental to a full causal explanation and understanding of human action. Lawyers, philosophers, and scientists argue about the definitions of mental states and theories of action, but that does not undermine the general claim that mental states are fundamental. Indeed, the arguments and evidence that disputants use to convince others presuppose the folk-psychological view of the person. Brains do not convince each other, people do. Folk psychology presupposes only that human action will at least be rationalizable by mental state explanations or will be responsive to reasons – including incentives – under the right conditions.

For example, the folk-psychological explanation for why you are reading this chapter is, roughly, that you desire to understand the relation of neuroscience to criminal responsibility or to law generally. You believe that reading the chapter will help fulfill that desire, so you formed the intention to read it. This is a practical, rather than a deductive, syllogism. Brief reflection should indicate that the law's psychology must be a folk-psychological theory, a view of the person as a conscious – and potentially self-conscious – creature who forms and acts on intentions that are the product of the person's other mental states. We are the sort of creatures who can act for and respond to reasons. The law treats persons generally as intentional creatures and not simply as mechanistic forces of nature.

Law is primarily action-guiding and is not able to guide people directly and indirectly unless people are capable of using rules as premises in their reasoning about how they should behave. Unless people could be guided by law, including by the law's influence on the formation of character and habits, it would be useless (and perhaps incoherent) as an action-guiding system of rules. Legal rules are action-guiding primarily because these rules provide an agent with good moral or prudential reasons for forbearance or action. Human behavior can be modified by means other than influencing deliberation, and human beings do not always deliberate before they act. Nonetheless, the law presupposes folk psychology even when we most habitually follow the legal rules. Unless people are capable of understanding and then using legal rules to guide their conduct, the law is powerless to affect human behavior.

The legal view of the person does not hold that people must always reason or consistently behave rationally according to some preordained, normative notion of rationality. Rather, the law's view is that people are capable of acting for reasons and are capable of minimal rationality according to predominantly conventional, socially constructed standards. The type of rationality the law requires is the ordinary person's common-sense view of rationality, not the technical notion that might be acceptable within the disciplines of economics, philosophy, psychology, computer science, and the like.

Virtually everything for which agents deserve to be praised, blamed, rewarded, or punished is the product of mental causation and, in principle, is responsive to reasons, including incentives. Machines may cause harm, but they cannot do wrong, and they cannot violate expectations about how people ought to live together. Machines do not deserve praise, blame, reward, punishment, concern, or respect because they exist or because they cause results that change the world. Only people, intentional agents with the potential to act, can do wrong and violate expectations of what they owe each other.

Many scientists and some philosophers of mind and action might consider folk psychology to be a primitive or prescientific view of human behavior. For the foreseeable future, however, the law will be based on the folk-psychological model of the person and behavior described. Until and unless scientific discoveries convince us that our view of ourselves is radically wrong, the basic explanatory apparatus of folk psychology will remain central. It is vital that scientific critics of the criminal law should understand that claims that our responsibility practices are not coherent and justified can only be demonstrated by showing that agency is an illusion. But as long as we have reason to believe, as we most assuredly do (Fodor, 1987; and see below), that human beings have the capacity to be guided by reason – a capacity fully consistent with the truth of determinism – neuroscience poses no general challenge to our responsibility doctrines and practices. If neuroscience is to have appropriate influence on current criminal law and legal decision-making, the science must be relevant to and translated into the law's folk-psychological framework.

Criminal responsibility doctrines

All of the law's doctrinal criteria for criminal responsibility are folk-psychological. Let us begin with the definitional criteria, the "elements" of crime. The "voluntary" act requirement is defined, roughly, as an *intentional* bodily movement – or omission in cases in which the person has a duty to act – done in a reasonably integrated state of consciousness. Other than crimes of strict liability, all crimes also require a culpable mental state, such as purpose, knowledge, or recklessness. All affirmative defenses of justification and excuse involve an inquiry into the person's mental state, such as the belief that self-defensive force was necessary or the lack of knowledge of right from wrong.

Our folk-psychological concepts of criminal responsibility follow logically from the action-guiding nature of law itself, from its folk-psychological concept of the person and action, and from the aim of achieving retributive justice, which holds that no one should be punished unless they deserve it and no more than they deserve. The general capacity for rationality is the primary condition for responsibility, and the lack of that capacity is the primary condition for excusing a person. If human beings were not rational creatures who could understand the good reasons for action and were not capable of conforming to legal requirements through intentional action or forbearance, the law could not adequately guide action and would not be just. Legally responsible agents are therefore people who have the general capacity to grasp and be guided by good reason in particular legal contexts (Wallace, 1994, considering responsibility generally).

In cases of excuse, the agent who has done something wrong acts for a reason but is either incapable of rationality generally or incapable on the specific occasion in question. This explains, for example, why young children and some people with mental disorders are not held responsible. The amount of lack of capacity for rationality that is necessary to find the agent not responsible is a moral, social, political, and, ultimately, legal issue. It is not a scientific, neuroscientific, medical, psychological, or psychiatric issue.

Compulsion or coercion is also an excusing condition. Literal compulsion exists when the person's bodily movement is a pure mechanism that is not rationalizable by reference to the agent's mental states. These cases defeat the requirement of a "voluntary act." For example, a tremor or spasm produced by a neurological disorder is not an action because it is not intentional and, therefore, defeats the ascription of a voluntary act. Metaphorical compulsion exists when an agent acts intentionally but in response to some hard choice imposed on the agent through no fault of his or her own. For example, if a miscreant holds a gun to an agent's head and threatens to kill her unless she kills another innocent person, it would be wrong to kill under these circumstances. Nevertheless, the law may decide as a normative matter to excuse the act of intentional killing because the agent was motivated by a threat so great that it would be supremely difficult for most citizens to resist. Cases involving internal compulsive states are more difficult to conceptualize because it is difficult to define and assess "loss of control" (Morse, 1994, 2002, 2011a). The cases that most fit this category are "disorders of desire," such as addictions and sexual disorders. The question is why these acting agents lack control, but other people with strong desires do not. If an agent frequently yields to his or her apparently very strong desires at great social, medical, occupational, financial, and legal cost, the agent will often say or observers will infer the agent was "out of control," and an excuse or mitigation is therefore warranted. But why mitigation or excuse should obtain is difficult to understand.

All the distinctions criminal responsibility criteria draw – act/no act; culpable mental state/no culpable mental state; rational capacity/lack of rational capacity; compulsion/no compulsion – are consistent with retributive and consequential theories of just blame and punishment that we endorse and with the truth of determinism. For example, a person whose bodily movement is a spasm that causes harm does not deserve blame and punishment for the harm because the spasm was not the agent's action and such harms cannot be deterred by the action-guiding function of the criminal law. Now assume that determinism is true. It is simply also true that some bodily movements are actions and others are not; that some people form culpable mental states and others don't; that some people commit crimes while they are psychotic and most other people who commit crimes are not psychotic; and that some people commit crimes because they are threatened with death or grievous bodily harm if they don't commit the crime and most other people who commit crimes are not so threatened. Wittgenstein famously asked: "when 'I raise my arm', my arm goes up. And the problem arises: what is left over if I subtract the fact that my arm goes up from the fact that I raise my arm?" (1991, para. 621). This is the question of agency. To dismantle this folk-psychological structure, neuroscience would have to demonstrate that the bodily movement produced by a muscular spasm and an identical movement that was intentional are indistinguishable metaphysically or should be treated morally the same. Neuroscience does not remotely indicate the former and it is the naturalistic fallacy to claim that it can do the latter.

Lost in translation? Legal relevance and the need for translation

What in principle is the possible relation of neuroscience to law? We must begin with a distinction between internal relevance and external relevance. An internal contribution or critique accepts the general coherence and legitimacy of a set of legal doctrines, practices, or institutions and attempts to explain or alter them. For example, an internal contribution to criminal responsibility may suggest the need for doctrinal reform of, say, the insanity defense, but it would not suggest that the notion of criminal responsibility is itself incoherent or illegitimate. By contrast, an externally relevant critique suggests that the doctrines, practices or institutions are incoherent, illegitimate, or unjustified. Because a radical, external critique has little possibility of success at present (as is explained below), I make the simplifying assumption that the contributions of neuroscience will be internal and thus will need to be translated into the law's folk-psychological concepts.

As we have seen, the law's criteria for responsibility and competence are essentially behavioral – acts and mental states. The criteria of neuroscience are mechanistic – neural structure and function. Is the apparent chasm between those two types of discourse bridgeable? This is a familiar question in the field of mental health law (Stone, 1984), but there is even greater dissonance in neurolaw. Psychiatry and psychology sometimes treat behavior mechanistically, sometimes treat it folk-psychologically, and sometimes blend the two. Neuroscience, in contrast, is purely mechanistic and eschews folk-psychological concepts and discourse. Neurons and neural networks do not act intentionally for reasons. They have no sense of past, present, and future, and no aspirations. They do not recognize that they will die. Thus, the gap will be harder to bridge.

The brain does enable the mind (even if we do not know how this occurs). Therefore, facts we learn about brains in general or about a specific brain could, in principle, provide useful information about mental states and about human capacities in general and in specific cases. Some believe that this conclusion is a category error (Bennett & Hacker, 2003; Pardo & Patterson, 2013). This is a plausible view, and perhaps it is correct. If it is, then the whole subject of neurolaw is empty, and there was no point writing this chapter in the first place. Let us therefore bracket this pessimistic view and determine what follows from the more optimistic position that what we learn about the brain and nervous system can be potentially helpful to resolving questions of criminal responsibility if the findings are properly translated into the law's psychological framework.

The question is whether the new neuroscience is legally relevant because it makes a proposition about responsibility or competence more or less likely to be true. Any legal criterion must be established independently, and biological evidence must be translated into the criminal law's folk-psychological criteria. That is, the expert must be able to explain precisely how the neuroevidence bears on whether the agent acted, formed the required *mens rea*, or met the criteria for an excusing condition. If the evidence is not directly relevant, the expert should be able to explain the chain of inference from the indirect evidence to the law's criteria. At present, as I explain below in the "Limits of neurolaw" section, few such data exist, but neuroscience is advancing so rapidly that such data may exist in the near or medium term.

Dangerous distractions concerning neuroscience and criminal responsibility

This section considers a number of related issues that are often thought to be relevant to criminal responsibility but that are in fact irrelevant, confusing, and distracting: free will, causation as an excuse, causation as compulsion, prediction as an excuse, dualism, and the non-efficacy of mental states. It is important to correct these errors because much of the unjustified legal exuberance about the contributions of neuroscience flow from them. The legal exuberance also flows, however, from unrealistic expectations about the scientific accomplishments of neuroscience. The next section of this chapter addresses the scientific exuberance.

Contrary to what many people believe and what judges and others sometimes say, free will in the strong sense of metaphysical libertarian freedom is not a legal criterion that is part of any doctrine, and it is not even foundational for criminal responsibility (Morse, 2007b). As discussed above, criminal law doctrines are fully consistent with the truth of determinism or universal causation that allegedly undermines the foundations of responsibility and they are consistent with moral and legal theories of responsibility and justice that we have reason to endorse. Criminal law addresses folk-psychological issues genuinely related to responsibility, including consciousness, the formation of mental states such as intention and knowledge, the capacity for rationality, and compulsion. But the law never addresses the presence or absence of free will understood as libertarian freedom.

When most people use the term "free will" in the context of legal responsibility, they are typically using it loosely as a synonym for the conclusion that the defendant was or was not criminally responsible. They typically have reached this conclusion for reasons that do not involve free will – for example, that the defendant was legally insane or acted under duress – but such use of the term free will only perpetuates misunderstanding and confusion. Once the legal criteria for excuse have been met – and no excuse includes lack of free will as a criterion – the defendant will be excused without any reference whatsoever to free will as an independent ground for excuse.

There is a genuine metaphysical problem regarding free will, which is whether human beings have the capacity to act uncaused by anything other than themselves and whether this capacity is a necessary foundation for holding anyone legally or morally accountable for criminal conduct. Philosophers and others have debated these issues in various forms for millennia. This is a philosophical issue, but it is not a problem for the law, and neuroscience raises no new challenge to this conclusion. Solving the free will problem would have profound implications for responsibility doctrines and practices, such as blame and punishment, but having or lacking libertarian freedom is not a criterion of any civil or criminal law doctrine.

The majority of experts on this question are "compatibilists," people who think that responsibility is genuinely possible even if determinism is true. Contrary to what philosophically naïve critics may think, compatibilism is not an illusion or sleight of hand definitional trick, it does not presuppose substance dualism, and it has powerful moral and metaphysical support (e.g., Vihvelin, 2013). Admittedly, there is no resolution in sight for the metaphysical problem, but compatibilism cannot simply be waved away. Its arguments must be met by responsibility skeptics who can try to show either that it is metaphysically unsound or that the model of the person and freedom it presupposes – roughly, a reasons-responsive creature like us – is simply wrong as a scientific matter. If the arguments cannot be successfully met – and I believe they cannot be at present or for the foreseeable future – the responsibility skeptic would do well to accept the more limited conception of freedom that compatibilist responsibility adopts, especially given the importance to our moral and social lives of responsibility practices.

In short, neuroscience is simply the most recent, mechanistic causal science that appears deterministically to explain behavior. Neuroscience thus joins social structural variables, behaviorism, genetics, and other scientific explanations that have also been deterministic explanations for behavior. In principle, however, neuroscience adds nothing new, even if neuroscience is a better, more persuasive science than some of its predecessors. No science, including neuroscience, can demonstrate that libertarian free will does or does not exist. As long as free will in the strong sense is not foundational for just blame and punishment and is not a criterion at the doctrinal level – which it is not – the truth of determinism or universal causation poses no threat to legal responsibility. Neuroscience may help shed light on folk-psychological excusing conditions, such as automatism or legal insanity, but the truth of determinism is not an excusing condition. The law will be fundamentally challenged only if neuroscience or any other science can conclusively demonstrate that the law's psychology is wrong, and that we are not the type of creatures for whom mental states are causally effective. This is a different question from whether determinism undermines responsibility, however, and this article returns to the more radical challenge below.

A related confusion is that behavior is excused if it is caused, but causation per se is not a legal or moral mitigating or excusing condition. I termed this confusion the "fundamental psycholegal error" (Morse, 1994). At most, causal explanations can only provide evidence concerning whether a genuine excusing condition, such as lack of rational capacity, was present. For example, suppose a life marked by poverty and abuse played a predisposing causal role in a defendant's criminal behavior or that an alleged new mental syndrome played a causal role in explaining criminal conduct. The claim is often made that such causes – for which the agent is not responsible – should be an excusing or mitigating position per se, but this claim is false.

All behavior is the product of the necessary and sufficient causal conditions without which the behavior would not have occurred, including brain causation, which is always part of the causal explanation for any behavior. If causation were an excusing condition per se, then no one would be responsible for any behavior. Some people might welcome such a conclusion and believe that responsibility is impossible, but this is not the legal and moral world we inhabit. The law holds most adults responsible for most of their conduct, and genuine excusing conditions are limited. Thus, unless the person's history or mental condition, for example, provides evidence of an existing excusing or mitigating condition, such as lack of rational capacity, there is no reason for excuse or mitigation.

Even a genuinely abnormal cause is not per se an excusing condition. For example, imagine an armed robber who suffers from intermittent hypomania and who robs only when clinically hypomanic because only then does he or she feel sufficiently energetic and confident. In other words, the hypomania is a "but for" cause of these robberies. Nevertheless, the robber would not be excused for an armed robbery because hypomania seldom compromises rational capacity sufficiently to warrant an excuse. If an armed robbery were committed under the influence of a delusional belief the robber's mania produced, then he or she might be excused by reason of legal insanity. In that case, the excusing condition would be compromised rationality and not the mania per se. In short, a neuroscientific causal explanation for criminal conduct, like any other type of causal explanation, does not per se mitigate or excuse. It only provides evidence that might help the law resolve whether a genuine excuse existed, or it may in the future provide data that might be a guide to prophylactic or rehabilitative measures.

Compulsion is a genuine mitigating or excusing condition, but causation –including brain causation – is not the equivalent of compulsion. Compulsion may be either literal or metaphorical and normative. It is crucial to recognize that most human action is not plausibly the result of either type of compulsion, but all human behavior is caused by its necessary and sufficient causes – including brain causation. Even abnormal causes are not necessarily compelling. To illustrate, suppose that a person has weak pedophilic urges and weak sexual urges in general. If this person molested a child, there would be no ground for a compulsion excuse. If causation was the equivalent of compulsion, all behavior would be compelled and no one would be responsible. Once again, this is not a plausible account of the law's responsibility conditions. Causal information from neuroscience might help us resolve questions concerning whether legal compulsion existed, or it might be a guide to prophylactic or rehabilitative measures when dealing with plausible legal compulsion. Causation, however, is not per se compulsion.

Causal knowledge, whether from neuroscience or any other science, can enhance the accuracy of behavioral predictions, but predictability is also not a per se excusing or mitigating condition – even if the predictability of the behavior is perfect. To understand this, consider how many things we do that are perfectly predictable but for which there is no plausible excusing or mitigating condition. If the variables that enhance prediction also produce a genuine excusing or mitigating condition, then excuse or mitigation is justified for the latter reason and independent of the prediction.

For example, recent research demonstrates that a history of childhood abuse coupled with a specific, genetically caused enzyme abnormality that produces a neurotransmitter deficit vastly increases the risk that a person will behave antisocially as an adolescent or young adult (Caspi et al., 2002). Does this mean that an offender with this gene by environment interaction is not responsible or less responsible? No. The offender may not be fully responsible or responsible at all, but not because there is a strong but partial causal explanation. What is the intermediary excusing or mitigating principle? Are these people, for instance, more impulsive? Are they lacking rationality? What is the actual excusing or mitigating condition?

Again, causation is not compulsion, and predictability is not an excuse. Just because an offender is caused to do something or is predictable does not mean that the offender was compelled to do the crime charged or is otherwise not responsible. Brain causation – or any other kind of causation – does not mean that we are automatons, not really acting agents at all, or otherwise excused.

Most informed people are not "dualists" concerning the relation between the mind and the brain. That is, they no longer think that our minds – or souls – are independent of our brains and bodies more generally and can somehow exert a causal influence over our bodies. It may seem as if law's emphasis on the importance of mental states as causing behavior is based on a prescientific, outmoded form of dualism, but this is not the case. Although the brain enables the mind, we have no idea how this occurs and have no idea how action is possible. It is clear that, at the least, mental states are dependent upon or supervene on brain states, but neither neuroscience nor any other science has demonstrated that mental states do not play an independent and partial causal role. Simply because we now know that water is divisible into two hydrogen and one oxygen atoms does not mean that it doesn't have the property of wetness that none of its component parts has individually. This is, of course, the issue of emergence and reductionism in philosophy and science. Applied to our context, even if mental states depend crucially on brain states, mental states may have independent causal properties that brain states alone may not have, and they may not be reducible to brain states. These are immensely thorny issues and the responsibility skeptics need to address them in detail rather than simply assume that science has demonstrated that mental states are just brain states or that mental states do no work.

Despite our lack of understanding of the mind–brain–action relation, some scientists and philosophers question whether mental states have any causal effect, thus treating mental states as "psychic appendixes" that evolution has created but that have no genuine function. These claims are not strawpersons. They are made by serious, thoughtful people (e.g., Greene & Cohen, 2006). As discussed below, if accepted, they would create a complete and revolutionary paradigm shift in the law of criminal responsibility and competence (and more widely). Thus, this claim is an external critique and must be understood as such. Moreover, as the section "The radical neurochallenge" suggests, given our current state of knowledge, there is little scientific or conceptual reason to accept it (Morse, 2011a).

The limits of neurolaw: the present limits of neuroscience

Most generally, the relation of brain, mind, and action is one of the hardest problems in all science. Again, we have no idea how the brain enables the mind or how action is possible. The brain–mind–action relation is a mystery, not in the sense that it depends on anything magical, but simply in the sense that it is so difficult to understand the relation. For example, to return to the Wittgensteinian example raised previously, we would like to know the difference between a neuromuscular spasm and intentionally moving one's arm in exactly the same way. The former is a purely mechanical motion, whereas the latter is an action, but we cannot explain the difference between the two. We know that a functioning brain is a necessary condition for having mental states and for acting. After all, if your brain is dead, you have no mental states, are not acting, and indeed are not doing much of anything at all. Still, we do not know how mental states and action are caused.

Despite the astonishing advances in neuroimaging and other neuroscientific methods, we still do not have sophisticated causal knowledge of how the brain works generally, and we have little information that is legally relevant. This is unsurprising. The scientific problems are fearsomely difficult. Only in the last fifteen years have researchers begun to accumulate much data from functional magnetic resonance imaging (fMRI), which is the technology that has generated most of the legal interest. Moreover, virtually no studies have been performed to address specifically legal questions.

Before turning to the specific reasons for neuromodesty, a few preliminary points of general applicability must be addressed. The first and most important is contained in the message of the prior section. Causation by biological variables, including abnormal biological variables, does not per se create an excusing or mitigating condition. Any excusing condition must be established independently. The goal is always to translate the biological evidence into the criminal law's folk-psychological criteria.

Assessing criminal responsibility involves a retrospective evaluation of the defendant's mental states at the time of the crime. No criminal wears a portable scanner or other neurodetection device that provides a measurement at the time of the crime, at least not yet. Further, neuroscience is insufficiently developed to detect specific, legally relevant mental content or to provide a sufficiently accurate diagnostic marker for even a severe mental disorder (Frances, 2009). Notably, the newest (fifth) edition,of the American Psychiatric Association's *Diagnostic and Statistical Manual of Mental Disorders* (American Psychiatric Association, 2013) neither contains any biological criterion nor identifies any biomarker for mental disorders with just a few exceptions (e.g., neurocognitive disorders). Nonetheless, certain aspects of neural structure and function that bear on legally relevant capacities, such as the capacity for rationality and control, may be temporally stable in general or in individual cases. If they are, neuroevidence may permit a reasonably valid retrospective inference about the defendant's rational and control capacities and their impact on criminal behavior. This will, of course, depend on the existence of adequate science to do this. We currently lack such science, but future research may provide the necessary data.

Questions concerning competence or predictions of future behavior are based on a subject's present condition. Thus, the problems besetting the retrospective responsibility analysis do not apply to such issues. The criteria for competence are functional. They ask whether the subject can perform some task – such as understanding the nature of a criminal proceeding or understanding a treatment option that is offered – at a level the law considers normatively acceptable to warrant respecting the subject's choice and autonomy.

Now, let us consider the specific grounds for neuromodesty in cognitive, affective, and social neuroscience, the sub-disciplines most relevant to law. At present, most neuroscience studies on human beings involve very small numbers of subjects, although this phenomenon is starting to change. Most of the studies have been done on college and university students, who are hardly a random sample of the population generally and of criminal offenders specifically. There is also a serious question of whether findings based on subjects' behavior and brain activity in a scanner would apply to real-world situations (the issue of "ecological validity"). Further, most studies average the neurodata over the subjects, and the average finding may not accurately describe the brain structure or function of any actual subject in the study. Replications are few, which is especially important for law. Policy and adjudication should not be influenced by findings that are insufficiently established, and replications of findings are crucial to our confidence in a result. Finally, the neuroscience of cognition and interpersonal behavior is largely in its infancy and what is known is quite coarse-grained and correlational, rather than fine-grained and causal (Miller, 2010). What is being investigated is an association between a condition or a task in the scanner and brain activity. These studies do not demonstrate that the brain activity is a sensitive diagnostic marker for the condition or either a necessary, sufficient, or predisposing causal condition for the behavioral task that is being done in the scanner. Any language that suggests otherwise – such as claiming that some brain region is the neural substrate for the behavior – is simply not justifiable based on the methodology of most studies. Moreover, activity in the same region may be associated with diametrically opposite behavioral phenomena – for example, love and hate.

There are also technical and research design difficulties. It takes many mathematical transformations to get from the raw fMRI data to the images of the brain that are increasingly familiar. Explaining these transformations is beyond me, but I do understand that the likelihood that an investigator will find a statistically significant result depends on how the researcher sets the threshold for significance. There is dispute about this, and the threshold levels are conventional. If the threshold changes, so does the outcome. I have been convinced by neuroscience colleagues that many such technical difficulties have largely been solved, but research design and potentially unjustified inferences from the studies are still an acute problem. It is extraordinarily difficult to control for all conceivable artifacts. Consequently, there are often problems of over-inference. Finally, it is also an open question whether accurate inferences or predictions about individuals are possible using group data when that group includes the individual (Faigman et al., 2014). This is a very controversial topic, but even if it is difficult or impossible now, it may become easier in the future. Over time, however, all these problems may ease as imaging and other techniques become less expensive and more accurate, research designs become more sophisticated, and the sophistication of the science increases generally.

Virtually all neuroscience studies of potential interest to the law involve some behavior that has already been identified as of interest, and the point of the study is to identify that behavior's neural correlates. Neuroscientists do not go on general "fishing" expeditions (but see Bennett et al., 2009, for an amusing counterexample). There is usually some bit of behavior – such as addiction, schizophrenia, or impulsivity – that investigators would like to understand better by investigating its neural correlates. To do this properly presupposes that the researchers have already identified and validated the behavior under neuroscientific investigation. Thus, neurodata can be no more valid than the behavior with which it is correlated.

On occasion, the neuroscience might suggest that the behavior is not well-characterized or is neurally indistinguishable from other, seemingly different, behavior. In general, however, the existence of legally relevant behavior will already be apparent before the neuroscientific investigation is begun. For example, some people are grossly out of touch with reality. If, as a result, they do not understand right from wrong, we excuse them because they lack such knowledge. We might learn a great deal about the neural correlates of such psychological abnormalities, but we already knew without neuroscientic data that these abnormalities existed, and we had a firm view of their normative significance. In the future, however, we may learn more about the causal link between the brain and behavior, and studies may be devised that are more directly legally relevant. I suspect that we are unlikely to make substantial progress with neural assessment of legally relevant mental content, but we are likely to learn more about capacities that will bear on excuse or mitigation. Again, however, the neurodata must be genuinely and not rhetorically relevant to the law's folk-psychological criteria.

The criteria for both responsibility and competence are behavioral; therefore, actions speak louder than images. This is a truism for all criminal responsibility and competence assessments. If the finding of any test or measurement of behavior is contradicted by actual behavioral evidence, then we must believe the behavioral evidence because it is more direct and probative of the law's behavioral criteria. For example, if the person behaves rationally in a wide variety of circumstances, the agent is rational even if the brain appears structurally or functionally abnormal. We also confidently knew that some people were behaviorally abnormal – such as being psychotic – long before there were any psychological or neurological tests for such abnormalities.

An analogy from physical medicine may be instructive. Suppose someone complains about back pain, a subjective symptom, and the question is whether the subject actually does have back pain. We know that many people with abnormal spines do not experience back pain, and many people who complain of back pain have normal spines. If the person is claiming a disability and the spine looks dreadful, evidence that the person regularly exercises on a trampoline without difficulty indicates that there is no disability caused by back pain. If there is reason to suspect malingering, however, and there is not clear behavioral evidence of lack of pain, then a completely normal spine might be of use in deciding whether the claimant is malingering. Unless the correlation between the image and the legally relevant behavior is very powerful, however, such evidence will be of limited help.

If actions speak louder than images, however, what room is there for introducing neuroevidence in legal cases? Is criminal law completely immune to neuroscientific findings? Let us begin with cases in which the behavioral evidence is clear and permits an equally clear inference about the defendant's mental state. For example, lay people may not know the technical term to apply to people who are manifestly out of touch with reality, but they will readily recognize this unfortunate condition. No further tests of any sort will be necessary to prove that the subject suffers from seriously impaired rationality. In such cases, neuroevidence will be at most convergent and increase our confidence in what we already had confidently concluded. Determining if it is worth collecting the neuroevidence will depend on whether the cost-benefit analysis justifies obtaining convergent evidence.

Roper v. *Simmons* (2005) is the most striking example of a case in which the behavioral evidence was clear. In *Roper* the United States Supreme Court categorically excluded the death penalty for capital murderers who killed when they were 16 or 17 years old on the grounds that adolescents do not deserve the death penalty. The amicus briefs were replete with neuroscience data showing that the brains of late adolescents are not fully biologically mature, and advocates used this data to suggest that adolescent killers could not fairly be put to death. Now, we already knew from common-sense observation and from rigorous behavioral studies that juveniles are on average less rational than adults. What did the neuroscientific evidence about the juvenile brain add? It was consistent with the undeniable behavioral data and perhaps provided a partial causal explanation of the behavioral differences. The neuroscience data was therefore merely additive and only indirectly relevant, and the Supreme Court did not cite it, except perhaps by implication when it referred vaguely to "other" scientific evidence. In two later cases dealing with the punishment of juvenile offenders, *Graham* v. *Florida* (2010) and *Miller* v. *Alabama* (2013), the Court did cite neuroscience in a general, conclusory way, but I believe these cases were fully controlled by the reasoning in *Roper* and that the use of neuroscience was dictum.

Whether adolescents are sufficiently less rational on average than adults to exclude them categorically from the death penalty is a normative legal question and not a scientific or psychological question. Advocates claimed, however, that the neuroscience confirmed that adolescents are insufficiently responsible to be executed, thus confusing the positive and the normative. The neuroscience evidence in no way independently confirms that adolescents are less responsible. If the behavioral differences between adolescents and adults were slight, it would not matter if their brains were quite different. Similarly, if the behavioral differences were sufficient for moral and constitutional differential treatment, then it would not matter if the brains were essentially indistinguishable.

If the behavioral data are not clear, then the potential contribution of neuroscience is large. Unfortunately, it is in just such cases that neuroscience at present is not likely to be of much help. I term the reason for this the "clear cut" problem (Morse, 2011b). Recall that neuroscientific studies usually start with clear cases of well-characterized behavior. In such cases, the neural markers might be quite sensitive to the already clearly identified behaviors precisely because the behavior is so clear. Less clear behavior is simply not studied, or the overlap in data about less clear behavior is greater between experimental and control subjects. Thus, the neural markers of clear cases will provide little guidance to resolve behaviorally ambiguous cases of legally relevant behavior, and they are unnecessary if the behavior is sufficiently clear

For example, suppose that in an insanity defense case the question is whether the defendant suffers from a major mental disorder, such as schizophrenia. In extreme cases, the behavior will be clear, and no neurodata will be necessary. Investigators have discovered various small but statistically significant differences in neural structure or function between people who are clearly suffering from schizophrenia and those who are not. Although there is reason to be cautious about the validity of such studies (Ioannidis, 2011), let us assume their validity for purposes of argument. In a behaviorally unclear case, however, the overlap between data on the brains of people with schizophrenia and people without the disorder is so great that a scan is insufficiently sensitive to be used for diagnostic purposes. In short, at present, in those cases in which the neuroscience would be most helpful, it has little to contribute. Again, this situation may change if neural markers become more diagnostically sensitive for legally relevant criteria.

Some people think that executive capacity – the congeries of cognitive and emotional capacities that help to plan and regulate human behavior – is going to be the Holy Grail to help the law determine an offender's true culpability. After all, there is an attractive moral case that people with a substantial lack of these capacities are less culpable, even if their conduct satisfied the prima facie case for the crime charged. Perhaps neuroscience can provide specific data previously unavailable to identify executive capacity differences more precisely.

There are two problems, however. First, significant problems with executive capacity are readily apparent without testing, and criminal law simply will not adopt fine-grained culpability criteria. Second, the correlation between neuropsychological tests of executive capacity and actual real-world behavior is not terribly strong (Barkley & Murphy, 2010). Only a small fraction of the variance is accounted for, and the scanning studies will use the types of tasks the tests use. Consequently, we are far from able to use neuroscience accurately to assess non-obvious executive capacity differences that are valid in real-world contexts.

The radical neurochallenge: are we victims of neuronal circumstances?

This section addresses the claim and hope alluded to earlier that neuroscience will cause a paradigm shift in criminal responsibility by demonstrating that we are "merely victims of neuronal circumstances" (or some similar claim that denies human agency). This claim holds that we are not the kinds of intentional creatures we think we are. If our mental states play no role in our behavior and are simply epiphenomenal, then traditional notions of responsibility based on mental states and on actions guided by mental states would be imperiled. But is the rich explanatory apparatus of intentionality simply a post hoc rationalization that the brains of hapless *Homo sapiens* construct to explain what their brains have already done? Will the criminal justice system as we know it wither away as an outmoded relic of a prescientific and cruel age? If so, criminal law is not the only area of law in peril. What will be the fate of contracts, for example, when a biological machine that was formerly called a person claims that it should not be bound because it did not make a contract? The contract is also simply the outcome of various "neuronal circumstances."

Given how little we know about the brain–mind and brain–action connections, to claim that we should radically change our conceptions of ourselves and our legal doctrines and practices based on neuroscience is a form of neuroarrogance. Although I predict that in the future we will see far more numerous attempts to use neuroscience in adjudication and law reform, I have elsewhere argued that for conceptual and scientific reasons, there is no reason at present to believe that we are not agents (Morse, 2008a, 2011b, 2013a). It is possible that we are not agents, but the current science does not remotely demonstrate that this is true. The burden of persuasion is firmly on the proponents of the radical view.

What is more, the radical view entails no positive agenda. Suppose we are convinced by the mechanistic view that we are not intentional, rational agents after all. (Of course, the notion of being "convinced" would be an illusion too. Being convinced means that we are persuaded by evidence or argument, but a mechanism is not persuaded by anything. A mechanism is simply neurophysically transformed.) What should we do now? We know that it is an illusion to think that our deliberations and intentions have any causal efficacy in the world. We also know, however, that we experience sensations – such as pleasure and pain – and care about what happens to us and to the world. We cannot just sit quietly and wait for our brains to activate, for determinism to happen. We must and will deliberate and act.

Even if we still thought that the radical view was correct and standard notions of genuine moral responsibility and desert were therefore impossible, we might still believe that the law would not necessarily have to give up the concept of incentives. Indeed, Greene and Cohen (2006) concede that we would have to keep punishing people for practical purposes.

Such an account would be consistent with "black box" accounts of economic incentives that simply depend on the relation between inputs and outputs without considering the mind as a mediator between the two. For those who believe that a thoroughly naturalized account of human behavior entails complete consequentialism, this conclusion might be welcomed.

On the other hand, this view seems to entail the same internal contradiction just explored. What is the nature of the agent that is discovering the laws governing how incentives shape behavior? Could understanding and providing incentives via social norms and legal rules simply be epiphenomenal interpretations of what the brain has already done? How do we decide which behaviors to reward or punish? What role does reason – a property of thoughts and agents, not a property of brains – play in this decision? And why would we call the intervention "punishment," a term that has immense normative connotation?

If the truth of pure mechanism is a premise in deciding what to do, no particular moral, legal, or political conclusions follow from it (see Berman, 2008, which first suggested this line of thought to me). The radical view provides no guide as to how one should live or how one should respond to the truth of reductive mechanism. Normativity depends on reason and, thus, the radical view is normatively inert. If reasons do not matter, then we have no reason to adopt any particular morals, politics or legal rules, or to do anything at all.

Given what we know and have reason to do, the allegedly disappearing person remains fully visible and necessarily continues to act for good reasons, including the reasons currently to reject the radical view. We are not Pinocchios, and our brains are not Geppettos pulling the strings.

The case for cautious neurolaw optimism

Despite having claimed that we should be exceptionally cautious about the current contributions that neuroscience can make to criminal law policy, doctrine, and adjudication, I am modestly optimistic about the near and intermediate term contributions neuroscience can potentially make to our ordinary, traditional, folk-psychological legal system. In other words, neuroscience may make a positive contribution even though there has been no paradigm shift in thinking about the nature of the person and the criteria for criminal responsibility. The legal regime to which neuroscience will contribute will continue to take people seriously as people – as autonomous agents who may fairly be blamed and punished based on their mental states and actions.

In general, my hope is that over time there will be feedback between the folk-psychological criteria and the neuroscientific data. Each might inform the other. Conceptual work on mental states might suggest new neuroscientific studies, for example, and the neuroscientific studies might help refine the folk-psychological categories. The ultimate goal would be a reflective, conceptual-empirical equilibrium.

More specifically, there are four types of situations in which neuroscience may be of assistance: (1) data indicating that the folk-psychological assumption underlying a legal rule is incorrect, (2) data suggesting the need for new or reformed legal doctrine, (3) evidence that helps adjudicate an individual case, and (4) data that help efficient adjudication or administration of criminal justice.

Many criminal law doctrines are based on folk-psychological assumptions about behavior that may prove to be incorrect. If so, the doctrine should change. For example, it is commonly assumed that agents intend the natural and probable consequences of their actions. In many or most cases, it seems that they do, but neuroscience may help in the future to demonstrate that this assumption is true far less frequently than we think. In that case, the rebuttable presumption used to help the prosecution prove intent should be softened or used with more caution.

Second, neuroscientific data may suggest the need for new or reformed legal doctrine. For example, control tests for legal insanity have been disfavored for some decades because they are ill understood and hard to assess. It is at present impossible to distinguish "cannot" from "will not." Perhaps neuroscientific information will help to demonstrate and to prove the existence of control difficulties that are independent of cognitive incapacities. If so, then perhaps independent control tests are justified and can be rationally assessed after all. More generally, perhaps a larger percentage of offenders than we currently believe have such grave control difficulties that they deserve a generic mitigation claim that is not available in criminal law today. Neuroscience might help us discover that fact. If that were true, justice would be served by adopting a generic mitigating doctrine. On the other hand, if it turns out that such difficulties are not so common, we could be more confident of the justice of current doctrine.

Third, neuroscience might provide data to help adjudicate individual cases. Consider the insanity defense again. As in *United States* v. *Hinckley* (1981), there is often dispute about whether a defendant claiming legal insanity suffered from a mental disorder, which disorder the defendant suffered from, and how severe the disorder was. At present, these questions must be resolved entirely behaviorally, and there is often room for considerable disagreement about inferences drawn from the defendant's actions, including utterances. In the future, neuroscience might help resolve such questions if the clear-cut problem difficulty can be solved. As mentioned previously, however, in the foreseeable future, I doubt that neuroscience will be able to help identify the presence or absence of specific *mens reas*.

Finally, neuroscience might help us to implement current policy more efficiently. For example, the criminal justice system makes predictions about future dangerous behavior for purposes of bail, sentencing, including capital sentencing, and parole. If we have already decided that it is justified to use dangerousness predictions to make such decisions, it is hard to imagine a rational argument for doing it less accurately if we are in fact able to do it more accurately. Validated behavioral prediction techniques already exist and should be used because they are more accurate than pure clinical judgment (Skeem & Monahan, 2011). The question is whether neuroscientific variables can add value by increasing the accuracy of such predictions considering the cost of gathering such data. Very recently, two studies have been published showing the potential usefulness of neural markers for enhancing the accuracy of predictions of antisocial conduct (Aharoni et al., 2013; Pardini et al., 2014). Although these must be considered preliminary, "proof of concept" studies, and a reanalysis of the Aharoni study demonstrated that the increase in accuracy beyond the behavioral measures was very small (Poldrack, 2013), it is perfectly plausible that in the future genuinely valid, cost-benefit justified neural markers will be identified, and thus, prediction decisions will be more accurate and just.

Responses to other chapters

Some of the chapters in this volume have addressed issues relevant to the argument I have presented. At the editor's suggestion, I will comment briefly on most of these chapters in light of the argument my chapter presents. I will focus more heavily on Steven Hyman's contribution, which addresses arguments that I have made specifically. My focus is on how one should think about the issues and about what the neuroscience contributes, if anything, to sensible resolution of them.

The central themes of my comments on all these chapters are, first, that they all deal with the folk-psychological concept of freedom rather than the metaphysical debate (although some are not entirely clear about the difference); second, the meanings of will and self-control are unsettled in both philosophy and science; and, third, neuroscience is unlikely in the near future to play a large role in resolving questions concerning folk-psychological freedom, the will, self-control, and responsibility.

De Haan et al.

Let us begin with the interesting contribution by de Haan et al. on the phenomenology of obsessive-compulsive disorder and what it teaches us about freedom of the will. The chapter is a contribution to the folk-psychological concept of freedom and not to the metaphysical debate. The metaphysical debate is all or none: either we have libertarian freedom or we don't as a result of how the universe "really is." How much conscious control – the authors' term – we have over our actions (and thoughts) is a folk-psychological issue. Conscious control is almost surely distributed on a continuum and how much we would need to be responsible is a normative question. Relatedly, I do not believe that neuroscience has demonstrated any worrisome limits on what we can consciously control if we have reason to exercise that control and no other excusing or mitigating condition is present.

The chapter's most general claim is that the extreme conscious control that sufferers from OCD exercise paradoxically diminishes their sense of agency and experience of freedom. But having such subjective self-impressions is a different issue from whether and how their freedom is in fact impaired. As I freely concede, genuine compulsion clearly diminishes freedom and people with OCD say that they are compelled to think certain thoughts or to do certain deeds. But "compelled" is a normative conclusion because OCD sufferers are not literally compelled. Suppose that a person whose major sign of OCD is compulsive handwashing were threatened with death if they yielded to a particular desire to wash. My hunch is that they wouldn't wash and thus that they could bring the action, although presumably not the desire, under conscious control if they had a good enough reason to exercise it. For all we know, it might be "easy" to control the impulse under these cruel conditions or it might be supremely difficult, but the action would be controlled. In most cases, however, we have very little valid, objective knowledge of how much conscious control an OCD sufferer has over his or her behavioral signs. Moreover, OCD sufferers are a heterogeneous lot. Are they compelled because the desire is so strong, the control mechanisms so weak, the motivation to control is lacking, or some combination of the three. It is almost impossible to tease out these variables independently and almost certainly the mix varies substantially among those with the disorder.

An interesting question is how much conscious control we could fairly expect OCD sufferers to have under what circumstances. In the following three examples, hold constant the intensity of the OCD. Imagine that a "compulsive" handwasher is with his or her spouse. They are enjoying quality time together – say, watching a television show they both like – when he gets up to wash, thus disrupting the quality time. Now, imagine that they are having the "make it or break it conversation" about potentially ending the marriage. In the midst of this intense discussion, he gets up to wash, interrupting his spouse in the midst of an important issue. In the third example, they are having dinner together and a chicken bone becomes lodged in her esophagus and threatens to asphyxiate her. The handwasher knows the Heimlich maneuver but gets up to wash and she dies. Remember: hold everything about the disorder and the sufferer otherwise constant. I think we would have a very different set of reactions. In the first case, the spouse would be disappointed but forgiving. In the second, the spouse might be genuinely indignant. In the third, we would expect much more from the handwasher and might indeed morally and legally condemn him for failing to exercise a capacity he should have exercised, albeit it would have been very hard for him to do so.

My preference is to treat impulse control problems as rationality problems. For the OCD sufferers, the intrusiveness of unwanted thoughts or the urgency of unwanted, strong desires interferes with their ability to bring reason to bear. In fact, in my view, this is the best explanation for "self-control" problems in most cases, but I am special pleading.

A last general observation about this chapter is a question about how far we can generalize about conscious control based on an analysis of the folk-psychological phenomenology of people with OCD.

Foquaert et al.

I have little to say about the excellent psychopathy chapter that uses a reasons-responsive model pioneered by Fischer and Ravizza to consider whether psychopaths should be held morally and legally responsible. This model is very close to the one I proposed in the main part of this chapter and therefore is a contribution to the folk-psychological conception of freedom rather than to the metaphysical debate.

In the chapter's introduction, they do imply that new discoveries about the neuroscience and genetics of psychopathy cast doubt on free will, but this is not true about either the metaphysical or the folk-psychological/compatibilist view. The metaphysical debate is, well, metaphysical, and scientific discoveries are not going to prove or disprove that we have libertarian freedom. As I said in the main body of my chapter, neurodeterminism or genodeterminism are simply the newest kids on the incompatibilist block. Nor will such discoveries cast doubt on the folk-psychological account of freedom and responsibility. We now have genetic and neuroscientific understanding of psychopathy because the condition was already well-characterized behaviorally and it is the behavior – mental states and actions – that are crucial for assessing freedom and responsibility. We know that some psychopaths totally lack empathy and conscience. Whether this should be a responsibility diminishing condition because it is a type of rational incapacity that bears on responsibility is a normative, not a scientific, question. And, since actions speak louder than images, even if we cannot find the neural correlates of empathy or its lack, we must believe the behavioral evidence.

For the record, I do argue elsewhere in agreement with this chapter that the psychological features of psychopathy, including lack of genuine moral sense, conscience, and empathy, should be responsibility diminishing because psychopaths lack rational moral agency (Morse, 2008b). These functional incapacities are doing the moral work, whether or not they are signs or symptoms of a disorder. Simply finding neural or genetic correlates or even causes for these incapacities does not entail that the condition is a disease. All behavior has brain and genetic causes. Although I believe that psychopathy is best characterized as a mental disorder and not a bad moral character, the moral argument is not hostage to a disease model and thus is not undermined by those who claim psychopathy is not a disorder. Even if it is not, some people have these functional incapacities through no fault of their own, and I believe their responsibility should be mitigated or excused if they commit immoral acts.

Meynen

This chapter is concerned with the question of how mental disorder affects the will. Although it gestures at the metaphysical problem, it is really a contribution to the folk-psychological account because if we don't have libertarian freedom, we don't, and no specific condition such as mental disorder affects this outcome. The chapter also claims that it is a matter of debate whether "free will has to do with criminal responsibility," but, with respect, it is not a matter of debate at the doctrinal level because libertarian freedom or its lack is not a criterion of any criminal law doctrine. At the most, one can argue that this type of freedom is foundational, but as the main body of the chapter demonstrates, criminal responsibility doctrines and practices are fully consistent with the truth of determinism.

The chapter's main difficulty is that it fails to provide an adequate conceptual or empirical account of what the will is. But this is a notoriously difficult problem in the philosophy of mind and action. Still more clarity on this point would have aided a reader's engagement with the arguments. In any case, the concept of the will envisioned is folk-psychological, and not a reduced neurophysiological mechanism. Of course, depression can make a sufferer generally avolitional, but specifiy-ing how this is different from not forming a desire in the first place is important.

Most of the examples the chapter uses to show how mental disorder can affect responsibility involve problems with rationality, e.g., psychosis, failure to integrate information in patients with delirium, alteration of decision-making rationality among some drug addicts. If the will is treated as an executory capacity, a volition in Michael Moore's terms (Moore, 1993), then a psychotic person who acts in response to his or her delusional beliefs or in response to a hallucination or who yields to a compulsive desire has a fully functioning will that executes their intentions (Fingarette & Hasse, 1979). The problem is not the will; it is rational capacity. If one wants to talk about failures of self-control, then the folk-psychological process by which this occurs needs to be specified. Saying that the person's will was undermined is simply a definitional stop that doesn't explain why the person "cannot" as opposed to "will not" control himself when there is apparently good reason to do so, as in cases of addiction. When the noted addiction researcher, Nora Volkow, whom the chapter quotes, claims that changes in the addict's brain undermine free will, what she is really referring to is the rationality of folk-psychological decision-making. One could do the same type of analysis with virtually all the clinical conditions the chapter reviews.

Most psychiatric conditions do not deprive the agent of the choice of how to act. People who experience command hallucinations do not have to obey them, and if they do, the will executes their intention very well. Suppose someone heard a voice tell them to commit a mass murder? How do we know that they could not but obey? If they complied, then the excusing condition would be lack of rational capacity, not a problem with the will. Even the absence of genuine choice does mean an action is necessarily "unfree." When Martin Luther said, "Here I stand; I can do no other," it was true that he believed he had no option and that tacking the theses to the church door was nonetheless a magnificent exercise of freedom. There was no lack of rational capacity and no normative compulsion.

I understand why coercion and manipulation may be excusing conditions, but it is unclear why not being "oneself" should also excuse or why any of these is a problem of the will. The chapter uses the example of a hypomanic person who is different from who he or she is when not in the hypomanic state. I applaud this example because I have written, including in the main body of this chapter, about the hypomanic armed robber in which the psychiatric condition plays a but-for role in producing armed robbery. Again, there is no problem with executory intentions, and I suggest that rational incapacity is doing the excusing work if it should be done at all. After all, many people do things "out of character" when they are stressed or the like, but we would not excuse them for wrongful behavior unless they became functionally impaired. It is the functional impairment that is crucial.

Hall & Carter

This chapter concerning the responsibility of addicts, by two distinguished addiction researchers, accurately covers the debate between those who claim that addiction is a chronic and relapsing brain disease and those who claim that it is best understood as a condition marked by voluntary but difficult choices. It also usefully surveys the literature on whether involuntary treatment for addiction is justified. I have written extensively on the question of the responsibility of addicts for actions related to their addiction (Morse, 2000, 2011c, 2013c) and wish in this brief comment to address only problems related to the central themes of this volume.

This chapter is once again addressed to the folk-psychological conception of freedom and responsibility, but it blurs the distinction between the metaphysical and the folk-psychological accounts by referring to the views of leading "voluntarists" such as Gene Heyman and Herbert Fingarette as "libertarian." This seems to suggest that these writers have a position requiring libertarian freedom in the metaphysical debate, but this is not true. Neither enters the metaphysical jousting. Their analyses are firmly folk-psychological, suggesting only that addicts do have the capacity to make uncompelled decisions in the folk-psychological sense about whether and how much to use substances and they are not "slaves" to their addictive desires to use substances. Neither relies on a metaphysical libertarianism.

The chapter is straightforwardly concerned with folk-psychological responsibility, so the folk-psychological facts about addicts are important. If addicts lack rational capacities or have control difficulties, they may seem less responsible than if these characterizations are false. Heyman's book on addiction (2009) pointed out that the epidemiological evidence about remission from addiction *without* treatment is inconsistent with the brain disease model of addiction. The vast majority of addicts simply stop using substances and no longer meet the criteria for addiction, albeit often after failed attempts, when they have a subjectively good enough reason to do so. The findings were criticized on numerous grounds, but Heyman effectively answered his critics in a more recent reanalysis (2013). His findings stand.

It is true that many addicts ruin their lives and the lives of others they profess to care about and that they have had multiple failed attempts to quit. The inference is that they are unable to quit, a conclusion bolstered by the neuroscientific finding that the reward circuits in addicts are negatively altered and by self-report that they can't help themselves. The problem, however, is that the studies of relapse and the neuroscientific studies are all done on addicts who are in treatment for addiction, and these addicts are not a representative sample of addicts. They are disproportionately co-morbid. That is, they suffer from other mental disorders as well as addiction, and it is impossible to know from this sample of addicts whether relapse is a product of addiction alone, the other disorder, or an interactive combination of the two.

The relation between addiction and responsibility is extremely complicated on any account, and it may vary according to the actions an addict performs. As Steven Hyman notes in an article the chapter quotes, addicts are not automatons. They are acting people. For example, one might argue that there is a more justifiable theory for mitigation and excuse for possession for personal use than for committing serious crimes against others to obtain the money needed to buy the substances. The reasons to forgo the latter crimes are much stronger than the reasons to forgo personal use, and addicts are responsive to reason. Rates of use and addiction vary with availability and price.

I believe that it is often the case that addicts cannot be adequately guided by reason at moments of peak desire when they can think of virtually nothing else except satisfying their desires. This may be especially true when their illegal actions are simply purchase or possession for personal use, when other-regarding reasons to abstain may be less strong. This is a rationality problem, which is a classic mitigating or excusing condition, and I find it very attractive. Nonetheless, the case for mitigation and excuse founders on the shoals of diachronous responsibility. When addicts are quiescent and not assaulted by persistent, intense urges, they are capable of rational thought unless their rational capacities are disabled for some other reason. At that point, they are capable of taking the steps necessary to avoid future trouble when they are in the state of peak desire again. The addict's self-assurance that he won't use today or anymore can only work a few times before the "denial" excuse can no longer obtain. He will have to take stronger steps to avoid trouble, and if he doesn't, he will be responsible for what he irrationally does later because he was responsible for failing to take those steps when he was capable of rational action.

Hyman

If I understand it correctly, this chapter suggests that science has demonstrated that agency is an illusion, but that this illusion is so central to our experienced lives that it cannot be abandoned. It recommends that we adopt "double vision," recognizing when we are in the lab that agency is an illusion, but ignoring this hard fact when we are outside the lab. It suggests that we do this without resorting to the comforts of compatibilism, which is treated as a sleight of hand. Thus, the chapter claims both that science has demonstrated that we do not have libertarian freedom and that we really are not agents who act for and can be guided by reasons. I fully agree that libertarian freedom is theoretically impossible, although science has not proven that this is so.

As is apparent from the main body of the chapter, however, I firmly disagree with the claims that compatibilism is a sleight of hand and that agency is an illusion. As Vargas argues (2013), rejecting compatibilism requires a lot of very hard philosophical work; it simply cannot be waved away. Indeed, the metaphysical arguments in its favor become ever more nuanced and sophisticated (e.g., Vihvelin, 2013). I concede that the truth of compatibilism has not been conclusively demonstrated – and cannot be – but it is the dominant view of experts in the field who are well-acquainted with the scientific worldview and with the empirical advances in biology and other sciences relevant to human behavior. Now, any writer is entitled to reject compatibilism as an asserted premise, but that isn't an argument. It is not contracausal freedom that is "saved" by compatibilism, as the chapter incorrectly suggests. What is saved is the possibility of robust responsibility as long as it is true that people have agency.

The chapter is on firmer argumentative ground in denying the truth of agency, but the science doesn't remotely support this assertion and it denies common sense. Perhaps we all truly are mere victims of neuronal circumstances, as Greene and Cohen assert (2006) but do not prove (and why is the neuronal level of explanation the right one if one is being reductionist?). But given common sense and the importance of agency to experienced living, the burden of persuasion is clearly on the agency-skeptics and they haven't begun to meet it. It seems to me that the more sensible scientific stance towards agency is to try to explain how it is possible rather than to explain it away reductionistically. After all, to date, the inter-theoretic reductionist project has been a dismal failure, even in the allegedly easiest cases such as the reduction of chemistry to physics. And, again, why should the biological level be the most sensible reduction? Why isn't everything reducible to physics? Why is there a field of chemistry or biology? If the answer is that the biological level is the most explanatory and useful to explain human behavior, then it's not reduction that is doing the work, but a pragmatic argument about levels of explanation. In that case, it is an open empirical and conceptual questions about which level of explanation is the most valuable for any particular phenomenon.

The chapter's section on punishment misconstrues retributivism. Although it may have its "evolutionary" roots in the expression of moral outrage and the suppression of free riding (Oldenquist, 1988), retributivism is fundamentally a theory of deontological justice. It is good in itself to give people what they deserve. Numerous studies, some of which the chapter cites, confirm that people are "instinctive" retributivists, but retributive theorists can take scant comfort from this because it does not provide a theoretical, normative justification. "Instincts" may be erroneous or undesirable. Further, it is not clear that ordinary people are metaphysical libertarians who believe that blame and punishment are foundationally based on strong free will. Most people have no clear understanding of what they mean by free will, including many educated people such as lawyers and judges.

The chapter is correct to conclude, however, that moral judgment is central to our lives and consistent with what we know neurobiologically and psychologically. Indeed, this conclusion seems inconsistent with the prior claim that agency is an illusion.

The section of the chapter devoted to neurobiology and the law flatteringly uses my work as an exemplar for the position that at present neuroscience has little to add to adjudication of criminal responsibility and legal policy. This section is admirably cautious about how much we know today that is legally relevant, and it properly recognizes the importance of genuine blaming doctrines and practices within the criminal law if justice is to be done. The underlying assumption, however, is that the increasing discovery of biological causal mechanisms is inconsistent with agency and at some point will cause our sense of agency to wither away, although not just yet. But this assumption raises the question of what science will demonstrate. If my claim is correct that the task of science is to explain how genuine agency is possible, then the discoveries of science may reinforce our sense of agency and the moral and legal practices that flow therefrom.

The chapter misreads my position to some degree. I do think that current doctrine and practice is consistent with the findings of neuroscience (and other sciences), but I do not think that legal doctrine and practice are insulated from the causal understanding science produces. As I have argued repeatedly in my writings, if science indicates that factual premises used in our moral and legal responsibility ascriptions are false, then the doctrines and practices should change. Moreover, neuroscience and other sciences might help us better characterize the folk-psychological capacities relevant to responsibility. Recall that in the main body of the chapter and in many previous writings, I argued for an interactive process between the psychological and biological realms of explanation to help refine both and to achieve a conceptual-empirical equilibrium. Thus, I agree with the chapter in this regard. But responsibility is about actions and mental states, so the science will have to demonstrate, for example, that offenders in individual cases do not have the agentic capacities we may otherwise think they have or that people in general do not have certain capacities crucial to current responsibility ascriptions. If this occurs, the science will help the law become more just in individual cases and more generally.

Contra the chapter's assertion, my position does not secretly adopt dualism to wall off responsibility practices from science. I do assume that mental states play a partial but crucial role in explaining human action and that mental states are enabled by the brain in interaction with the environment (Noe, 2009), although at present we have almost no idea how this happens. Science is of course relevant to legal doctrine and practice, but only if it teaches us something about the acting human person. Mental states and actions are the stuff of responsibility and actions speak louder than images.

Of course the criminal law should pay the closest attention to the new, causal discoveries being made by many of the mechanistic sciences, such as neuroscience, but discovering causes does not entail that we are not agents as the chapter seems to suggest (and most of what we know neuroscientifically about behavior is correlational, not causal). Once again, until and unless science demonstrates that we do not have the agentic capacities we are fully entitled to believe we have, criminal responsibility doctrines and practices have a firm foundation without any magical assumptions being made.

Conclusion

At present, neuroscience has little to contribute to more just and accurate criminal law decision-making concerning policy, doctrine, and individual case adjudication. This was the conclusion reached when I tentatively identified "Brain Overclaim Syndrome" eight years ago, and it remains true today. In the future, however, as the philosophies of mind and action and neuroscience mutually mature and inform one another, neuroscience will help us understand criminal behavior. Although no radical transformation of criminal justice is likely to occur, neuroscience can inform criminal justice as long as it is relevant to law and translated into the law's folk-psychological framework and criteria.

REFERENCES

PRIMARY MATERIALS

Graham v. *Florida*, 130 S. Ct. 2011 (2010).
Miller v. *Alabama*, 132 S. Ct. 2455 (2013).
Roper v. *Simmons* 543 US 551 (2005).
United States v. *Hinckley*, 525 F Supp 1342 (DDC 1981).

SECONDARY MATERIALS

Aharoni, Eyal, G. Vincent, C. Harenski, V. Calhoun, W. Sinnott-Armstrong, et al. (2013). "Neuroprediction of Future Arrest," *PNAS* 110, 6223–6228.

American Psychiatric Association (2013). *Diagnostic and Statistical Manual of Mental Disorders* (5th edn. DSM-5). Arlington, VA: American Psychiatric Association.

Barkley, Russell A., and Kevin R. Murphy (2010). "Impairment in Occupational Functioning and Adult ADHD: The Predictive Utility of Executive Function (EF) Ratings versus EF Tests," *Archives of Clinical Neuropsychology* 25, 157–173.

Bennett, C. M., A. Baird, M. Miller, and G. Wolford (2009). "Neural Correlates of Interspecies Perspective Taking in the Post-mortem Atlantic Salmon: An Argument for Multiple Comparisons Correction," *Journal of Serendipitous and Unexpected Results* 1, available at http://citeseerx.ist.psu.edu/viewdoc/summary?doi=10.1.1.161.8384.[order.

Bennett, Max R., and Peter M. S. Hacker (2003). *Philosophical Foundations of Neuroscience.* Maiden, MA: Blackwell.

Berman, Mitchell (2008). "Punishment and Justification," *Ethics* 118, 258–290.

Caspi, Avshalom, J. McClay, T. Moffitt, J. Mill, J. Martin, et al. (2002). "Role of Genotype in the Cycle of Violence in Maltreated Children," *Science* 297, 851–854.

Doherty, Brian (2007). "You Can't See Why on an FMRI: What Science Can and Can't Tell Us About the Insanity Defense," *Reason* (July), available at http://reason.com/archives/2007/06/19/you-cant-see-why-on-an-fmri.

The Economist (2002). "The Ethics of Brain Sciences: Open Your Mind," *The Economist* 23 (May 23), available at www.economist.com/node/1143317/print.

Faigman, David L., John Monahan, and Christopher Slobogin (2014). "Group to Individual Inference (G2i) in Scientific Expert Testimony," *University of Chicago Law Review* 81, 417–480.

Feldman, Robin (2009). *The Role of Science in Law.* New York: Oxford University Press.

Fingarette, Herbert, and Ann Fingarette Hasse (1979). *Mental Disabilities and Criminal Responsibility.* Berkeley: University of California Press.

Fodor, Jerry A. (1987). *Psychosemantics: The Problem of Meaning in the Philosophy of Mind.* Cambridge, MA: MIT Press.

Frances, Allen (2009). "Whither DSM-V?" *British Journal of Psychiatry* 195, 391–392.

Greene, Joshua, and Jonathan Cohen (2006). "For the Law, Neuroscience Changes Nothing and Everything," in *Law and the Brain* (S. Zeki and O. Goodenough eds.). New York: Oxford University Press, 207–226.

Heyman, Gene (2009). *Addiction: A Disorder of Choice.* Cambridge, MA: Harvard University Press.

(2013). "Quitting Drugs: Qualitative and Quantitative Features," *Annual Review of Clinical Psychology* 9, 29–59.

Ioannidis, John P. A. (2011). "Excess Significance Bias in the Literature on Brain Volume Abnormalities, *Archives of General Psychiatry* 68, 773–780.

McHugh Paul R., and Phillip R. Slavney (1998). *The Perspectives of Psychiatry* (2nd edn.), Baltimore, MD: Johns Hopkins University Press.

Miller, Gregory A. (2010). "Mistreating Psychology in the Decades of the Brain," *Perspectives on Psychological Science* 5, 716–743.

Monahan, John, H. Steadman, E. Silver, P. Appelbaum, P. Clark Robbins, et al. (2001). *Rethinking Risk Assessment: The MacArthur Study of Mental Disorder and Violence.* Cambridge, MA: Oxford University Press.

Moore, Michael S. (1993). *Act and Crime: The Theory of Action and Its Implications for Criminal Law.* Cambridge, MA: Oxford University Press.

Morse, Stephen J. (1994). "Culpability and Control," *University of Pennsylvania Law Review* 142, 1587–1660.

(2000). "Hooked on Hype: Addiction and Responsibility," *Law & Philosophy* 19, 3–49.

(2002). "Uncontrollable Urges and Irrational People," *Virginia Law Review* 18, 1025–1078.

(2004). "New Neuroscience, Old Problems," in *Neuroscience and the Law: Brain, Mind and the Scales of Justice* (B. Garland ed.). New York: Dana Press, 157–198.

(2006a). "Brain Overclaim Syndrome: A Diagnostic Note," *Ohio State Journal of Criminal Law* 3, 397–412.

(2006b). "Moral and Legal Responsibility and the New Neuroscience," in *Neuroethics in the 21st Century: Defining the Issues in Theory, Practice and Policy* (J. Illes ed.). Oxford University Press, 33–50.

(2007a). "Criminal Responsibility and the Disappearing Person," *Cardozo Law Review* 28, 2545–2575.

(2007b). "The Non-Problem of Free Will in Forensic Psychiatry and Psychology," *Behavioral Sciences & the Law* 25, 203–220.

(2008a). "Determinism and the Death of Folk Psychology," *Minnesota Journal of Law, Science & Technology* 9, 1–36.

(2008b). "Psychopathy and Criminal Responsibility," *Neuroethics* 1, 205–212.

(2009). "Neuroethics," in *Psychiatric Ethics* (4th edn., S. Bloch and S. Green eds.). Oxford University Press, 309–335.

(2011a). "Lost in Translation?: An Essay on Law and Neuroscience," in *Law and Neuroscience* (Michael Freeman ed.). Oxford University Press, 529–562.

(2011b). "Neuroscience and the Future of Personhood and Responsibility," in *Constitution 3.0: Freedom and Technological Change* (J. Rosen and B. Wittes eds.). Washington, DC: Brookings Institution, 113–129.

(2011c). "Addiction and Criminal Responsibility," in *Addiction and Responsibility* (J. Poland & G. Graham eds.). Cambridge, MA: MIT Press, 159–199.

(2012). "Neuroimaging Evidence in Law: A Plea for Modesty and Relevance," in *Neuroimaging in Forensic Psychiatry* (J. Simpson ed.). Chichester, West Sussex: Wiley-Blackwell, 341–357.

(2013a). "Brain Overclaim Redux," *Law & Inequality* 31, 509–534.

(2013b). "Preventive Detention of Psychopaths and Dangerous Offenders," in *Handbook on Psychopathy and Law* (K. Kiehl and W. P. Sinnott-Armstrong eds.). New York: Oxford University Press, 321–345.

(2013c). "A Good Enough Reason: Addiction, Agency and Criminal Responsibility," *Inquiry* 156, 490–518.

Noe, Alva. (2009). *Out of Our Mind: Why You Are Not Your Brain, and Other Lessons from the Biology of Consciousness.* New York: Hill & Wang.

Oldenquist, Andrew. (1988). "An Explanation of Retribution," *Journal of Philosophy* 85, 464–478.

Pardini, Dustin A., A. Raine, K. Erickson, and R. Loeber (2014). "Lower Amygdala Volume in Men Is Associated with Childhood Aggression, Early Psychopathic Traits, and Future Violence," *Biological Psychiatry* 75, 73–80.

Pardo, Michael S., and Dennis Patterson. (2013). *Minds, Brains and Law: The Conceptual Foundations of Law and Neuroscience.* New York: Oxford University Press.

Poldrack, Russell. (2013). "How Well Can We Predict Future Criminal Acts from fMRI Data?," *Russpoldrack.org* (April 6), available from www.russpoldrack.org/search?q=aharoni.

Skeem, Jennifer, and John Monahan. (2011). "Current Directions in Violence Risk Assessment," *Current Directions in Psychological Science* 20, 38–42.

Stone, Alan A. (1984). *Law, Psychiatry, and Morality.* Washington, DC: American Psychiatric Press.

Vargas, Manuel. (2013). "If Free Will Doesn't Exist, Neither Does Water," in *Exploring the Illusion of Free will and Moral Responsibility* (G. D. Caruso, ed.). Lanham MD: Lexington Books, 177–202.

Vihvelin, Kaadri. (2013). *Causes, Laws, and Free Will: Why Determinism Doesn't Matter.* Oxford University Press.

Wallace, Jay. (1994). *Responsibility and the Moral Sentiments.* Cambridge, MA: Harvard University Press.

Wittgenstein, Ludwig. (1991). *Philosophical Investigations* (3rd edn.). Somerset, NJ: Wiley-Blackwell.

Index

Locators in **bold type** refer to figures and tables

For EU product safety concerns, contact us at Calle de José Abascal, 56–1°, 28003 Madrid, Spain or eugpsr@cambridge.org.

www.ingramcontent.com/pod-product-compliance
Lightning Source LLC
LaVergne TN
LVHW011525200926
848484LV00001B/155
9781107036031